The General Surgeon's Guide to Passing the Oral Boards

The General Surgeon's Guide to Passing the Oral Boards

EDITORS:

Shelby Reiter, MD
General Surgery
Swedish Medical Center
Edmonds, Washington

Danielle Hayes, MD
General Surgery
Swedish Medical Center
Seattle, Washington

New York   Chicago   San Francisco   Lisbon   London   Madrid   Mexico City
New Delhi   San Juan   Seoul   Singapore   Sydney   Toronto

1 2 3 4 5 6 7 8 9   DSS   28 27 26 25 24 23

ISBN 978-1-265-08285-7
MHID 1-265-08285-5

This book was set in Minion Pro by MPS Limited.
The editors were Sydney Keen Vitale and Christie Naglieri.
The production supervisor was Richard Ruzycka.
Project management was provided by Poonam Bisht, MPS Limited.
The text designer was Mary McKeon; the cover designer was W2 Design.
This book is printed on acid-free paper.

Library of Congress Cataloging-in-Publication Data

Names: Reiter, Shelby, editors. | Hayes, Danielle, editors.
Title: The general surgeon's guide to passing the oral boards / editors,
   Shelby Reiter, Danielle Hayes.
Description: New York : McGraw Hill, 2023. | Includes bibliographical
   references and index. | Summary: "Each year, general surgery residents across the county
   spend hundreds of hours studying for the American Board of Surgery certifying exam, also
   known as general surgery oral boards. This test is the final obstacle for general surgery
   residents on their journey to become board certified, practicing general surgeons in an easy
   to reference study guide with information covering the most commonly tested topics. This
   book is compiled based on ACS curriculum outlie making it helpful for medical students
   interested in surgery, general surgery residents, and practicing general surgeons. For each
   disease process, we include the relevant points of the history and physical, work-up, staging,
   treatment options, key surgical steps, and post-operative care. The unique format we use
   makes this book optimal for quick referencing and self-study. While this book was initially
   designed as a tool to study for the oral boards, it will also be extremely useful for residents
   and practicing surgeons as a quick reference guide in daily practice to brush up on procedural
   steps or the work up of complex conditions"—Provided by publisher.
Identifiers: LCCN 2022058686 (print) | LCCN 2022058687 (ebook) | ISBN 9781265082857
   (paperback ; alk. paper) | ISBN 9781265084677 (ebook)
Subjects: MESH: Surgical Procedures, Operative | General Surgery | Study Guide
Classification: LCC RD37.2 (print) | LCC RD37.2 (ebook) | NLM WO 18.2 |
   DDC 617.0076—dc23/eng/20230501
LC record available at https://lccn.loc.gov/2022058686
LC ebook record available at https://lccn.loc.gov/2022058687

McGraw Hill books are available at special quantity discounts to use as premiums and sales
promotions, or for use in corporate training programs. To contact a representative please visit the
Contact Us pages at www.mhprofessional.com.

To our partners, Gary and Patrick. To the general surgeons who trained us, we are forever grateful.
And to those in training, this book is for you.

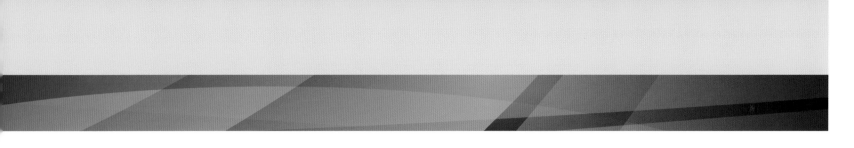

Contents

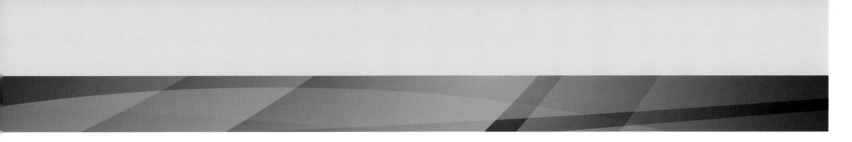

Contributors

Mohamed Alassas, MD, FACS
General Surgery, Surgical Oncology
Swedish Medical Center
Seattle, Washington

Andrew Feczko, MD
Thoracic and Cardiovascular Surgery
Cleveland Clinic
Cleveland, Ohio

Melinda Hawkins, MD
Colon and Rectal Surgery
Swedish Medical Center
Seattle, Washington

Danielle Hayes, MD
General Surgery
Swedish Medical Center
Seattle, Washington

Richy Lee, MD
Pediatric Surgery
Swedish Medical Center
Seattle, Washington

Gary Lucas, MD
General Surgery
Multicare Allenmore Hospital
Tacoma, Washington

Katherine Mandell, MD, MPH, FACS
General Surgery, Surgical Critical Care
Swedish Medical Center
Seattle, Washington

Michelle Marieni, MD
Obstetrics and Gynecology
California Pacific Medical Center –
    Mission Bernal Women's Clinic
San Francisco, California

Xuan-Binh (Ben) Pham, MD
Vascular Surgeon
Vascular and Interventional Specialists of
    Orange County
Orange, California

Shelby Reiter, MD
General Surgery
Swedish Medical Center
Edmonds, Washington

Joseph Sniezek, MD, MBA, FACS
Head & Neck Endocrine Surgery
Swedish Medical Center
Seattle, Washington

Sean Wells, MD, FACS
General Surgery
Swedish Medical Center
Seattle, Washington

David White, MD, FACS
General Surgery
Pacific Medical Center
Seattle, Washington

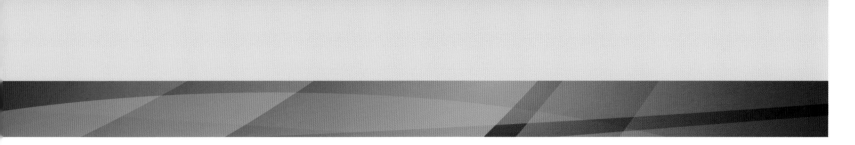

Preface

Dear Reader:

We created this book because we felt we needed a comprehensive study resource like this to help us prepare for our oral boards and none existed at the time. In terms of subject matter, this book aims to cover the majority of the topics on the SCORE curriculum and present them in a format that is practical for group study and self-quizzing.

Topics on the SCORE curriculum are categorized as either core or advanced. In this book, each chapter begins with a list of topics. Core topics and operations are denoted with a "c," while advanced topics are labeled with an "a." Additionally, you will see some topics that do not have a "c" or an "a" – these are topics that weren't explicitly listed on the SCORE curriculum but that we thought could potentially be useful.

General tips to prepare for the oral boards:
-   Give yourself at least 2–3 months to study. Make a plan and stick to it, so you are not stressed and cramming in the last 1–2 weeks before your exam.
-   Focus on mastering the core topics initially, and then once you have those covered, start working on the advanced topics.

-   Incorporate multiple different studying formats into your study plan including practicing scenarios with a peer, study books, podcasts, and/or a review course.
-   Complications will often arise in scenarios – it does not necessarily mean you made a mistake, so don't let this rattle you.
-   In this book, we describe the steps of operations the way we learned to do them, however there are often multiple other acceptable ways to perform them.
-   Hopefully your program is helping to prepare you by administering mock oral exams. Take these mock oral exams seriously and study hard. If your program doesn't coordinate formal mocks orals, then meet up with your co-residents and practice together on a regular basis throughout your residency.
-   Please refer to the American Board of Surgery website for the most up to date information and a copy of the SCORE curriculum.

We hope that you will find this book to be helpful in your oral boards studying endeavors as well as for preparing for daily life as a surgical resident.

Sincerely,
Shelby Reiter, MD
Danielle Hayes, MD

General Surgery

Sean Wells, MD, FACS

DISEASES AND CONDITIONS

- Elective inguinal hernia (c), open and laparoscopic repair (c)
- Incarcerated inguinal and femoral hernias (c), McVay repair
- Umbilical and epigastric hernias (c)
- Umbilical hernia in cirrhotic patient
- Ventral hernias (c), ventral hernia repair (c)
- Rectus sheath hematoma (c)
- Biliary colic (c), cholecystitis (c), cholecystectomy (c), surgical cholecystostomy (c)
- Benign biliary obstruction (c), common bile duct exploration (c), choledochoenteric anastomosis (a)

- Peptic ulcer disease (c), gastroduodenal perforation repair (c), vagotomy and drainage (c)
- Appendicitis (c), appendectomy (c)
- Appendiceal neoplasms
- Small bowel obstruction (c), adhesiolysis (c)
- Gallstone ileus
- Adynamic ileus (c)
- Small bowel neoplasms (c), small bowel resection (c)
- Small bowel neuroendocrine tumor
- Enteral feeding access (c), gastrostomy (c), jejunostomy (c)
- Enterocutaneous fistulas (c)

- Ileostomy creation and closure (c)
- Adrenal incidentaloma (c), laparoscopic transabdominal adrenalectomy (a)
- Hyperaldosteronism (c)
- Hypercortisolism (c)
- Pheochromocytoma (c)
- Adrenal cortical carcinoma (a), open adrenalectomy (a)
- Peritoneal dialysis catheter insertion (c)
- Desmoid tumor (a)
- Peritoneal neoplasms (a)

(c) = core topic   (a) = advanced topic

Disease Process	Relevant H&P	Work-up/Staging	Treatment	Key Surgical Steps	Post-op Care	Tips & Tidbits
Inguinal hernia, elective (core)	Groin bulge, groin pain Ask about obstructive symptoms, incarceration events, enlargement over time Examine patient and look for inguinal hernia while standing and sitting	Typically diagnosed on exam but can get groin U/S if diagnosis is unclear	Repair symptomatic inguinal hernias Watchful waiting is safe for asymptomatic or minimally symptomatic inguinal hernias in male patients; however, symptoms often progress and patients seek repair - Watchful waiting is not appropriate for femoral hernias, these should be repaired on a semi-urgent basis Repair can be done open or minimally invasive - Open preferable in patients who will not tolerate general anesthesia and/or pneumoperitoneum - Laparoscopic repair may be preferable in morbidly obese patients, patients with bilateral hernias, and female patients due to higher risk of femoral hernia (not addressed by Lichtenstein repair) - If patient has recurrent hernia, typically prefer to fix it with a method that was not previously used Minimally invasive options for repair include TAPP (transabdominal preperitoneal) vs TEP (totally extraperitoneal)	**Open Lichtenstein repair (core):** - Inguinal incision made between pubic symphysis and ASIS, overlying the cord, dissect down to external oblique - Open external oblique aponeurosis to superficial ring - Preserve or sacrifice ilioinguinal nerve - Encircle the cord with a Penrose drain - Locate indirect hernia sac and dissect it off the cord, ligate or reduce sac - Examine floor of canal for direct defect - Secure mesh to pubic tubercle then run this stitch along the shelving edge of the inguinal ligament - Lay tails of mesh on either side of the cord and then tuck tails of mesh under the external oblique - Place interrupted sutures medially in the conjoint tendon - Close tails of the mesh around the cord by suturing them together (tight enough to accommodate only a fingertip) - Close external oblique aponeurosis, Scarpa's, and skin **Laparoscopic TEP inguinal hernia repair:** - Start with an infra-umbilical incision - Incise anterior rectus sheath transversely just lateral to the linea alba, retract rectus muscle laterally and access retromuscular space, place 12-mm trocar - Dissect retromuscular space toward pubic symphysis, some use balloon dissector - Place 2 additional 5-mm ports in the lower midline - Identify Coopers ligament, then work laterally, pushing peritoneum down, staying clear of iliac vessels, and keeping epigastric vessels up - Identify and reduce hernias, fully separate indirect sac from the cord, reduce cord lipoma if present - Place mesh so that it covers entire myopectineal orifice and is below the parietalized peritoneum - Repeat on contralateral side if bilateral hernias are present	Complications: - Genital edema and hematoma—common, resolves with time - Urinary problems— urinary retention is common, catheterization as needed, resolves with time - Wound infection—if concern for mesh infection, may need to remove mesh - Chronic groin pain— pain >3 months after repair occurs in 5-15% - Ischemic Orchitis— testicular pain and swelling, may result in testicular atrophy - Vas deferens damage— repair in the OR if noted at the time - Bladder injury—repair primarily if seen intra-op and place Foley, get cystogram in 7-10 d	Additional reading: Fitzgibbons RJ, et al. Long-term results of a randomized controlled trial of a nonoperative strategy (watchful waiting) for men with minimally symptomatic inguinal hernias. *Ann Surg*. 2013; 258(3):508-515

Disease Process	Relevant H&P	Work-up/Staging	Treatment	Key Surgical Steps	Post-op Care	Tips & Tidbits
Incarcerated inguinal or femoral hernia (core)	Patient may present with painful unreducible groin bulge, N/V, obstipation, may have skin changes Consider other potential etiologies including abscess, pseudoaneurysm, and lymphadenopathy	Full labs Can sometimes diagnose on exam alone Consider CT	Attempt reduction—pain medication/sedation, Trendelenburg positioning, and ice pack may aid in reduction - Consider immediate operation without reduction if incarcerated for > 8 h or clinical signs of bowel ischemia If able to reduce, then observe patient for 12-24 h and trial PO prior to discharge to ensure there was no irreversible bowel ischemia, plan for elective repair prior to discharge or in near future If unable to reduce, take to OR - Place NGT prior to intubation to prevent aspiration - McVay repair—this is a good repair to know, it is a tissue repair that can be used in the setting of hernias with contamination, and it fixes inguinal and femoral hernias - If the bowel is viable and no contamination, can do typical mesh repair	**McVay repair:** - Open inguinal canal and dissect out the spermatic cord, same as with Lichtenstein repair (see elective inguinal hernia section) - Open floor of the inguinal canal from deep inguinal ring to pubic tubercle to enter the preperitoneal space and examine for femoral hernias (watch out for the inferior epigastric vessels) ◦ If having issues reducing a femoral hernia, can divide lacunar ligament and/or inguinal ligament - Identify hernia, open sac, and inspect the incarcerated bowel. If viable, reduce back into the abdomen. If nonviable, will have to do bowel resection, which can be done through the groin or convert to laparotomy - Sew conjoint tendon to Cooper's ligament starting medially on tubercle, working laterally - Eventually have to make a transition stitch, which includes conjoint tendon, inguinal ligament, Cooper's ligament - Sew conjoint tendon to inguinal ligament working out laterally to the level of the deep inguinal ring. If too much tension, can make relaxing incision medially on the anterior rectus sheath - Close the external oblique and skin	Tissue repairs have a higher risk of recurrence	There are many different acceptable approaches to an incarcerated groin hernia, just make sure your logic is safe Major missteps: While in real life it may be acceptable to place synthetic mesh in the setting of minimal contamination, you should not do this on the oral boards

Disease Process	Relevant H&P	Work-up/Staging	Treatment	Key Surgical Steps	Post-op Care	Tips & Tidbits
Umbilical and epigastric hernias (core)	History of prior repair? Obstructive symptoms? On exam, see if hernia is reducible, size of defect, skin changes Umbilical hernias are more common in pregnant and cirrhotic patients	Can get U/S if diagnosis is unclear but can usually be diagnosed based on exam	Hernia with strangulated bowel → emergent repair Don't have to repair small, asymptomatic umbilical hernias Primary vs mesh repair— typically use mesh if > 2 cm fascial defect and not contaminated In women of childbearing age, usually wait to repair until woman is done having children, unless it is very symptomatic, in which case you could do a primary repair	**Umbilical/epigastric hernia repair (core):** - Identify defect and make overlying incision - Dissect and define hernia sac - Open sac, evaluate viability of contents, reduce contents into the abdomen - Define fascial edges - Close fascia primarily vs place mesh - Tac the umbilical stalk down - Close incision in layers	- Pain control - Respiratory hygiene - Watch for mesh infections/wound complications	
Umbilical hernia in cirrhotic patient	Relatively common, higher risk for complications (incarceration, strangulation, rupture)		Elective—medically optimize treatment, including management of ascites, prior to repair ○ Hepatology referral, sodium restriction, diuretics, intermittent paracentesis, TIPS ○ In patients with advanced cirrhosis (MELD > 15), wait to repair at time of liver transplant Incarcerated/strangulated → forced to operate	**Tips for hernia in cirrhotic patient:** - Have blood products available - Avoid mesh - Close peritoneum and close incision in layers to avoid post-op leakage	In cirrhotic patients: - Control ascites with medical management and intermittent paracentesis to optimize wound healing and minimize risk of wound dehiscence - Continue antibiotics for SBP prophylaxis for 14 d post-op	

Disease Process	Relevant H&P	Work-up/Staging	Treatment	Key Surgical Steps	Post-op Care	Tips & Tidbits

Ventral hernia (core)	Bulging mass, pain
	
	Can present with incarcerated bowel leading to obstruction and strangulation
	
	Palpate hernia and fascial defect, attempt to reduce
	
	Ask about comorbidities, smoking, prior MRSA or MDR bacterial infections, and medical issues that can be optimized prior to elective repair
		Often diagnosed on physical exam
		
		Can consider U/S or CT if diagnosis is unclear or if it is a complex hernia—determine hernia defect size, location, and contents
			Minimally invasive vs open procedure, there are many different options for hernia repair, operation depends on acuity, size, prior operations, etc
			
			If elective, optimize the patient pre-op (smoking-cessation, weight loss, diabetes control) to optimize results
			
			Type of repair depends on multiple factors including size of hernia, condition of patient, and prior repairs:
			- Primary repair
			- Repair with underlay mesh in pre-peritonteal or intraperitoneal location
			- Retrorectus repair (Rives-Stoppa) +/- transversus abdominis release (TAR)—can get significant medial advancement with retrorectus/TAR dissection, releases 8-12 cm on each side
				Retrorectus repair +/- TAR (core) (Figure 1.1):
				- Midline incision, excise redundant skin and hernia sac
				- Access the abdomen, lyse any adhesions to the anterior abdominal wall
				- Open retrorectus space by incising posterior sheath 1 cm lateral to the linea alba
				- Develop retromuscular plane out to the linea semilunaris
				- If you would also like to do a TAR, expose the transversus abdominis muscle near the linea semilunaris and incise it ~0.5 cm medial to the perforating neurovascular bundles, which supply the rectus
				  ○ It is easiest to start in upper 1/3 of the abdomen and work inferiorly (Figure 1.2)
				  ○ This will allow entry into the space between the transversus abdominus and transversalis fascia
				  ○ This space can be extended laterally all the way back to the psoas muscle, allowing the posterior sheath to advance medially
				- Once this dissection is complete, close the posterior sheath and place a large mesh in the space
				- Close the anterior sheath and skin over the top, +/- drains
				
				Anterior component separation:
				- Midline incision, excise redundant skin and hernia sac
				- Get into the abdomen, lyse any adhesions to the anterior abdominal wall
				- Expose external oblique aponeurosis 2 cm lateral to linea semilunaris bilaterally (can do by raising skin flaps, small paramedian incisions, or tunneling), preserve periumbilical perforators
				- Incise the external oblique fascia and bluntly dissect it from underlying internal oblique from costal margin down to inguinal ligament and laterally out to anterior axillary line
				- Should be able to close fascia with minimal tension after this mobilization
				- Can also mobilize the retrorectus space if further advancement is needed
				- Can place mesh intra-abdominally or within rectus sheath
					Avoid heavy lifting for 4-6 wk
					
					Complications:
					- Skin necrosis, seroma, and hematoma are fairly common after anterior component separation due to large skin flaps
					- Wound dehiscence—large gush of serosanguinous fluid, need to take back to OR for reclosure
					- Mesh infection
					  ○ May present as wound infection or persistent drainage
					  ○ Initially treat with antibiotics, wound care, IR drain if needed
					  ○ Occasionally mesh infections can be salvaged with antibiotics, depends on type of mesh
					- It is never an emergency to excise infected mesh so do not rush the patient to the OR
					- Once patient is stabilized and optimized, take back for mesh excision and typically primarily close hernia defect or use absorbable mesh and delay definitive reconstruction
						If a patient presents with ventral hernia with strangulated bowel:
						- Avoid placing synthetic mesh and performing a fascial release in a contaminated setting because you don't want to "burn bridges"
						- Close the fascia primarily if possible
						- If you cannot close the defect primarily, use a Vicryl or synthetic mesh, knowing that the patient will develop a hernia down the road

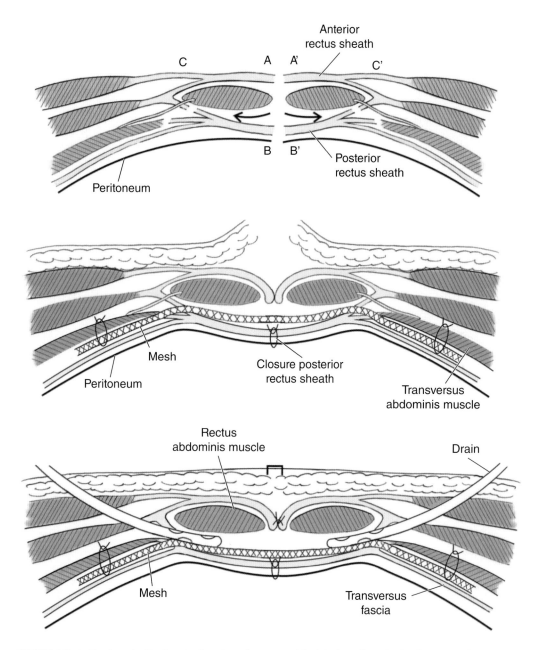

FIGURE 1.1: Ventral hernia repair with retrorectus dissection and transversus abdominis release. (Reproduced with permission from Ellison EC, Zollinger Jr RM, Pawlik TM, et al. *Zollinger's Atlas of Surgical Operations,* 11th ed. New York, NY: McGraw Hill; 2022, Figure 9 E-G.)

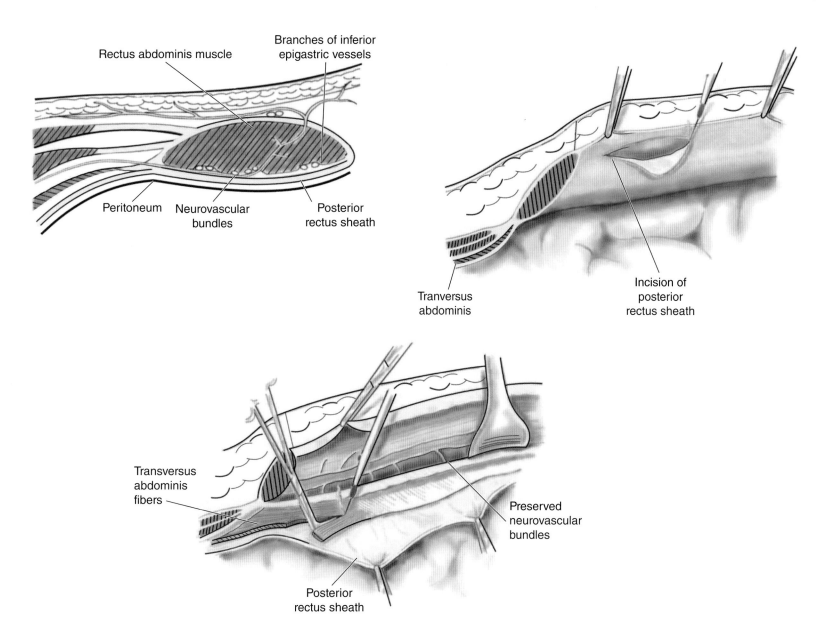

FIGURE 1.2: Retrorectus dissection and transversus abdominis release. (Reproduced with permission from Ellison EC, Zollinger Jr RM, Pawlik TM, et al. *Zollinger's Atlas of Surgical Operations,* 11th ed. New York, NY: McGraw Hill; 2022, Figure 9 B-D.)

Disease Process	Relevant H&P	Work-up/Staging	Treatment	Key Surgical Steps	Post-op Care	Tips & Tidbits

Rectus sheath hematoma (core)	Occurs due to injury to the epigastric artery or its branches within the rectus muscle
	
	Typically related to therapeutic anticoagulation and/or trauma, can occur spontaneously
	
	Common scenario—elderly patient on anticoagulation develops abdominal pain and mass after vigorous coughing
	
	On exam, patient will have palpable abdominal mass that does not cross the midline, remains palpable with abdominal wall flexion
		CBC, INR, CT/CTA
		
		Type I—small, confined within rectus, does not cross midline or dissect fascial plans
		
		Type II—within the rectus muscle but can dissect across midline or along the transversalis fascia
		
		Type III—large, usually below the arcuate line, extends into the peritoneum and/or the prevesical space
			Majority of patients managed with no invasive intervention, just rest, ice, compression, and analgesia
			
			+/- anticoagulation reversal depending on severity
			
			Patients with significant anemia or hemodynamic instability should have transfusion as needed
			
			If patient has persistent evidence of bleeding, despite supportive measures, then consider IR embolization
			
			It is rare for rectus sheath hematoma to require surgical intervention, only if unstable with ongoing bleeding and embolization unsuccessful/ unavailable
				Surgical management of rectus sheath hematoma:
				- Paramedian or midline incision to access rectus sheath in the area of the largest component of the hematoma
				- Evacuate the hematoma
				- Identify and ligate any bleeding vessels
				  ○ Ligation of epigastric vessel is well tolerated due to collateral flow
				  ○ Inferior epigastric may be ligated where if comes off the external iliac artery via groin cut down, if unable to ligate via initial abdominal incision
				  ○ Irrigate, leave drain, close
					Remove drain when <30 mL/d
					
					Lump from hematoma may last up to 3-6 mo if managed nonoperatively	

Disease Process	Relevant H&P	Work-up/Staging	Treatment	Key Surgical Steps	Post-op Care	Tips & Tidbits

Biliary colic, cholecystitis (core)	Risk factors for cholelithiasis: female, increased age, obesity, pregnancy, rapid weight loss
	- Biliary colic: episodic, often postprandial, RUQ pain
	- Cholecystitis: persistent RUQ pain, fever, N/V
	- Chronic cholecystitis: recurrent attacks of biliary colic lead to chronic inflammatory change
	- Acalculous cholecystitis: occurs in critically ill patients, may have abdominal pain, fever
		CBC
		LFT—elevated T bili, alk phos, lipase should raise concern for possible ductal obstruction
		Lipase—elevated lipase should raise concern for gallstone pancreatitis and possible ductal obstruction
		RUQ U/S—look for gallstones, gallbladder wall thickening, pericholecystic fluid, CBD dilation
		HIDA scan—can be used if diagnosis unclear or to make diagnosis of acalculous cholecystitis, failure to fill gallbladder after 2 h suggests cholecystitis
			Antibiotics
			Laparoscopic cholecystectomy (LC), open cholecystectomy if needed
			Percutaneous cholecystostomy tube for critically ill patients with acalculous cholecystitis
			- Can also be used for patients with cholecystitis who are not appropriate for cholecystectomy at time of presentation
			- Get drain check in 6 wk to evaluate for patent cystic duct, remove tube if gallbladder is no longer obstructed, consider lap chole in reasonable operative candidates
			For patients with gallstone pancreatitis, LC prior to discharge encouraged due to high recurrence rate
				Laparoscopic cholecystectomy (core):
				- Place ports and retract gallbladder cephalad and lateral
				- Open peritoneum on both sides of the gallbladder, dissect out cystic artery and duct
				- Obtain critical view of safety:
				  1. Hepatocystic triangle cleared of fatty and fibrous tissue
				  2. The lower 1/3 of the gallbladder separated from the liver to expose the cystic plate
				  3. Only 2 structures seen entering the gallbladder
				- Obtain a cholangiogram, if indicated
				- Clip and divide cystic duct and artery
				- Separate gallbladder from gallbladder fossa and place in endocatch bag
				- Check for bleeding or bile leakage, remove gallbladder and close
				
				Open cholecystectomy (core):
				- Perform right subcostal incision and divide the falciform
				- Dissect adhesions off the gallbladder and pack the colon down for exposure
				- Grasp gallbladder fundus with clamp and place a second clamp on the infundibulum
				- Incise peritoneum on either side of gallbladder, and take gallbladder off liver, dome down
				- Identify and control cystic duct and artery (get IOC, if needed)
				- Complete dissection of gallbladder off cystic plate, ligate and divide cystic duct and artery
				- Check for bile leak and hemostasis, close
				
				Surgical cholecystostomy (core):
				- Bail out maneuver if terrible gallbladder encountered or if IR not available to place percutaneous cholecystostomy
				- Make hole in fundus, decompress gallbladder, try to remove stone stuck in neck if possible
				- Place purse string suture around hole, insert Foley balloon and tie down suture around Foley
				- Bring foley balloon out of skin in RUQ, suture to skin to prevent dislodgement
					Complications:
					- Iatrogenic bile duct injury—occurs in 0.3-0.6% of cases
					- Cystic duct leak—percutaneous drainage, ERCP to determine location of the leak and place stent, which usually resolves the leak
					- Dropped gallstones—can cause abscess, fistula, wound infection, SBO
					- Retained CBD stone—treat with ERCP
						Consider performing a subtotal cholecystectomy, converting to open cholecystectomy or cholecystostomy tube placement in cases of difficult LC when unable to get critical view
						Biliary dyskinesia—presents as classic biliary pain w/o evidence of stones or other pathology
						- Work-up: LFT, lipase, U/S, +/- CT
						- HIDA scan with low EF (<35%) may be associated with gallbladder dysfunction
						- Consider LC, as long as patient knows it is not guaranteed to resolve their pain
						  ○ >60% patients diagnosed with functional gallbladder disorder have symptom improvement after LC
						Additional reading:
						Strasberg SM, et al. Subtotal cholecystectomy-"fenestrating" vs "reconstituting" subtypes and the prevention of bile duct injury: definition of the optimal procedure in difficult operative conditions. *J Am Coll Surg.* 2016 Jan;222(1):89-96

Disease Process	Relevant H&P	Work-up/Staging	Treatment	Key Surgical Steps	Post-op Care	Tips & Tidbits
Benign biliary obstruction (core)	May present with abdominal pain, jaundice, fever, N/V	CBC, CMP, lipase U/S—dilated CBD Consider MRCP if further anatomical info needed May present with simple choledocholithiasis, cholangitis, and/or gallstone pancreatitis	Common bile duct stones can be removed via common bile duct exploration (CBDE) or ERCP Transgastric ERCP may be required for patients with choledocholithiasis and history of RNY gastric bypass If patient has cholangitis and unable to perform ERCP, may need to do percutaneous transhepatic cholangiocatheter (PTC) for biliary decompression Patient may need sphincteroplasty or choledochoduodenostomy if issues with recurrent stones	**Laparoscopic transcystic common bile duct exploration (core):** - Place cholangiocatheter, and attempt to flush stones by giving 1mg glucagon IV and flush duct with saline and 1% lidocaine - If stones persist, thread hydrophilic wire through cholangiocatheter, use fluoro to confirm wire is in duodenum - Remove cholangiocatheter and thread sheath over wire into cystic duct - Remove wire and insert choledochoscope into cystic duct via sheath - Drive choledochoscope down into the distal CBD and find stone, use wire basket to extract stone ◦ If unable to pull stone back, may be able to dilate the sphincter and push stone through the ampulla into the duodenum - Once stone is removed, repeat cholangiogram to ensure duct is now clear - Complete LC in typical fashion **Open common bile duct exploration +/- transduodenal sphincteroplasty:** - Right subcostal incision - Remove gallbladder, do cholangiogram through cystic stump to evaluate for stone disease - Dissect out CBD, avoid vessels at 3 and 9 o'clock - Place 4-0 Prolene stay sutures on either side of duct and make longitudinal incision on the anterior surface of CBD just above the duodenum - Extract stones, use Fogarty catheter proximally and distally - Place T tube in CBD and secure with 4-0 PDS, obtain cholangiogram to ensure CBD clearance and check for leak, leave drain - If residual stones, perform transduodenal removal or choledochoduodenostomy - Kocherize the duodenum - Identify location of ampulla (can pass Fogarty or Bakes dilator down CBD) and make ~5 cm longitudinal duodenostomy over this area - Open the ampulla ~5 mm in the 11 o'clock position and then suture the cut edge of the ampulla to the duodenum using 5-0 PDS - Extract residual stones through opened sphincter - Close duodenotomy in 2 layers without narrowing it, leave drain **Choledochoduodenostomy (advanced) (Figure 1.3):** - Right subcostal incision - Cholecystectomy - Dissect out the anterior surface of CBD from cystic duct insertion down - Kocherize duodenum so that it can be elevated to CBD without tension - Make longitudinal ductotomy on CBD below cystic duct as distal as possible to minimize sump syndrome - Extract stones - Make longitudinal duodenotomy on adjacent anterior aspect of duodenum - Create anastomosis with 4-0 PDS, placing corner sutures first (3 and 9 o'clock), then back row, then front row - Leave drain		

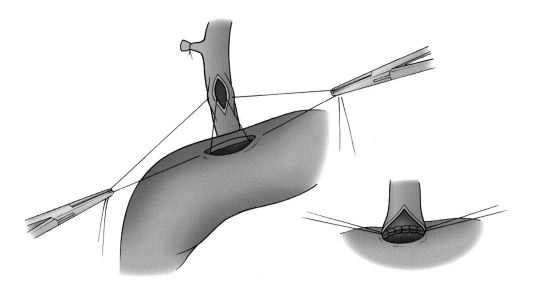

FIGURE 1.3: Creation of choledochoduodenostomy. (Modified with permission from Minter RM, Doherty GM. *Current Procedures: Surgery*. New York, NY: McGraw Hill; 2010, Figure 12-7.)

Disease Process	Relevant H&P	Work-up/Staging	Treatment	Key Surgical Steps	Post-op Care	Tips & Tidbits

Peptic ulcer disease (core)	Ulcer may present as GI bleed or free perforation
	
	- If perforated, patient will typically have abrupt onset of diffuse abdominal pain
	- Posterior ulcers tender to cause bleeding and anterior ulcers tend to cause perforation
	
	Risk factors: *H. pylori*, NSAID use, Zollinger-Ellison, anticoagulation
		Significant bleeding can occur with posterior duodenal ulcers that erode into the GDA
		
		- If bleeding: place NGT, get full labs including CBC, CMP, coags, type and screen, serial Hgb, EGD, transfuse as needed
		
		If perforated: get full labs, imaging (upright CXR vs CT depending on patient stability)
			Bleeding ulcer:
			- EGD is first step
			- Consider repeat EGD or interventional radiology if initial EGD unsuccessful or patient rebleeds
			- Surgery only if unstable or refractory to prior attempts at endoscopy and IR not successful/available
			
			Perforated ulcer: antibiotics, resuscitation, OR
			- Consider acid reducing procedure if patient is stable and has ulcer disease refractory to medical management
			
			Patients should have *H. pylori* testing and treatment, PPI
				Surgical management of bleeding duodenal ulcer:
				- Upper midline laparotomy, Kocher maneuver
				- Longitudinal duodenotomy
				- Use UR-6 needle to ligate vessel (GDA) at 12, 3, 6 o'clock
				- Close duodenotomy transversely, +/- drain
				
				Surgical management of perforated ulcer (core):
				- Upper midline laparotomy
				- Biopsy ulcer and debride back to healthy tissue
				- Repair with Graham patch vs modified Graham patch
				  ○ For large perforations not amenable to Graham patch, consider jejunal sucker patch vs Thal patch (serosal patch) vs distal gastrectomy
				- Consider truncal vagotomy and pyloroplasty in stable patient with refractory ulcer disease
				  ○ Truncal vagotomy:
				    ■ Mobilize left lobe of the liver to expose hiatus
				    ■ Mobilize the esophageal hiatus, open phrenoesophageal ligament
				    ■ Get Penrose drain around esophagus
				    ■ Identify anterior and posterior vagus nerves
				    ■ Clip nerves 4-6 cm above GEJ (to include criminal nerve of Grassi)
				    ■ Excise 2-3 cm and send for frozen to confirm
				    ■ Pyloroplasty— ~5cm incision from antrum to proximal duodenum, close transversely
				
				Distal gastrectomy:
				- Kocherize the duodenum and mobilize the distal stomach
				- Take the omentum off the greater curve halfway to the GEJ, ligate right gastroepiploic artery near GDA
				- Open the gastrohepatic ligament and divide right gastric artery
				- Free the first part of the duodenum from the pancreas
				- Divide stomach and first portion of duodenum with stapler, oversew duodenal staple line
				- Reconstruct with Billroth I/II or Roux-en-Y gastrojejunostomy
				- Leave NGT in place
					Empiric *H. pylori* treatment—amoxicillin, clarithromycin, omeprazole for 10-14 d	When ligating the GDA, do not place a stitch at 9 o'clock (risk of injuring CBD)
						
						Perforated ulcers should be biopsied and tested for *H. pylori* and malignancy

Disease Process	Relevant H&P	Work-up/Staging	Treatment	Key Surgical Steps	Post-op Care	Tips & Tidbits
Appendicitis (core)	Periumbilical pain that migrates to right lower quadrant	CBC, CMP CT A/P with IV contrast	Acute, uncomplicated appendicitis—laparoscopic appendectomy versus antibiotics, discuss pros and cons of each approach with the patient Complicated appendicitis (perforated, phlegmon, abscess)—typically treat with antibiotics +/- IR drain and interval appendectomy in ~8 wk Pregnant patient—appendectomy should be performed regardless of trimester, port placement will have to be adjusted, depending on trimester	**Laparoscopic appendectomy (core):** - Position supine with left arm tucked - Place 12-mm port at umbilicus and 5-mm ports in the LLQ and suprapubic areas - Identify the appendix - Make window in mesoappendix at the base of the appendix - Use separate staple loads to transect the appendix and mesoappendix **Open appendectomy:** - Oblique RLQ incision over McBurney's point - Dissect down in a muscle splitting fashion by dividing each muscle/aponeurotic layer parallel to its fibers - Enter the peritoneum and identify the cecum - Identify the appendix and deliver it into the wound - Make a hole in the mesoappendix at the base of the appendix, ligate and transect the mesoappendix - Ligate and transect the appendix at the base, invaginate the stump with a purse string suture placed in the wall of the cecum - Washout as needed - Close incision in layers		Additional reading: CODA Collaborative, Flum DR, et al. A randomized trial comparing antibiotics with appendectomy for appendicitis. *N Engl J Med.* 2020 Nov 12;383(20):1907-1919 Hayes D, et al. Is interval appendectomy really needed? A closer look at neoplasm rates in adult patients undergoing interval appendectomy after complicated appendicitis. *Surg Endosc.* 2021 Jul;35(7):3855-3860

Disease Process	Relevant H&P	Work-up/Staging	Treatment	Key Surgical Steps	Post-op Care	Tips & Tidbits
Appendiceal neoplasms	Can present with abdominal pain, appendicitis, or be incidentally noted on imaging or colonoscopy	Colonoscopy recommended in any patient with appendiceal mass Staging: - Appendiceal neuroendocrine tumor (NET) (carcinoid)—CT A/P if > 2 cm, positive margins, or positive LN - Low grade appediceal mucinous neoplasm (LAMN)—CT A/P, tumor markers (CEA, Ca 19-9, Ca-125), colonoscopy, consider diagnostic laparoscopy - Adenocarcinoma/goblet cell—CT C/A/P, colonoscopy, tumor markers (CEA, Ca 19-9, Ca-125, chromogranin A)	Appendiceal mass → appendectomy Appendiceal NET: - If less than <1 cm and margins negative, then appendectomy sufficient - 1-2 cm—consider right hemicolectomy, discuss with multidisciplinary team, consider grade and Ki67, invasion of mesoappendix - > 2 cm, margin +, or LN + then do right hemicolectomy LAMN—no further surgery if proximal appendectomy margin is negative - If proximal margin has mucinous epithelium, perform resection to negative margin (cecectomy vs right hemicolectomy) - Patients with pseudomyxoma peritonei (PP) may be candidates for cytoreduction and HIPEC Adenocarcinoma/goblet cell—right hemicolectomy if M0	See key surgical steps in appendectomy and right hemicolectomy sections	Surveillance: Appendiceal NET—yearly H&P, CT C/A/P, consider biochemical testing such as 24-h urine or plasma 5-HIAA LAMN—regular surveillance with CT A/P and tumor markers Adenocarcinoma/goblet cell—H&P, CEA q3mo x 2y then q6mo through 5 y, annual CT C/A/P x 3 y, colonoscopy at 1y post-op	Risk of nodal metastasis in patients with appendiceal NET based on tumor size: • <1 cm: 0% • 1-2 cm: ~7% • >2 cm: 33% Additional reading: Chicago Consensus Working Group. The Chicago Consensus on peritoneal surface malignancies: management of appendiceal neoplasms. *Cancer*. 2020 Jun 1; 126(11):2525-2533

Disease Process	Relevant H&P	Work-up/Staging	Treatment	Key Surgical Steps	Post-op Care	Tips & Tidbits
Small bowel obstruction (SBO) (core)	Patient presents with abdominal distention, nausea, vomiting, and obstipation Ask about prior surgical history, prior obstructions Most common causes of SBO: - Adhesions - Hernia - Malignancy Perform abdominal exam, look for incarcerated hernia	Full set of labs including lactate CT—look for transition point, signs of ischemia or perforation - SBO vs ileus: SBO will have discrete transition point - Concerning findings include free fluid, free air, mesenteric edema, pneumatosis, volvulus, or closed-loop obstruction Consider small bowel follow through (gastrograffin challenge) in patients with SBO and no indication for immediate surgical intervention - If contrast has not reached colon by 24 h, obstruction unlikely to resolve nonoperatively	Nonoperative SBO management appropriate for patients without peritonitis or other signs of ischemia or perforation—bowel rest, NGT, IVF Surgical intervention required for patients with peritonitis, signs of perforation or ischemia, closed loop bowel obstructions, and those who fail trial of nonoperative management Diagnostic laparoscopy vs exploratory laparotomy with lysis of adhesions, bowel resection as needed	**Diagnostic laparoscopy/laparotomy with lysis of adhesions (core):** - Begin with diagnostic laparoscopy vs laparotomy - Run the bowel starting at LOT or terminal ileum and find the transition point, lyse adhesions - Assess bowel viability, resect if needed	Complications: - Early post-op bowel obstruction: supportive care and delay re-operation until at least 4 wk out, if possible	Even in patients without prior abdominal surgeries, 50% of SBO are due to adhesions, only 4-13% due to malignancy (Amara et al) Additional reading: Amara Y, et al. Diagnosis and management of small bowel obstruction in virgin abdomen: a WSES position paper. *World J Emerg Surg*. 2021 Jul 3;16(1):36 Zielinski MD, et al. Multi-institutional, prospective, observational study comparing the Gastrografin challenge versus standard treatment in adhesive small bowel obstruction. *J Trauma Acute Care Surg*. 2017 Jul;83(1):47-54
Gallstone ileus	N/V, abdominal distention, pain	CT scan—may show pneumobilia, foreign body in RLQ (intraluminal gallstone usually stuck at IC valve), fistula between gallbladder and bowel	NGT decompression, resuscitation OR for stone removal when stabilized	**Surgical management of gallstone ileus:** - Laparotomy - Make longitudinal enterotomy upstream from where gallstone is lodged and milk it back to remove it - Palpate the bowel for any additional stones - Close enterotomy transversely - If stable, can consider cholecystectomy with take down of fistulous tract and repair of duodenum, but if patient is unwell, return to do that later - During fistula take down, perform cholecystectomy and repair duodenal defect in 2 layers	Recurrent obstruction can occur if there are remaining sizeable gallstones and fistula was not taken down	Major misstep: Rushing unwell patient with gallstone ileus to the OR and attempting fistula takedown at that time

Disease Process	Relevant H&P	Work-up/Staging	Treatment	Key Surgical Steps	Post-op Care	Tips & Tidbits
Adynamic ileus (core)	Patients present with abdominal distention, nausea, vomiting, and obstipation Functional issue- stoppage of the flow of intestinal contents without mechanical cause Small bowel ileus is most common after open intra-abdominal surgery, can also occur in critically ill patients, and patients with intra-abdominal infection Ogilvie's syndrome (acute colonic pseudo-obstruction) most common in patients with advanced age, many comorbidities, electrolyte imbalance, polypharmacy, opioid use, and/or poor underlying functional status Examine abdomen Perform DRE in cases of Ogilvie's to rule out rectal mass/stricture causing obstruction	Full set of labs including lactate KUB Consider CT scan - look for transition point, signs of ischemia or perforation - SBO vs ileus: SBO will have a discrete transition point Ogilvie's Syndrome: typically warrants colonoscopic evaluation to rule out mechanical obstruction and provide decompression	Small bowel ileus almost always managed nonoperatively with supportive care - Bowel rest, NGT, IV hydration, address underlying cause, correct electrolytes, minimize narcotics Ogilvie's treated with supportive care as long as there are no signs of perforation - Bowel rest, NGT, IV hydration, correct electrolytes, minimize narcotics and anti-cholinergics, decompression with colonoscopy/rectal tube - Neostigmine indicated for some patients—must have cardiac monitoring during administration due to risk of bradycardia Perforation or full thickness ischemia suspected → OR			Do not rush these patients to the OR, unless concerned for perforation or full thickness ischemia

Disease Process	Relevant H&P	Work-up/Staging	Treatment	Key Surgical Steps	Post-op Care	Tips & Tidbits
Small bowel neoplasms (core)	May be noted incidentally or present with bleeding, obstruction, abdominal pain, and/or weight loss Patients with Crohn's disease are at increased risk of small bowel adenocarcinoma Patients with celiac disease and AIDS are at increased risk of small bowel lymphoma	Differential for small bowel mass: - Adenoma - Neuroendocrine tumor (carcinoid) - Adenocarcinoma - Lymphoma: most commonly found in terminal ileum - GIST - Metastatic disease CT scan Capsule endoscopy Stage patient appropriately once cancer diagnosis is made	Neuroendocrine tumor—see small bowel neuroendocrine tumor section Small bowel adenocarcinoma: - SBR and wide mesenteric lymphadenectomy - Adenocarcinoma of terminal ileum → right hemicolectomy - If M1 disease and not obstructed, give chemo (FOLFOX) before operating Small bowel lymphoma—conservative SBR to remove gross disease if obstructing, bleeding, or perforated - Survival dictated by response to systemic therapy, not the extent of surgical resection - Tend to be chemo responsive, in absence of symptoms they do not mandate surgery GIST—SBR, no lymphadenectomy needed	**Small bowel resection (core):** - Create mesenteric defect and transect bowel with GIA stapler proximally and distally - Clamp and tie or LigaSure to divide the mesentery associated with the specimen, take a wedge of mesentery with the specimen, if indicated - Line up the bowel side by side, functional end-to-end and cut off the corner of the staple line on both limbs - Insert the GIA stapler and fire to create a common enterotomy along the antimesenteric border - Close the bowel with another fire of the stapler - Close the mesenteric defect - Can also do hand sewn anastomosis with inner layer of running 3-0 Vicryl and outer layer of interrupted 3-0 silk	Small bowel adenocarcinoma 5-y survival 14-33% Small bowel lymphoma 5-y survival 50-60%	For all cancer cases, remember to identify the type of cancer, stage if needed, and then treat
Small bowel neuroendocrine tumor (carcinoid)	May be found incidentally or present with bleeding, obstruction, abdominal pain, and/or weight loss Once disease is metastatic to the liver it may present as carcinoid syndrome (flushing, wheezing, diarrhea, palpitations)	Full labs including chromogranin A 24-h urine 5-HIAA CT—small bowel mass, obstruction, "spoke-like" mass with spiculated borders and linear strands in the mesentery DOTATATE scan About 45% of patients with small bowel NET have metastasis at presentation	Small bowel resection of affected segment Even if patient has wide-spread disease, surgical debulking may provide symptomatic relief Liver disease: - Surgical resection if possible - Liver directed therapy (TACE, RFA) if unable to resect - Octreotide/lantreotide → symptomatic relief, delay progression	**Surgical management of small bowel neuroendocrine tumor:** - Examine abdomen for signs of metastasis - Perform small bowel resection including wide wedge of mesentery to get lymph nodes - Be sure to run all of the bowel because 20-30% of patients have multicentric disease	Follow chromogranin A levels	Carcinoid crisis: flushing, labile blood pressure, arrhythmia - Tx: octreotide

Disease Process	Relevant H&P	Work-up/Staging	Treatment	Key Surgical Steps	Post-op Care	Tips & Tidbits
Enteral feeding access (core)	Reason for enteral access? Prior abdominal surgeries? Avoid G-tube in patients who may eventually need esophagectomy with gastric conduit	If planning to do PEG, can look at CT scan to assess for "window"	Options for more durable enteral access include gastrostomy vs jejunostomy Gastrostomy can be placed a variety of ways,—PEG vs surgical G-tube vs lap-assisted PEG placement	**Percutaneous endoscopic gastrostomy tube (pull method):** - Advance endoscope into stomach and insufflate, look for transillumination and 1:1 movement with abdominal wall palpation - Pick a spot several centimeters below the costal margin, make small stab incision, and insert needle while aspirating and watching endoscopically (you should not get air back into the syringe until you see needle in the stomach) - Once in the stomach, insert guidewire through needle, which is snared by the endoscope and pulled out through the mouth - Loop the PEG tube onto the guide-wire that was pulled up through the mouth, and pull guidewire back out of abdominal wall until the PEG tube is pulled up and the bumper is against gastric wall **Open Stamm gastrostomy (core):** - Upper midline laparotomy - Select spot on stomach 2/3 distance from GEJ to pylorus where there is no tension when brought up to the anterior abdominal wall and place purse string x2 at chosen site - Make hole in abdominal wall ~2 fingerbreadths below costal margins and pull G-tube through - Make gastrotomy and insert G-tube in the center of the purse string sutures and tie them down, inflate G-tube balloon - Place 4 tacking sutures around tube between stomach and abdominal wall - Secure G-tube to abdominal wall and close abdomen **Open jejunostomy tube placement (core):** - Small upper midline incision - Use loop of jejunum ~30cm distal to LOT that reaches abdominal wall easily - Bring J tube through abdominal wall at chosen site - Place purse string suture at chosen tube site and create enterotomy in center of purse string - Thread J tube into the bowel, making sure it threads distally and then tie down purse string - Create Witzel tunnel around the tube - Tack the bowel to the abdominal wall in 4 quadrants around the tube and place "anti-swivel" stitch	Complications: - Tube dislodgement: can attempt to replace at bedside if it goes easily, if successful get tube check to confirm intraluminal location ○ If PEG tube is dislodged early in post-op course prior to tract maturing (requires 2-4 wk), will likely require operative intervention - Typically less problematic if surgical feeding tube is dislodged because stomach is sutured to the abdominal wall - Over inflation of feeding tube balloon can cause obstruction	

Disease Process	Relevant H&P	Work-up/Staging	Treatment	Key Surgical Steps	Post-op Care	Tips & Tidbits
Enterocutaneous fistula (ECF) (core)	Most commonly occurs after abdominal surgery Typically presents as signs of sepsis, succus drainage from incision site FRIEND - reasons for persistent fistula - Foreign body - Radiation - Infection/ inflammation - Epithelization - Neoplasm - Distal obstruction	Full labs CT with contrast—look for source, undrained collections May need to get fistulogram to determine anatomy of the fistula Large bowel fistula—consider colonoscopy to rule out underlying malignancy, IBD	Use S.N.A.P. to take care of ECF patients: - Sepsis, skin care—treat with antibiotics and IR drainage to manage infection, take excellent care of patient's skin - Nutrition—optimize nutrition, measure fistula output, replace electrolytes and fluid as needed, ideally can feed enterally but if high output will likely need to be NPO with TPN - Anatomy—determine course of the fistula, can do CT with enteral contrast or fistulogram - Patience and planning—do not rush back to the OR, stabilize and optimize the patient ○ Postpone surgery for at least 3-6 mo, some will wait 6-12 mo Medications that may decrease fistula output—PPI, H2 blocker, somatostatin analogues	**Surgical management of ECF:** - Exploratory laparotomy - Resect involved bowel and fistula tracts - Remove foreign material/mesh, if present - Consider placement of feeding tube		Major misstep: Do not prematurely take patients with an ECF back to the OR. Follow the S.N.A.P. principles and delay surgery as long as fistula output is decreasing and wound is showing signs of healing ~30% ECF will heal spontaneously with time, which usually occurs in first 6 wk. If they do not heal in first 6 wk, unlikely to heal spontaneously High output fistulas and fistulas from small bowel source less likely to heal spontaneously (stomach and large bowel more likely to close)

Disease Process	Relevant H&P	Work-up/Staging	Treatment	Key Surgical Steps	Post-op Care	Tips & Tidbits
Ileostomy creation, management, and closure (core)	Ileostomy may be required for a variety of reasons—temporary diversion after colorectal surgery, distal obstruction, Crohn's, etc	Preoperative stoma marking—should go through the patient's rectus, should be on a flat surface, not in skin crease, above belt line. Can involve stoma therapist "Stoma triangle"—ASIS, pubic tubercle, umbilicus	End vs loop ileostomy, depending on why it is needed Stoma reversal in 6-12 wk, depending on patient condition and why the ileostomy was created in the first place (ie, completion of chemo/XRT, healing of anastomosis)	**Ileostomy creation (core):** - Excise circular area of skin 2-3 cm in diameter at chosen site - Dissect down to the anterior sheath - Make cruciate cut in the anterior rectus sheath, split the rectus, and then incise the posterior sheath, aperture should accommodate ~2 fingers - Bring up ileum through opening so that 4-5 cm is above the skin - When making loop ileostomy, need to use ileum 10-15 cm proximal to IC valve so that you will have room to make anastomosis when ileostomy is reversed - Open the ileum and place Brooking sutures in 3-4 quadrants, with interrupted sutures in between - Brooking sutures are done with a full thickness bite at the open end of the bowel, a seromuscular bite ~2cm more proximal on the bowel wall, and then a bite of dermis can be done in similar fashion but aperture may need to be wider and only Brooke the proximal limb of bowel **Loop ileostomy reversal (core):** - Can usually be done locally, without re-laparotomy - Suture stoma closed with purse string to prevent leakage - Use Bovie to cut through mucocutaneous junction all the way around the ileostomy - Dissect ileostomy away from the subcutaneous tissues until you enter the abdomen and loop ileostomy is free circumferentially - Make sure bowel appears viable, then insert stapler (one side into afferent limb and one side in efferent limb) and fire to create common enterotomy, then staple bowel closed - Reduce new anastomosis back into the abdomen and close the fascia - Purse string the skin with 2-0 Vicryl and leave small opening with betadine-soaked Telfa that can be removed in 2-3 d	Ideal ileostomy output is <1.2 L/d - Can give fiber, Imodium, Lomotil, and/ or tincture of opium for high ileostomy output Ileostomy complications: - High output ileostomy (>1.2 L/d)—can lead to dehydration, AKI - Stoma ischemia—if just superficial, can usually observe but if it extends below the fascia take patient back for revision - Stoma prolapse—not an emergency unless bowel becomes necrotic - Parastomal hernia is very common, need for repair is based on symptoms	For diverting ileostomies, get contrast enema to evaluate distal anastomosis prior to reversal

Disease Process	Relevant H&P	Work-up/Staging	Treatment	Key Surgical Steps	Post-op Care	Tips & Tidbits

Adrenal incidentaloma (core)	Adrenal incidentalomas seen on 1-4% of abdominal imaging
	History of malignancy?
		Two key questions to ask when presented with adrenal incidentaloma:
		- Is it functional or nonfunctional?
		- Is it benign or malignant?
		Biochemical work-up
		- BMP, renin, aldosterone
		- Plasma metanephrines
		- 24 h urine cortisol, ACTH level, dexamethasone suppression test if cortisol elevated
		- +/- androgen measurement (DHEA-sulfate)
		Adrenal protocol CT
		- Features of benign adrenal lesion: <4 cm, homogeneous, <10 HFU, >50% washout on delayed images
		- Features concerning for ACC: >4cm, heterogeneous, irregular borders, >20 HFU, delayed contrast washout (<50% washout at 10 min)
		Do not biopsy unless there is diagnostic uncertainty and concerned for metastatic disease
		- Always rule out pheochromocytoma prior to biopsy of adrenal mass
			Nonfunctional and < 4 cm: surveillance
			- Repeat imaging at 3-6 mo, then annually for 2 y
			- Repeat biochemical testing with plasma fractionated metanephrines and overnight dexamethasone test annually for 5 y
			Functional and/or >4-6 cm: adrenalectomy
			- 25% risk of malignancy in tumors >6 cm (4-6 cm is a gray area)
			Perform open adrenalectomy, rather than laparoscopic, if malignancy suspected
				Laparoscopic transabdominal adrenalectomy (advanced):
				- Positioning is key
				  ○ Lateral decubitus with lesion side up
				  ○ Flex the bed → widen space between costal margin and iliac crest
				  ○ Place ports
				    ■ Insert 3 ports ~2 cm below costal margin, with the posterior port placed as far lateral-posterior as possible
				    ■ Leave at least 5 cm between each port
				- Left adrenalectomy:
				  ○ Take down splenic flexure of the colon
				  ○ Take down lateral attachments to the spleen, rotate the spleen and tail of pancreas anteromedially
				  ○ Use left crus of diaphragm as landmark that leads to left inferior phrenic vein, which runs along medial aspect of left adrenal gland and joins with left adrenal vein (typically gland has sizable vein that needs to be identified and ligated and multiple small arteries that can be taken with the LigaSure)
				  ○ Left adrenal vein clipped and divided
				  ○ Dissect adrenal gland off superior pole of the kidney and posterior abdominal wall
				- Right adrenalectomy:
				  ○ Right triangular ligament of the liver mobilized and liver rotated anteromedially
				  ○ On the right side, colon usually lies inferior to the operative field
				  ○ Develop space between adrenal gland and IVC from superior to inferior
				  ○ Right adrenal vein is dissected out, clipped, and divided—watch out for aberrant vein anatomy
				  ○ Mobilize and remove adrenal
					Reevaluate need for preoperative medications	Major misstep—forgetting to check metanephrines to rule out pheochromocytoma prior to biopsy or surgery

Disease Process	Relevant H&P	Work-up/Staging	Treatment	Key Surgical Steps	Post-op Care	Tips & Tidbits

Hyperaldosteronism (core)	Presents with difficult to control hypertension and hypokalemia
	
	Conn syndrome
		Biochemical work-up:
		- Check plasma renin and aldosterone
		  ◦ Plasma aldosterone to renin ratio >20 suggestive of hyperaldosteronism
		  ◦ If the ratio is >20, then perform confirmatory test
		    ▪ Suppression test—give oral or IV salt load and measure 24-h urine aldosterone
		    ▪ High aldosterone after salt load is confirmatory
		Localize with adrenal protocol CT
		- If mass seen, confirm with adrenal vein sampling prior to proceeding with surgery
		Rule out pheochromocytoma with serum/urine metanephrines
			Aldosteronoma—open vs laparoscopic adrenalectomy
			
			If patient has bilateral adrenal hyperplasa or is not a good surgical candidate → medical treatment with spironolactone
				See adrenal incidentaloma section for surgical steps	Re-evaluate need for pre-operative medications	Left adrenal vein drains into left renal vein
						
						Right adrenal vein drains directly into the IVC

Hypercortisolism (core)	Symptoms of Cushing disease: easy bruising, muscle wasting, hypertension, moon facies, stria, buffalo hump, diabetes, and central obesity
	
	Differential diagnosis for hypercortisolism:
	- Exogenous steroid use
	- Cushing disease—ACTH-hypersecreting pituitary adenoma
	- Primary adrenal Cushing syndrome
	- Ectopic ACTH syndrome, ie, small-cell lung cancer
		Biochemical work-up:
		- Check 24-h urine free cortisol and ACTH level
		  ◦ If cortisol elevated, get low dose dexamethasone test to confirm
		    ▪ Give 1 mg dexamethasone at 11 PM and check serum cortisol at 8 AM the next morning
		    ▪ Cortisol high, ACTH low → suggests adrenal source, get adrenal protocol CT
		    ▪ Cortisol high, ACTH high → suggests ACTH-dependent source (pituitary vs ectopic source), get high dose dexamethasone suppression test
			Laparoscopic vs open adrenalectomy
			
			- Open adrenalectomy if concerned for ACC
				See adrenal incidentaloma section for surgical steps	At risk of post-op adrenal insufficiency—treat with hydrocortisone, eventually taper, and transition to PO steroid
					
					Signs and symptoms of Cushing syndrome take 2-12 mo to dissipate	

Disease Process	Relevant H&P	Work-up/Staging	Treatment	Key Surgical Steps	Post-op Care	Tips & Tidbits
Pheochromocytoma (core)	Headache, diaphoresis, palpitations, HTN Can be associated with MEN 2A/B	Biochemical work-up: - Plasma metanephrines $\rightarrow$ if positive, check 24-h urine metanephrines (more specific) Localize—CT adrenal protocol - If cannot find with CT, then do MRI or MIBG scan Genetic testing if concerned for inherited genetic syndrome—MEN IIA/B, RET mutation	Preoperative volume expansion and alpha blockade with phenoxybenzamine, prazosin, or doxazosin - Start alpha blocker 2 wk pre-op, titrate to orthostatic hypotension - Add beta-blockade and/or CCB as needed Adrenalectomy	**Surgical management of pheochromocytoma:** - Can usually do laparoscopic adrenalectomy, unless concerned for malignancy (See adrenal incidentaloma section for surgical steps) - Make sure anesthesia has vasopressors and antihypertensives immediately available - Ligate adrenal vein first to avoid spillage of catecholamines with tumor manipulation	Monitor closely post-op for HTN, hypoglycemia, hypotension, bronchospasm, arrythmias	Major misstep: Placing patient with pheochromocytoma on a beta-blocker prior to an alpha-blocker. This will result in dangerous unopposed alpha receptor stimulation Multiple endocrine neoplasia syndromes: - MENI—pituitary adenoma, pancreatic tumors, parathyroid hyperplasia - MEN IIA—medullary thyroid cancer, pheochromocytoma, parathyroid hyperplasia - MEN IIB—medullary thyroid cancer, pheochromocytoma, marfanoid habitus, mucosal neuromas

Disease Process	Relevant H&P	Work-up/Staging	Treatment	Key Surgical Steps	Post-op Care	Tips & Tidbits

Adrenal cortical carcinoma (ACC) (advanced)	Hormonal symptoms? Cushing syndrome? Virilization? History of prior malignancy? Family history of malignancy?	Biochemical work-up:
		- Plasma/urine catecholamines, ACTH, cortisol, BMP, aldosterone, renin, DHEA-S, testosterone
		- ACC can be functional (usually cortisol producing) or nonfunctional
		Imaging with adrenal protocol CT abdomen or MRI
		Imaging features concerning for ACC: >6 cm, heterogeneous, irregular borders, >20 HFU, delayed contrast washout (<50% washout at 10 min)
		Additional staging for ACC
		- Chest CT
		- PET scan
		Avoid percutaneous biopsy, unless patient has history of prior malignancy and there is concern the adrenal mass may be metastasis
			If concerned for ACC → open adrenalectomy, not MIS
			Locoregional: can resect tumors with N+ or local invasion if R0 possible
			- Intracaval extension of tumor thrombus is not a contraindication to surgery
			M1 disease → chemoXRT for symptoms control
				Open anterior transabdominal adrenalectomy (advanced):
				- Position supine with ipsilateral side bumped
				- Midline laparotomy vs subcostal incision
				• Right side
				  ○ Mobilize hepatic flexure
				  ○ Kocherize to expose IVC
				  ○ Retract liver superior and kidney inferior to expose adrenal gland
				  ○ Ligate vessels and resect adrenal en bloc with surrounding adipose tissue, avoid rupture
				• Left side
				  ○ Mobilize the splenic flexure, spleen, and tail of pancreas to expose the adrenal
				  ○ Superior retraction on pancreas and inferior retraction on kidney exposes adrenal
				  ○ Ligate vessels and resect adrenal en bloc with surrounding adipose tissue, avoid rupture
					Watch out for adrenal insufficiency post-op in patients with cortisol secreting tumor—will present as fatigue, hypotension, hyponatremia, and hyperkalemia
					Consider adjuvant mitotane and XRT
					Surveillance: CT C/A/P q3mo x 2 y, then q6mo x 5 y
						Major misstep: Getting biopsy of an adrenal mass that appears consistent with ACC on imaging Biopsy of ACC can lead to seeding and biopsy of pheochromocytoma can lead to hypertensive crisis

Disease Process	Relevant H&P	Work-up/Staging	Treatment	Key Surgical Steps	Post-op Care	Tips & Tidbits
Peritoneal dialysis	Good candidates: GFR 20-30, motivated and able to perform exchanges at home Patients with extensive abdominal surgical history are not good candidates Examine patient for any hernias that may need to be fixed prior to PD	Basic labs	Peritoneal dialysis catheter can be placed with open cut down, laparoscopically, or under fluoroscopic guidance If the patient has any hernias, those should be repaired prior to or at the time of PD catheter placement	**Open peritoneal dialysis catheter placement (core):** - Make supraumbilical paramedian skin incision overlying the rectus muscle - Dissect down to fascia and make ~2 cm transverse incision in anterior sheath - Split the rectus, grasp, and incise the posterior sheath to enter the abdomen - Place purse string Vicryl suture around peritoneal opening - Insert the catheter into the abdomen, directing it down into the pelvis - Flush and make sure you get return - Tie the purse string suture - Tunnel the catheter 1-2 cm cephalad in subfascial plane and make a hole in the fascia and thread it into the subcutaneous tissue, there should be a cuff under the fascia - Close both fascial incisions - Tunnel the catheter in the subcutaneous tissue down into the left lower quadrant and make a small skin nick to bring the catheter out, there should be a cuff in the subcutaneous tissue - Close skin - Flush the catheter with heparinized saline	Wait 2 wk to use PD catheter dysfunction: - Get KUB - Most common cause is outflow issue from constipation → bowel regimen - Clogged → try fibrinolytic therapy - Kinked → can try laparoscopic/ fluoroscopic manipulation of catheter PD catheter peritonitis - May present with abdominal pain, cloudy dialysate - Obtain culture and cell count of dialysate fluid, cell count >100 leukocytes with >50% PMN is diagnostic - Tx: intraperitoneal antibiotics with each peritoneal dialysis cycle x 5 d. If no response, have to remove catheter.	Peritoneal dialysis catheters can be placed many different ways. Make sure you know how to describe at least one reliable way

Disease Process	Relevant H&P	Work-up/Staging	Treatment	Key Surgical Steps	Post-op Care	Tips & Tidbits
Desmoid tumor (advanced)	Presenting symptoms depend on location of desmoid – abdominal vs intra-abdominal vs retroperitoneal - Abdominal wall mass - Intra-abdominal desmoid tumors can cause abdominal pain, pressure, and/or palpable mass - Retroperitoneal tumors can cause ureteral obstruction Most common in females in their thirties, during or after pregnancy Frequently noticed after an injury/trauma	CT/MRI Core needle biopsy—bundle of spindle cells Consider colonoscopy if family history suggestive of FAP	Desmoids have unpredictable clinical course—may grow, remain stable, or spontaneously regress Watchful waiting is the preferred strategy for stable, asymptomatic primary or recurrent desmoids, particularly if resection would entail major morbidity, repeat imaging in 3-6 mo Wide local excision of desmoids that are not appropriate for surveillance (growing, symptomatic, etc) Symptomatic but unresectable desmoids can sometimes be treated with XRT, NSAIDS (sulindac), tamoxifen, and/or chemo	Goal of surgery is complete resection with negative margin If resecting abdominal wall desmoid, will have to reconstruct abdominal wall to prevent hernia If resecting mesenteric desmoid, usually also have to resect involved bowel	Recurrence is very common	Most desmoids are sporadic but some are associated with Gardner syndrome (FAP + desmoids) Mesenteric desmoids are more lethal because they can cause local complications, including intestinal obstruction, ischemia, and perforation

Disease Process	Relevant H&P	Work-up/Staging	Treatment	Key Surgical Steps	Post-op Care	Tips & Tidbits

Peritoneal neoplasms (advanced)	Patients with pseudomyxoma peritonei (PMP) or peritoneal carcinomatosis may present with:
	
	- Abdominal pain
	- Increasing abdominal girth
	- Weight gain
	- New inguinal hernia
	- Early satiety
	- Symptoms of obstruction
	
	Sometimes incidentally discovered on imaging or surgery for another reason
	
	What is patient's functional status?
		Peritoneal malignancy differential
		- Peritoneal mesothelioma
		- Appendiceal origin
		  ○ Low grade appendiceal mucinous neoplasm (LAMN)
		  ○ Appendiceal adenocarcinoma
		- Colorectal cancer
		- Gastric cancer
		- Ovarian cancer
		
		PMP is usually from appendiceal or ovarian origin
		
		Tumor markers—CEA, CA 125, CA 19-9
		
		CT scan—may show peritoneal studding, intra-abdominal mucin causing scalloping of the liver and spleen edges
		
		Imaging has low sensitivity in cases of lower disease burden
		
		Diagnostic laparoscopy is the most accurate way to evaluate a patient's disease burden, can take biopsy
		
		Peritoneal cancer index (PCI)—method for quantifying disease burden based on the size and distribution of peritoneal disease, score range 0-39
			Cytoreductive surgery (CRS) and hyperthermic intraperitoneal chemotherapy (HIPEC) is an option for select patients with peritoneal malignancies
			
			- Surgically resect all disease >2 mm and then treat the rest with heated chemo
			- Typically involves stripping the peritoneum, omentectomy, possible bowel resection
			- May not be possible if there is extensive small bowel or porta hepatis involvement
			- Most common agents used for HIPEC are mitomycin-C, doxorubicin, and oxaliplatin
			- Typically only used for patients when complete cytoreduction is thought to be possible; however, LAMN patients are an exception, because incomplete cytoreduction may still be beneficial for symptom control
			- Gastric cancer - CRS + HIPEC only for very select patients (PCI < 6)
			
			May require palliative procedures such as intestinal bypass or decompressive G-tube
			
			+/- palliative chemo
					Surveillance depends on type of cancer	Additional reading:
						
						Chicago Consensus Working Group. The Chicago Consensus on peritoneal surface malignancies: management of peritoneal mesothelioma. *Cancer.* 2020 Jun 1;126(11): 2547-2552
						
						Quénet F, et al. Cytoreductive surgery plus hyperthermic intraperitoneal chemotherapy versus cytoreductive surgery alone for colorectal peritoneal metastases (PRODIGE 7): a multicentre, randomised, open-label, phase 3 trial. *Lancet Oncol.* 2021 Feb;22(2):256-266

2

Foregut Surgery

Andrew Feczko, MD

DISEASES AND CONDITIONS

- GERD (c), hiatal hernia (c), antireflux procedures (c)
- Achalasia (c), Heller myotomy (a)
- Esophageal perforation (c), esophageal perforation repair/resection (a)
- Barrett's esophagus (c), upper endoscopy (c)

- Esophageal cancer (c), esophagectomy (a)
- Gastric adenocarcinoma (c), gastrectomy (c)
- GIST (c)
- Gastric volvulus
- Gastroparesis (c)

- Gastric foreign bodies (c), esophageal foreign bodies and caustic ingestion (a)
- Morbid obesity (c), sleeve gastrectomy (a), Roux-en-Y gastric bypass (a)
- Zenker diverticulum, cricopharyngeal myotomy with Zenker diverticulectomy (a)

GENERAL FOREGUT SURGERY TIPS

- Don't forget to restage cancer patients after they receive neoadjuvant treatment, prior to operating.
- Advanced endoscopic techniques, such as esophageal stenting, per-oral endoscopic myotomy

(POEM), and endoscopic submucosal dissection (ESD) may be applicable in certain foregut scenarios. Residents have variable exposure to these techniques during training. Avoid describing

them in depth unless you have experience in performing the procedure and the management of any complications that may arise.

(c) = core topic   (a) = advanced topic

Disease Process	Relevant H&P	Work-up/Staging	Treatment	Key Surgical Steps	Post-Op Care	Tips & Tidbits

GERD, hiatal hernia (core)	Typical GERD symptoms: heartburn, regurgitation
	
	Atypical GERD symptoms: cough, hoarseness, sore throat, SOB, chest pain
	
	Alarm symptoms: dysphagia, GIB, weight loss, anemia
		CBC, BMP
		
		Always get ECG in a patient with chest pain
		
		Recommended pre-op work-up for GERD:
		- UGI
		- EGD—biopsy with H. pylori testing
		- pH monitoring, impedance testing
		  ○ Demeester score > 14.7 is abnormal
		  ○ Must be off PPI for at least 5 d for accurate test
		- Manometry—evaluates motility
		  ○ Avoid 360° wrap in a patient with poor esophageal motility
		- Consider gastric emptying study to rule out gastroparesis if patient has bloating, N/V
		- pH monitoring and manometry are of limited utility in patients with large PEH
		
		Patients with GERD are frequently found to have a hiatal hernia
		
		Hiatal hernia types:
		- I: sliding (most common)—LES elevated into chest
		- II: paraesophageal (PEH)—fundus herniated through the hiatus, but LES remains in anatomic position
		- III: combined sliding and PEH
		- IV: other organs herniating through hiatus
			GERD:
			- First line = 6 to 8-wk trial of PPI, lifestyle modification (weight loss, smoking cessation)
			  ○ Alarm symptoms should prompt additional work-up immediately
			- If patient fails medical management, obtain further work-up, consider surgery
			
			Patients with symptomatic PEH should have them repaired
			
			Patients with asymptomatic PEH—decision to repair depends on size of hernia and if patient is good operative candidate
			- Strongly consider repair of type III and IV PEH to prevent incarceration/strangulation and need for emergent operation
			
			Fundoplication options:
			- Nissen—360° wrap
			  ○ Best acid control but highest risk for dysphagia, inability to belch or vomit
			- Toupet—270° posterior wrap
			  ○ Less dysphagia, can still belch
			- Dor—anterior 180° wrap
				Paraesophageal hernia repair with Nissen fundoplication (core):
				- Four fundamental steps of PEH repair:
				• Complete reduction and excision of hernia sac
				• Reduction of stomach and GEJ into abdomen without tension
				• Crural closure
				• Fundoplication and/or gastropexy
				- Position patient in split leg/lithotomy
				- Place ports, including liver retractor
				- Reduce herniated contents back into the abdomen
				- Dissect through gastrohepatic ligament to identify right crus
				  ○ Watch out for replaced left hepatic artery
				- Start dissection at right crus and work right to left to dissect out the hiatus, locate and protect the vagus nerves, get Penrose drain around the esophagus
				- Reduce and excise hiatal hernia sac
				- Perform thoracic esophageal mobilization
				  ○ Need at least 2-3 cm of intra-abdominal esophagus
				  ○ Consider Collis gastroplasty if unable to obtain sufficient intra-abdominal length
				- Take down short gastrics to free fundus
				- Close crura posteriorly with interrupted permanent sutures
				- Creation of Nissen fundoplication:
				  ○ Place 58-60 Fr bougie
				  ○ Bring fundus posteriorly around the esophagus so that it is symmetric, and the line of divided short gastric vessels is posterior (shoeshine maneuver)
				  ○ Suture wrap with full thickness bite of fundus, then partial thickness bite of esophagus, then full thickness bite of fundus on either side
				  ○ Wrap should be ~2-2.5 cm long and sit at 10-11 o'clock on the esophagus with 3 sutures ~1 cm apart
				- Intra-op EGD to assess repair
					Complications:
					Post-op pathway is heavily institution dependent
					- Typically, NPO on POD 0, UGI on POD 1, start liquids if UGI looks good
					- FLD for 2 wk, soft diet from 2-6 wk post-op, advance to regular diet at 6 wk post-op
					
					PACU capnothorax—usually of no consequence and will rapidly reabsorb, nothing to do unless patient is unstable
					
					Dysphagia—post-op swelling vs fundoplication is too tight
					- If patient cannot tolerate secretions, fundoplication is too tight, take patient back to OR for revision
					- If patient is able to tolerate liquids, can consider trial of conservative management and then repeat UGI in several weeks once post-op swelling resolved
					
					Any unexplained post-op tachycardia, SOB and/or chest or abdominal pain should be evaluated with UGI with gastrograffin to look for leak
						In patients with GERD and BMI > 35, Roux-en-Y gastric bypass is typically preferred over anti-reflux procedure/hiatal hernia repair alone
						
						Cameron's Ulcer—gastric ulcer associated with a hiatal hernia, can cause anemia, indication for hiatal hernia repair

Disease Process	Relevant H&P	Work-up/Staging	Treatment	Key Surgical Steps	Post-Op Care	Tips & Tidbits

Achalasia (core)	Dysphagia (usually to solids and liquids), regurgitation, chest discomfort, weight loss
	
	Eckardt score used to quantify symptoms
		CBC, BMP, ECG
		
		Barium Swallow—"bird's beak"
		
		EGD—rule out pseudoachalasia caused by tumor
		
		Manometry
		- Achalasia is defined by incomplete relaxation of LES (IRP >15 mm Hg) + aperistalsis of the body of the esophagus
		- Chicago classification used for diagnosis of achalasia and other esophageal motility disorders
			Medical therapy—CCB, nitrates
			- Can have intolerable side effects (headache, hypotension) and poor efficacy
			
			Botox injection—inhibits ACh release from nerve endings → temporary LES relaxation
			
			Pneumatic dilation—essentially an uncontrolled myotomy, effective but results may not last, 4% rate of perforation
			
			Per-oral endoscopic myotomy (POEM)—endoscopic alternative to surgical myotomy that has increased in popularity
			
			Heller myotomy with Dor fundoplication—traditional option
			
			Esophagectomy occasionally needed in severe cases with "burnt out" esophagus
				Laparoscopic Heller myotomy with Dor fundoplication (advanced):
				- Place ports
				- Divide phrenoesophageal membrane and dissect into the mediastinum
				  ○ Posterior dissection is not necessary
				  ○ Identify and preserve anterior vagus nerve
				- Use scissors or cautery to make myotomy 6 cm up from GEJ and 2 cm down onto stomach
				  ○ If there is a mucosal hole, repair mucosa and cover with fundoplication or repair in 2 layers and perform myotomy on the contralateral side
				- Perform EGD and leak test
				- Create Dor fundoplication
				  ○ Divide short gastrics
				  ○ Flap of fundus rotated over myotomy and secured to right crus to create anterior 180° wrap
					Obtain UGI on POD 1 to evaluate for leak, if appropriate, start liquid diet
					
					Consider POEM vs pneumatic dilation if patient develops recurrent dysphagia after Heller myotomy
						Other motility disorders:
						- Diffuse esophageal spasm—uncoordinated rigorous esophageal contractions, "corkscrew" esophagus on esophagram
						  ○ Tx: CCB, nitrates, avoid triggers
						- Nutcracker esophagus (hypercontractile esophagus)—characterized by hypercontractility of the esophagus
						  ○ Tx: CCBs, nitrates, antispasmodics
						- Ineffective esophageal motility—dampened esophageal contractility, > 50% of swallows ineffective on manometry
						  ○ Tx: acid suppression
						- Hypertensive LES—median IRP > 15 mm Hg but differs from achalasia by having evidence of effective peristalsis
						  ○ Tx: Botox injection, dilations, surgical myotomy for refractory cases

Disease Process	Relevant H&P	Work-up/Staging	Treatment	Key Surgical Steps	Post-Op Care	Tips & Tidbits
Esophageal perforation (core)	May present with recent emesis/wretching, chest pain, fever, pain with swallowing, hemoptysis, hematemesis On exam, patient may have crepitus of the neck or chest wall, blood in NGT Etiologies include iatrogenic (EGD, TEE, etc), trauma, Boerhaave syndrome, caustic injury, foreign body/food impaction, perforation related to underlying esophageal cancer or achalasia	Full labs, CXR, ECG CXR—may show pleural effusion, pneumomediastinum, or mediastinal contour changes UGI vs CT with PO contrast - UGI—first with gastrograffin, if study is negative but have a high suspicion, then repeat with thin barium, then regular barium - Determine if leak is contained or uncontained and where perforation is located EGD - Rigid esophagoscopy preferred for diagnosis of proximal injuries	Resuscitation, antibiotics, antifungal, PPI Operative management strategy depends on timing of presentation, degree of contamination, etiology of perforation, location of perforation, and patient stability - principles of management include: - Control of ongoing contamination (repair, stent, divert, and/or drain) - Drainage and debridement of contaminated/devitalized tissue - Distal feeding access Primary repair and drainage—should be performed whenever possible Resection and diversion with cervical esophagostomy may be needed for cases where perforation is associated with cancer, severe tissue loss, or presentation is significantly delayed T-tube drainage—for destructive injuries that cannot be primarily repaired, create controlled fistula Can consider esophageal stent in certain cases Don't forget to treat the underlying etiology 　○ If perforation is associated with achalasia, do myotomy Select patients who meet the following criteria (Cameron's criteria) may be managed nonoperatively: - Contained perforation—contrast flows out and back into esophagus - Minimal symptoms - No evidence of sepsis - No distal obstruction	**Repair of cervical esophageal perforation (advanced):** - Left neck incision along anterior border of SCM - Divide omohyoid muscle - Retract carotid sheath laterally - Bluntly dissect between trachea and esophagus, avoid injury to recurrent laryngeal nerve - Place Penrose drain around esophagus - Debride and expose full extent of the mucosal injury - Close defect in 2 layers (absorbable suture for mucosa, silk for muscularis) - Buttress with tissue flap (omohyoid, sternocleidomastoid, or strap muscles) - Irrigate and drain widely **Repair of thoracic esophageal perforation (advanced):** - Place in the lateral decubitus position, single lung ventilation - Thoracotomy 　○ Mid thoracic perforation → right posterolateral thoracotomy in 5th/6th intercostal space (ICS) 　○ Distal perforation → left posterolateral thoracotomy in the 7th ICS - Harvest intercostal muscle flap on the way in - Expose entire mucosal defect and debride any nonviable tissue - Repair in 2 layers and buttress with intercostal flap 　○ If intercostal flap unavailable, can use pleura, pericardium, thymus, or other vascularized rotational flap - Leave NGT or place G-tube for gastric decompression - Widely drain chest/mediastinum - Place J-tube for enteral access	NGT or gastrostomy for decompression of the stomach and jejunostomy for distal feeding should be used until the repair is healed Strict NPO until post-op esophagram confirms no leak (~POD 7) In cases where esophageal resection and diversion was necessary, consider reconstructing 6-12 mo post-op with gastric conduit or colonic interposition	In a trauma patient, if there is concern for traumatic esophageal injury based on mechanism, trajectory, or CTA findings, an EGD and esophagram should be performed - Perform direct laryngoscopy and neck exploration if concerned for cervical esophageal injury

Disease Process	Relevant H&P	Work-up/Staging	Treatment	Key Surgical Steps	Post-Op Care	Tips & Tidbits
Barrett's esophagus (core)	RF: GERD, obesity, smoking	EGD with biopsy - Salmon-colored mucosal extending proximally to GEJ (Figure 2.1) - Intestinal metaplasia of distal esophagus: squamous → columnar epithelium, goblet cells Patients with Barrett's have 30x higher risk of esophageal cancer - Nondysplastic → 0.25%/y progress to esophageal cancer - Low-grade dysplasia (LGD) → 0.5-1%/y progress to esophageal cancer - High-grade dysplasia (HGD) → 4-8%/y progress to esophageal cancer	PPI and lifestyle modification (weight loss, smoking cessation, diet modifications, head of bed up while sleeping) Surveillance of Barrett's: - Seattle protocol for endoscopic surveillance—4 quadrant biopsies q1-2 cm - Nondysplastic Barrett's → EGD q3-5y - Barrett's with LGD → EGD q6-12 mo - Barrett's with HGD → EGD q3 mo - White light endoscopy and chromoendoscopy may be used as adjuncts for better detection of dysplasia and invasive cancer Treatment of Barrett's: - Goal in patients with dysplasia is endoscopic eradication of all dysplastic/metaplastic tissue - Endoscopic mucosal resection (EMR) or endoscopic submucosal dissection (ESD) of visible lesions/mucosal irregularities - RFA of Barrett's areas without visible changes - Repeat EGD 6 wk after endoscopic treatment to assess response and evaluate for residual disease Consider fundoplication—does not necessarily result in Barrett's regression but can stop progression	EGD (core): - Can be done with general anesthesia or conscious sedation - If under conscious sedation, place patient on left side - Place endoscope into oropharynx - Keep scope in the center of the lumen and insufflate as scope is advanced down the esophagus into the stomach - Take note of location of squamocolumnar junction and GEJ, look for Barrett's - Retroflex to see GEJ, determine Hill grade of gastroesophageal valve - Pass scope into the duodenum - Biopsy any abnormal appearing tissue, take antral biopsies to test for H. pylori - Suction air out and withdraw scope	Complications: - Perforation during EMR → if seen, can treat with endoscopic clipping - Risk of stricture development after RFA treatment	Many elements of the management of Barrett's remain controversial and may vary between providers. HGD is equivalent to carcinoma in situ. In a study of patients with HGD who underwent esophagectomy, up to 13% were found to have invasive adenocarcinoma on final pathology. Additional reading: Shaheen NJ, et al. Diagnosis and management of Barrett's esophagus: an updated ACG Guideline. *Am J Gastroenterol*. 2022 Apr 1;117(4):559-587. Konda VJ, et al. Is the risk of concomitant invasive esophageal cancer in high-grade dysplasia in Barrett's esophagus overestimated? *Clin Gastroenterol Hepatol*. 2008 Feb;6(2):159-64.

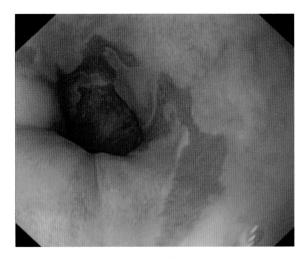

FIGURE 2.1: Barrett's esophagus seen on EGD. Salmon-colored mucosa extending proximal to GEJ. (Modified with permission from Hunter JG, Spight DH, Sandone C, et al. *Atlas of Minimally Invasive Surgical Operations*. New York, NY: McGraw Hill; 2018, Figure 22-16.)

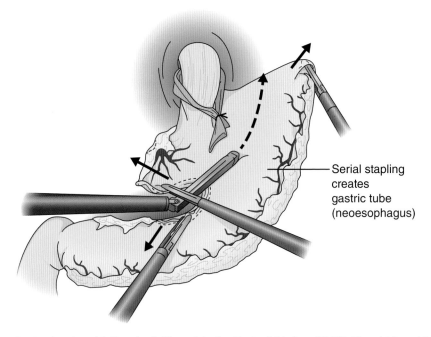

Serial stapling creates gastric tube (neoesophagus)

FIGURE 2.2: Creation of gastric conduit. (Reproduced with permission from Brunicardi F, Andersen DK, Billiar TR, et al. *Schwartz's Principles of Surgery,* 11th ed. New York, NY: McGraw Hill; 2019, Figure 25-16 B.)

Disease Process	Relevant H&P	Work-up/Staging	Treatment	Key Surgical Steps	Post-Op Care	Tips & Tidbits

Esophageal cancer (core)	Symptoms: dysphagia, odynophagia, weight loss, hematemesis
	
	Adenocarcinoma
	- Risk factors: Barrett's, GERD, obesity
	- More common in the distal esophagus and GEJ
	
	Squamous cell carcinoma (SCC)
	- Risk factors: alcohol use, tobacco
	- More common in cervical and mid-esophagus
		CBC, CMP, nutrition labs
		
		Staging work-up:
		- EGD with biopsy
		- EUS—can determine T and N stage
		- CT C/A/P—assess for metastasis
		- PET—assess for metastasis
		- +/- diagnostic laparoscopy—recommended for Siewert II/III tumors to assess for peritoneal involvement
		- If tumor is proximal to carina, bronchoscopy is recommended to assess for airway involvement
		
		TNM staging
		- T stage
		  ◦ Tis—HGD, has not broken through basement membrane
		  ◦ T1a—lamina propria, muscularis mucosae
		  ◦ T1b—into submucosa
		  ◦ T2—into muscular layer
		  ◦ T3—through muscular layer
		  ◦ T4—invading surrounding structures
		  ◦ T4a—invading resectable structures
		  ◦ T4b – invading unresectable structures
		- N stage—need 15 lymph nodes
		  ◦ N1—1-2 LN
		  ◦ N2—3-6 LN
		  ◦ N3—7+ LN
			Discuss patient at multidisciplinary tumor board
			
			Tis, T1a—EMR/ESD vs upfront esophagectomy
			
			T1b—upfront esophagectomy (or endoscopic resection if very high surgical risk)
			
			T2N0—upfront esophagectomy vs neoadjuvant chemoXRT
			
			T2-4a and/or N+—neoadjuvant chemoXRT, then restage, then possible esophagectomy
			
			T4b or M1—definitive chemoXRT
			
			Neoadjuvant treatment:
			- Paclitaxel + carboplatin + XRT (CROSS trial regimen)
			- Can also use FOLFOX + XRT
			
			Optimize nutrition, place feeding tube if needed
			- Avoid G-tube in patient who may eventually have esophagectomy
				Ivor Lewis esophagectomy (advanced):
				- Can be done open vs minimally invasive
				- Make upper midline laparotomy/place ports, look for metastasis
				- Perform lymphadenectomy and mobilize stomach taking care to preserve the right gastroepiploic artery
				- Dissect out the esophageal hiatus to mobilize the GEJ and distal esophagus
				- Kocherize the duodenum +/- pyloromyotomy
				- Create greater curve-based, tubularized gastric conduit, check that pylorus will reach the hiatus, ensuring sufficient length for the reconstruction (Figure 2.2)
				- Place J-tube
				- Reposition in left lateral decubitus
				- Right posterolateral thoracotomy in 5th ICS vs place ports for R VATS
				- Perform thoracic lymphadenectomy
				- Mobilize esophagus and transect at least 5 cm proximal to tumor
				- Pull specimen and conduit up, remove specimen
				- Make esophagogastric anastomosis using EEA stapler
				- Leave drains and NGT in place
				- Other options for esophagectomy:
				  ◦ Transhiatal
				  ◦ McKeown (3 hole)
					NGT, strict NPO, J-tube feeds
					
					Swallow study on POD 7
					
					Complications:
					- Respiratory complications common
					- Leak—presentation depends on location of anastomosis
					  ◦ Patient may present with fever, tachycardia, AMS, change in drain output
					  ◦ Check drain amylase, esophagram/CT with contrast, drain amylase, EGD to characterize leak
					  ◦ Treat with antibiotics, drainage, NPO, J-tube feeds
					    ▪ Cervical leak—open cervical incision, wound care
					    ▪ Intrathoracic leak—small contained leak may be treated with stent, large leak may require esophageal diversion
					
					- Anastomotic stricture—treat with dilation
					Surveillance:
					- H&P q3mo x 2 y, then q6mo through 5 y, then annually
					- CT chest/abdomen q12mo x 3 y
					- EGD as clinically indicated
						Leiomyomas are the most common type of benign tumor of the esophagus
						
						Additional reading: van Hagen P, et al; CROSS Group. Preoperative chemoradiotherapy for esophageal or junctional cancer. *N Engl J Med.* 2012 May 31;366(22):2074-2084.
						
						[Figure 2.2]

Disease Process	Relevant H&P	Work-up/Staging	Treatment	Key Surgical Steps	Post-Op Care	Tips & Tidbits

Gastric cancer (core)	May present with vague symptoms, epigastric pain, early satiety, anemia, GIB
	
	Examine abdomen, look for lymphadenopathy
		CBC, CMP, nutrition labs
		Staging work-up:
		- EGD with biopsy
		- EUS—helps determine T & N staging
		- CT C/A/P
		- PET—alters treatment in up to 20% of cases
		- Diagnostic laparoscopy with peritoneal washings for ≥ T1b
		  ○ Can place J-tube at the same time if indicated
		  ○ Positive peritoneal cytology = M1 disease, poor prognosis
		- Discuss at multidisciplinary tumor board
		
		TNM staging:
		- T stage
		  ○ T1a—invades lamina propria or muscularis mucosa
		  ○ T1b—submucosa
		  ○ T2—into muscular layer
		  ○ T3—through muscular layer
		  ○ T4—invades serosa or other structures
		- N stage (Need 15 LN)
		  ○ N1 1-2 LN
		  ○ N2 3-6 LN
		  ○ N3 7+ LN
			Tis, T1a → EMR (must be < 2 cm, no LVI, well-mod differentiated)
			
			T1bN0 +/- T2N0 → upfront surgery
			
			T3/4 and/or N+ (+/-T2N0) → neoadjuvant, then restage, then surgery
			
			M1 or unresectable → definitive chemo +/- targeted therapy (Her2, etc)
			
			Neoadjuvant chemo regimens:
			- FLOT—5-FU, leucovorin, oxaliplatin, docetaxel (MAGIC trial regimen)
			
			Unclear role for XRT
			
			Type of resection:
			- Proximal 1/3 gastric tumor → total gastrectomy with EJ vs esophagectomy
			- Distal 2/3 gastric tumor → distal/subtotal gastrectomy with BI, BII, or Roux-en-Y reconstruction
			- Aim for 5-cm gross margins from tumor
				Total gastrectomy (core):
				- Laparotomy
				- Mobilize stomach and perform D2 lymphadenectomy
				  ○ Mobilize the GEJ
				- Mobilize the greater curve, including ligation of right gastroepiploic, left gastroepiploic and short gastric arteries
				- Mobilize the lesser curve, open the gastrohepatic ligament, ligate right gastric vessels
				  ○ Kocherize the duodenum
				- Proximal duodenum divided with stapler
				- Retract stomach cephalad to expose and divide the left gastric artery
				- *Mobilize distal esophagus if needed for additional esophageal length* (ie, for margins on proximal gastric tumor)
				- Place stay sutures in distal esophagus to prevent retraction, distal esophagus transected and stomach removed
				- Reconstruction with Roux-en-Y esophagojejunostomy (Figure 2.3)
				  ○ Divide proximal jejunum ~20 cm distal to LOT
				  ○ Distal end of the transected jejunum brought up to esophagus as retrocolic Roux limb
				  ○ Create esophagojejunal anastomosis
				    ▪ Anvil of EEA stapler secured in distal end of esophagus with purse string
				    ▪ Stapled end of Roux limb opened so that EEA stapler can be inserted
				    ▪ Stapler positioned so that anastomosis will be ~3 cm from tip of Roux limb along antimesenteric border, fire stapler
				    ▪ Staple off open distal tip of Roux limb
				  ○ Place NGT through anastomosis, leak test
				  ○ Create JJ anastomosis ~50 cm distal to EJ anastomosis, close mesenteric defects
				- Place a J-tube and leave drains
					Remove NGT once output minimal and having bowel function, +/- UGI
					Surveillance: H&P q3mon x 2 y, then q6mo x 3-5 y
					CT C/A/P q6mo x 2 y, then annually until 5 y out
					Monitor for B12 and iron deficiency
						Hereditary diffuse gastric cancer—patients with CDH1 (e-cadherin) mutation
						- Prophylactic gastrectomy at 18-40 yo
						
						Additional reading:
						Cunningham D, et al; MAGIC Trial Participants. Perioperative chemotherapy versus surgery alone for resectable gastroesophageal cancer. *N Engl J Med.* 2006 Jul 6;355(1):11-20.
						
						[Figure 2.3]

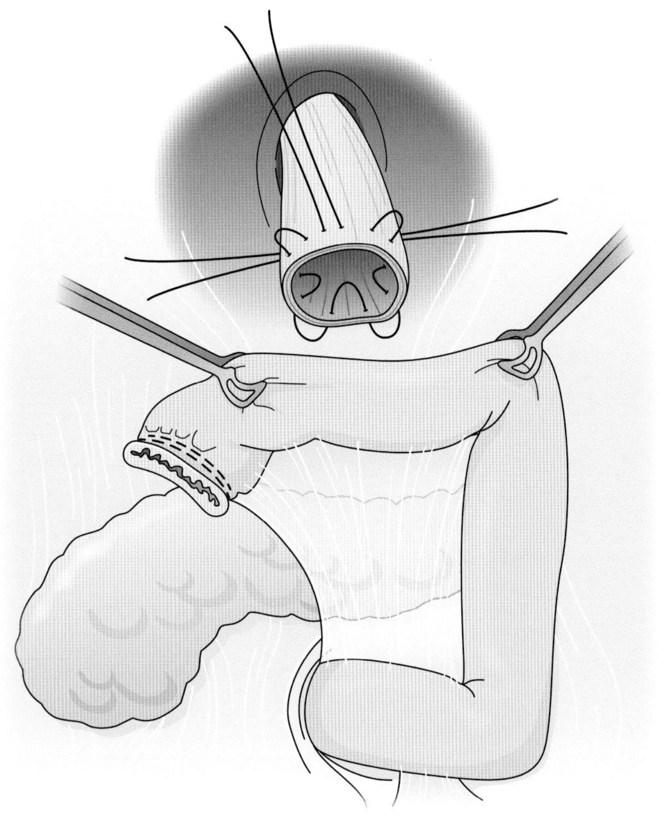

FIGURE 2.3: Set-up of gastrojejunostomy anastomosis follow-up total gastrectomy. (Modified with permission from Minter RM, Doherty GM. *Current Procedures: Surgery*. New York, NY: McGraw Hill; 2010, Figure 6-17 C.)

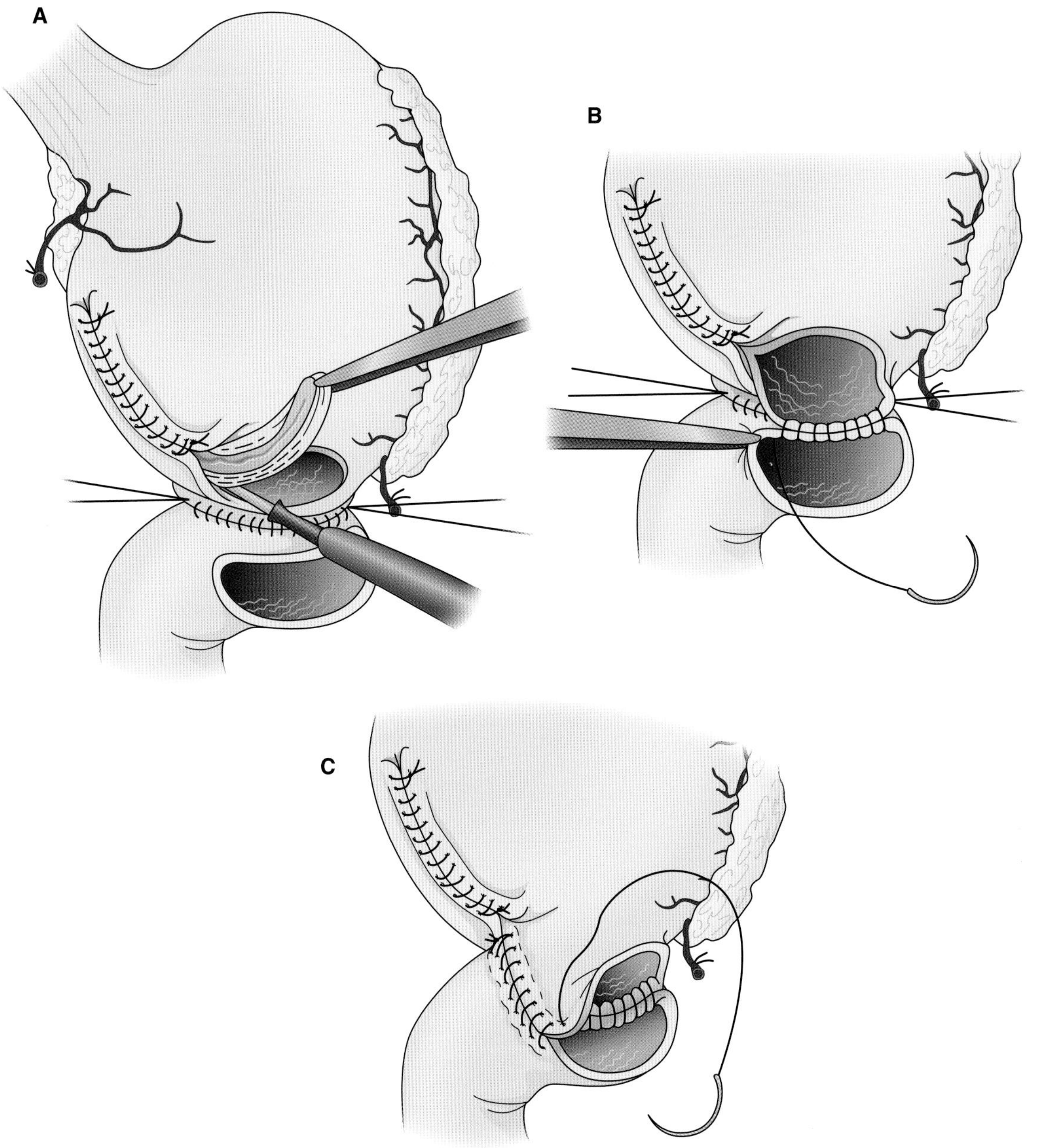

FIGURE 2.4: Creation of handsewn Billroth I gastrojejunostomy following distal gastrectomy. (Modified with permission from Minter RM, Doherty GM. *Current Procedures: Surgery*. New York, NY: McGraw Hill; 2010, Figure 6-10 A-C.)

Disease Process	Relevant H&P	Work-up/Staging	Treatment	Key Surgical Steps	Post-Op Care	Tips & Tidbits

Gastrointestinal stromal tumor (GIST) (core)	Often found incidentally, may also present with abdominal discomfort, early satiety, GIB, obstruction
	
	Most common locations:
	1. Stomach (60%)
	2. Small intestine
	3. Rectum
	4. Esophagus
		CT C/A/P for staging—GIST will appear exophytic and heterogenous
		
		EGD, EUS +/- biopsy
		- Submucosal mass, can be ulcerated
		- Do not necessarily need to biopsy if planning to do resection, can resect based on imaging appearance only
		- Biopsy needed prior to starting systemic therapy
		- Biopsy demonstrates spindle cells, CD117+, C-kit mutation
			If <2 cm and no high-risk features, can consider surveillance
			
			If >2 cm or presence of high-risk features, requires resection
			
			Gastric GIST → wedge resection vs distal gastrectomy vs total gastrectomy depending on size and location
			
			Small bowel GIST—en bloc resection
			- Aim for 1-cm gross margins, avoid capsule rupture
			- No lymphadenectomy needed, spreads via direct extension or hematogenously
			
			Imatinib indications:
			- Metastatic or unresectable disease
			- Recurrent disease
			- High risk patients: > 5 mitoses/50 hpf or tumor >3-5 cm
			- GIST in non-gastric location
			- Typically give GIST for 3 y
			
			Sunitinib is second line
			
			Select patients with metastatic disease that is resectable and responsive/stable on imatinib may be surgical candidates
				Distal gastrectomy:
				- Laparotomy
				- Kocher maneuver to mobilize duodenum
				- Taken down gastrocolic ligament beginning at the pylorus with ligation of the right gastroepiploic artery and continuing along the greater curvature until you reach point of planned gastric transection
				- Gastrohepatic ligament incised and lesser curvature is dissected, right gastric vessel ligated close to the stomach
				- Proximal duodenum divided with stapler
				- Stomach divided with stapler
				- Reconstruction with Billroth I, Billroth II, or Roux-en-Y gastrojejunostomy
				  ○ Billroth I
				    ■ Duodenal staple line and inferior portion of gastric staple lines apposed, staple lines excised, and GJ anastomosis created (Figure 2.4)
				  ○ Billroth II
				    ■ Proximal loop of jejunum brought up to remaining stomach (ante- or retrocolic), GJ anastomosis created
				- Leave NGT and drains		

Disease Process	Relevant H&P	Work-up/Staging	Treatment	Key Surgical Steps	Post-Op Care	Tips & Tidbits

Gastric volvulus	Borchardt's triad: retching without vomiting, epigastric pain and distention, inability to pass NGT
	
	May be acute or chronic
		Full labs
		CXR
		UGI vs CT
		Can have organo-axial volvulus or mesenteroaxial volvulus
			Need to de-torse volvulus and decompress stomach ASAP with NGT, EGD, or surgery
			- Early decompression with NGT/EGD can convert urgent operation into semi-elective operation, allows for resuscitation and resolution of gastric distention and edema prior to surgical repair
			  ◦ If patient is poor surgical candidate, can place 2 PEG tubes to fix stomach intra-abdominally, rather than surgical repair
			- If patient is unstable and/or unable to detorse with NGT and EGD, take to OR immediately
				Operative intervention for gastric volvulus:
				- Can be done open vs minimally invasive
				- Reduce stomach into abdomen
				- Manage paraesophageal hernia
				  ◦ In a stable patient, perform formal repair with crural closure and fundoplication
				  ◦ In an unstable patient, reduce the hernia, reapproximate the crura, and perform gastropexy +/- gastrostomy tube		

Gastroparesis (core)	May present with early satiety, N/V, abdominal pain Risk factors for gastric motility issues: diabetes, previous surgery (vagotomy, PEHR, partial gastrectomy), H. pylori infection, medications (ie, opioids, antidepressants, CCB), lung transplant, or idiopathic	CBC, BMP, HgbA1C, nutritional studies (albumin, prealbumin) Test for H. pylori EGD Gastric emptying study—abnormal if >60% of radiotracer remains in the stomach at 2 h or >10% at 4 h	Medical management—dietary modifications, promotility agents (metoclopramide, erythromycin), treat H. pylori if present If patient fails medical management, consider endoscopic/surgical intervention: - Pyloric botox, G-POEM - Pyloroplasty - Gastric pacemaker placement - Subtotal gastrectomy—salvage option Persistent gastroparesis post vagotomy can be managed with subtotal gastrectomy w/BII or Roux-en-Y reconstruction			

Disease Process	Relevant H&P	Work-up/Staging	Treatment	Key Surgical Steps	Post-Op Care	Tips & Tidbits
Gastric foreign bodies (core), esophageal foreign bodies and caustic ingestion (advanced)	Object and caustic ingestion most common in children, developmentally delayed, incarcerated, and psychiatric patients Find out what the patient ingested/ how much the patient drank In a patient with caustic ingestion or esophageal foreign body, evaluating airway and breathing is the first priority - Exam findings of airway compromise (i.e. drooling, stridor, hoarse-ness) may necessitate intubation	Two-view XR of neck, chest, and abdomen are initial diagnostic test of choice ○ Looking for metallic objects, bones, and mediastinal and/or peritoneal air CT—obtain if there is high suspicion for foreign body, but none identified on XR - May identify nonradiopaque objects (wood, glass, fish bones) Esophageal foreign body most likely to get lodged at 1 of 3 sites of physiologic narrowing: - Upper esophageal sphincter - Level of the aortic arch - Diaphragmatic hiatus Caustic ingestion obtain—UGI and/or endoscopy to evaluate for perforation and extent of injury	Gastric foreign bodies—80-90% pass without intervention, 10-20% require endoscopic removal, ~1% require surgical removal Ingested foreign objects that require endoscopic removal: - Sharp, pointed objects (ie, paper clips) - Object > 6 cm long or > 2 cm wide (unlikely to pass) - Object causing esophageal or gastric obstruction - 2+ magnets - Button batteries in some situations - Asymptomatic patient with object that remains in stomach for >3-4 wk Foreign body perforation may be managed with primary repair vs stent vs conservative management depending on characteristics of the perforation Caustic injury management: - Airway protection - Induction of vomiting and blind NGT placement contraindicated, may lead to additional injury - Monitor for signs of necrosis or perforation - If patient requires OR, often managed with esophagectomy and cervical esophagostomy, delayed reconstruction	See EGD in Barrett's section May have to use endoscopic forceps, snare, or retrieval net to remove foreign bodies	Patients with a history of severe caustic esophageal injury are at increased risk of stricture and malignancy, require surveillance	There is evidence in the literature that suggests some sharp gastric foreign bodies can be managed expectantly. Additional reading: Zamary KR, et al. This too shall pass: A study of ingested sharp foreign bodies. *J Trauma Acute Care Surg.* 2017 Jan;82(1):150-155. PMID: 27805997.

Disease Process	Relevant H&P	Work-up/Staging	Treatment	Key Surgical Steps	Post-Op Care	Tips & Tidbits

Morbid obesity (core)	Ask about comorbidities
	
	Smoking, NSAID use, and GERD history can influence choice of operation
		BMI > 25 → overweight
		
		BMI > 30 → obese
		
		BMI > 35 → morbid obesity
		
		BMI > 40 → super morbid obesity
			Medically supervised weight loss as part of a multidisciplinary weight-loss program
			- Typically required for 3-6 mo prior to bariatric surgery
			Criteria for bariatric surgery:
			- BMI > 35+ comorbidities
			- BMI > 40
			Surgical options:
			- Laparoscopic adjustable gastric band (LAGB)—not commonly performed anymore
			- Laparoscopic sleeve gastrectomy (LSG)
			  ◦ Typically avoid sleeve gastrectomy in patients with GERD or Barrett's
			- Laparoscopic Roux-en-Y gastric bypass (RNYGB)—avoid in patients with ongoing smoking and/or NSAID use
			- Duodenal switch
				Laparoscopic sleeve gastrectomy (LSG) (advanced):
				- Place ports, including liver retractor
				- Take down greater curve, starting several centimeters proximal to pylorus, working up to angle of His
				- Repair hiatal hernia if present
				- Insert 34-40 Fr bougie
				- Perform longitudinal gastrectomy along the greater curve with linear cutting stapler, typically starting 5-7 cm proximal to the pylorus
				- Remove specimen
				- +/- EGD
				
				Roux-en-Y gastric bypass (advanced):
				- Place ports, including liver retractor
				- Identify LOT, divide jejunum ~50 cm distal
				- Create J-J anastomosis
				  ◦ Typically make Roux limb ~100 cc, but if a very high BMI, make longer Roux limb (~150 cm)
				- Close mesentery at J-J
				- Bring up Roux limb (antecolic vs retrocolic)
				- Transect stomach to create ~30-mL lesser curve-based pouch
				- Create GJ anastomosis
				- EGD with leak test
					Complications:
					- Post-op tachycardia → wide differential
					  ◦ Need to consider leak → UGI or CT with oral contrast
					  ◦ PE is MCC of post-op mortality in bariatric patients
					- Marginal ulcer at gastrojejunal anastomosis after RNYGB
					  ◦ RF: smoking, NSAIDS
					  ◦ Diagnose on EGD, test for H. pylori
					  ◦ Treatment: PPI, Sucralfate, treat H. pylori, smoking and NSAID cessation
					  ◦ Can lead to GIB or perforation
					    ▪ Can usually manage marginal ulcer perforation with Graham patch
						Expected excess body weight loss (EBWL)
						- LAGB → 50-60% EBWL
						- RNYGB → 70-80% EBWL
						- LSG → 40-80% EBWL
						GERD after LSG
						- Manage initially with lifestyle modifications
						- UGI and EGD to evaluate for stricture or hiatal hernia
						- If refractory to medical management, consider conversion to Roux-en-Y or LINX placement

Disease Process	Relevant H&P	Work-up/Staging	Treatment	Key Surgical Steps	Post-Op Care	Tips & Tidbits

Zenker diverticulum	May present with regurgitation, coughing, dysphagia, halitosis
	
	More common in older patients
		Zenker diverticulum is a posterior, pulsion diverticulum located proximal to the cricopharyngeus muscle in the area of Killian's triangle
		
		Barium esophagogram
		
		CT scan of the neck
		
		EGD
			Surgical options include open cricopharyngeal myotomy with diverticulectomy/diverticulopexy vs transluminal cricopharyngeal myotomy
			- Can do endoscopic myotomy for diverticula 2-5 cm in size
				Open cricopharyngomyotomy with diverticulectomy (advanced):
				- Patient placed supine with shoulder roll, head is angulated backward and turned to the right
				- Left neck Incision along anterior border of the SCM, SCM retracted laterally
				- Posterior surface of the pharynx and esophagus exposed with blunt dissection and diverticulum identified (can insert rubber catheter into diverticulum via mouth to help identify it)
				  ○ Diverticulum will be located between the inferior constrictors of the pharynx and cricopharyngeal muscle below
				- Divide the cricopharyngeus muscle
				  ○ Avoid recurrent laryngeal nerves
				- If diverticulum is small (<2 cm), diverticulopexy can be performed by suturing diverticulum to prevertebral fascia
				- If diverticulum is large (>2 cm), resect it using a linear stapler, prevent esophageal narrowing by placing 45 Fr bougie
				- Close muscular defect between inferior constrictors and cricopharyngeus with row of horizontal sutures
				- Close incision in layers, leave drain
					Patients with fever, tachycardia, and chest, back, or neck pain should be evaluated for a leak with gastrograffin swallow
					If patient develops leak, reopen neck incision and place drains
					
					Other post-op complications: mediastinitis, vocal cord paralysis, fistula, esophageal stenosis, recurrent diverticula	

3

Colon and Anorectal Surgery

Melinda Hawkins, MD

DISEASES AND CONDITIONS

- Colon cancer screening, polyp management (c), colonoscopy (c)
- Colon cancer (c), right hemi-colectomy (c)
- Rectal cancer (c), low anterior resection (c), trans-anal resection (a)
- Diverticulitis (c), sigmoidectomy (c), colostomy creation and closure (c)
- Sigmoid volvulus (c)
- Cecal volvulus (c), ileocecectomy (c)

- Large bowel obstruction (c)
- Lower GI bleed (c), total abdominal colectomy (c)
- Anorectal abscess (c)
- Anorectal fistulae (c)
- Anal fissure (c), anal sphincterotomy (c)
- Hemorrhoids (c), hemorrhoidectomy (c)
- Anal cancer (c), abdominal perineal resection (a)
- Perianal condyloma and STDs (c), perianal condyloma removal (c)

- C. diff colitis (c)
- Ischemic colitis (c)
- Surgical management of ulcerative colitis (c)
- Surgical management of Crohn's disease (c)
- Rectal prolapse (a), rectal prolapse repair (a)
- Fecal incontinence (a)
- Polyposis syndromes (a)

GENERAL COLORECTAL TIPS

- Don't forget to give patients a bowel prep with oral antibiotics prior to elective colorectal resections.
- The ASCRS is an excellent resource for management guidelines of various colorectal topics.

(c) = core topic   (a) = advanced topic

Disease Process	Relevant H&P	Work-up/Staging	Treatment	Key Surgical Steps	Post-Op Care	Tips & Tidbits
Colon cancer screening, polyp management (core)	Colon cancer screening should start at 45yo for average-risk patients Patients with increased risk, specifically family history of colorectal cancer or polyps, known genetic syndromes, history of radiation to the abdomen or history of inflammatory bowel disease (IBD) need to start colonoscopies sooner	Colonoscopy is the ideal screening modality Other screening options: • Flex sig q5y or q10y with annual FOBT • FOBT annually • FIT annually • Stool DNA test q1-3y • CT colonography q5y • If any of these are positive, the patient should undergo colonoscopy	Preprocedure bowel prep with polyethylene glycol or magnesium citrate	**Screening colonoscopy (core):** - Position patient in left lateral decubitus with knees bent up - Sedation with propofol or fentanyl/versed - Inspect anal area for any irregularities and perform digital rectal exam - Insert scope - Use air insufflation or water irrigation, advance scope all the way to the cecum - May require transabdominal pressure or repositioning to advance past difficult areas - Withdraw the endoscope while looking for polyps, remove polyps if encountered should have (minimum 6-min withdrawal time) - Retroflex to view proximal rectal vault prior to scope removal Colonoscopy findings and recommended follow-up: • No polyps or small (< 10 mm) hyperplastic polyps ⟶ repeat in 10 y • 1-2 tubular adenomas <10 mm ⟶ repeat in 7-10 y • 1-2 sessile serrated polyps (SSP) <10 mm ⟶ repeat in 5-10y • 3-4 SSP <10 mm or hyperplastic polyps ≥ 10 mm ⟶ repeat in 3-5 y • 3-10 adenomas, adenoma or serrated polyp ≥10 mm, adenoma with villous features or high-grade dysplasia, SSP with dysplasia, or 5-10 SSP ⟶ repeat in 3 y • > 10 synchronous adenomas ⟶ repeat in 1y, consider genetic testing • Piecemeal resection of adenoma ≥20 mm ⟶ repeat in 6 mo	Complications: - Perforation—risk of perforation is 0.1% for diagnostic procedures, up to 3% for therapeutic procedures - Post-polypectomy bleeding	Examiners may give you a case of a malignant appearing polyp ⟶ criteria for endoscopic removal of malignant polyp: • T1 • Grade 1-2 • No lymphovascular invasion • Must be in one piece • Negative margin ≥ 2 mm Endoscopic surveillance for high-risk populations: • HNPCC ⟶ start at 20-25 yo, repeat q1-2y • FAP ⟶ start flex sig at 12 yo q1y, then full colonoscopy q1y once polyps are seen • IBD ⟶ start 8 y after diagnosis, q1-2y with screening biopsies every 10 cm

Disease Process	Relevant H&P	Work-up/Staging	Treatment	Key Surgical Steps	Post-Op Care	Tips & Tidbits

Colon cancer (core)	May present with obstructive symptoms, abdominal discomfort, change in stools, bloody stools, weight loss, anemia
	
	May be detected during screening colonoscopy
	
	Family history?
		Colon cancer staging:
		- CBC, CMP, CEA
		- Tissue biopsy
		  ○ All new colorectal cancers show be tested for MMR deficiency (Lynch syndrome)
		    ■ If positive for MMR deficiency, total abdominal colectomy should be recommended
		- Full colonoscopy
		  ○ 5% rate of synchronous cancer
		- CT C/A/P
		  ○ Can get MRI to further evaluate any concerning liver lesions
		TNM Staging:
		- T stage:
		  ○ T1—submucosa
		  ○ T2—into, muscularis
		  ○ T3—through muscularis
		  ○ T4—through colon wall, perforating cancer is automatically T4
		- N stage (12 LN needed for accurate staging):
		  ○ N1—1-3 +LN
		  ○ N2—≥ 4 +LN
		- M stage:
		  ○ M0—no metastasis
		  ○ M1—metastasis
		- Stage I—T1-2N0M0
		- Stage II—T3-4N0M0
		- Stage III—T1-4N+M0
		- Stage IV—T1-4N0-2M1
			Resectable, M0 → colectomy up front
			- Type of colectomy needed based on location of tumor (table 3.1)
			- Stage III/IV tumors should receive adjuvant chemo (FOLFOX or CAPEOX)
			Unresectable and/or M1—FOLFIRINOX (5-FU, leucovorin, irinotecan, oxaliplatin) + bevacizumab
			- In patient with stage IV colon cancer that is completely obstructing or bleeding, may need to resect primary so that patient can go on to get systemic therapy
			- Liver and lung metastasis—can potentially resect if R0 possible, can do staged or synchronous resection with colectomy + neoadjuvant or adjuvant chemo
			  ○ Can also use liver directed therapies (RFA, MWA, TACE) for liver metastases if resection not feasible
			- Peritoneal disease—debulking may be beneficial if amenable to complete macroscopic resection
			Obstructing colon cancer → resection/ostomy vs stent (depends on location)
				Open right hemicolectomy (core):
				- Laparotomy
				- Lateral to medial dissection—take down white line of Toldt from cecum to hepatic flexure
				- Take down hepatocolic ligament
				- Lift right colon and brush down thin areolar tissue on the lateral surface
				- Identify and preserve the right ureter and duodenum, gently dissect away from the colonic mesentery
				- Divide terminal ileum
				- Identify ileocolic pedicle and other vessels you plan to take (+/- middle colic)
				- Divide ileocolic pedicle high, divide mesentery to specimen
				- Determine distal transection point and divide colon and omentum
				- Primary anastomosis
				
				Laparoscopic right hemicolectomy:
				- Place ports
				- Identify cecum and lift to identify ileocolic artery
				- Skeletonize ileocolic pedicle for high ligation, make sure you visualize and protect duodenum
				- Divide ileocolic with tan stapler
				- Medial to lateral dissection
				- Visualize and protect the ureter and duodenum
				- Take down lateral attachments to colon
				- Divide bowel proximally and distally with at least 5-cm margins
				- Intracorporeal vs extracorporeal anastomosis, specimen extraction
					Anastomotic leak rate after right hemicolectomy 1-3%
					
					Adjuvant chemo (FOLFOX), if indicated—Stage III, IV, high risk stage II (LVI, perineural invasion, tumor budding, etc)
					
					Surveillance:
					- H&P and CEA q3mo x 2 y and then q6mo through 5 y (CEA surveillance not needed for stage I)
					- Annual CT C/A/P q6-12mo x 5 y
					- Colonoscopy at 1-y post-op
					- If not able to do full colonoscopy pre-op, do 6 mo post-op
					  ○ If adenomas found, repeat in 1 y
					  ○ If normal, repeat in 3 y
					  ○ If not able to do full colonoscopy pre-op, do one 6 mo post-op
						Liver and lungs are the most common sites of metastatic disease
						
						Half of patients with colorectal cancer will present with liver disease or will develop it at some point
						
						Typically stop bevacizumab 6-8 wk prior to surgery (impairs wound healing)

Table 3.1: Type of colectomy needed based on location of tumor	
Location of tumor	**Operation needed**
Cecum, ascending colon, hepatic flexure	Right hemicolectomy
Transverse colon	Extended right hemicolectomy • Extended right hemicolectomy with ileocolic anastomosis typically recommended for transverse colon mass because leak rate is only 2%, (lower than for colo-colonic anastomosis)
Splenic flexure	Extended right hemicolectomy or left hemicolectomy
Descending colon	Left hemicolectomy
Sigmoid colon	Sigmoidectomy

Disease Process	Relevant H&P	Work-up/Staging	Treatment	Key Surgical Steps	Post-Op Care	Tips & Tidbits

Rectal cancer (core)	May present with obstructive symptoms, abdominal discomfort, change in stools, bloody stools, weight loss, anemia
	
	May be detected during screening colonoscopy
	
	Family history?
		Rectal cancer staging:
		- Full colonoscopy
		- Rigid sigmoidoscopy—determine accurate distance from dentate line
		- CEA
		- CT C/A/P
		  ◦ Obtain liver MRI if any suspicious liver lesions seen on CT
		- Pelvic MRI vs endorectal U/S (EUS)—evaluate depth of tumor invasion, local invasion, involvement of the mesorectal envelope, and lymph node involvement
		  ◦ MRI preferred over EUS, although EUS can be better at differentiating early-stage tumors (T1-2)
		
		TNM staging is the same as colon cancer (see colorectal cancer section)
			T1N0 → some rectal polyps/early rectal cancers can be resected transanally
			- Criteria for transanal excision:
			  ◦ ≤3 cm
			  ◦ <30% of circumference
			  ◦ T1
			  ◦ No LVI, PNI
			  ◦ Well to moderately differentiated
			  ◦ No evidence of +LN on imaging
			  ◦ Able to get margin clear (>3 mm)
			T1-2N0 → upfront surgery
			- Surgery: Low anterior resection (LAR) vs abdominoperineal resection (APR) with TME
			  ◦ LAR typically preferrable but APR indicated for patients with tumor involving anal sphincters/levator ani, without distance from sphincters for adequate negative margin and/or in patients with poor continence
			Locally advanced (T3-4 and/or LN+) → total neoadjuvant therapy (TNT), then surgery
			- TNT—Induction chemotherapy (FOLFOX or CAPOX), then chemoXRT, then restage 6 wk after XRT completion, surgery 6-12 wk after completion of XRT
			M1 and/or unresectable → definitive chemo
			- FOLFOX, FOLFIRINOX, or CAPEOX + bevacizumab
			- Liver and lung mets—can potentially resect if R0 resection possible, can do staged or synchronous resection
			  ◦ Can also use liver directed therapies (RFA, MWA, TACE) for liver metastases
			
			Pelvic exenteration indicated for patients with rectal cancer with unreconstructable involvement of other pelvic organs (urethra, prostate, bladder)
				Transanal resection (advanced):
				- Patient should have pre-op bowel prep or enemas
				- Position in prone jackknife or lithotomy, depending on location of pathology
				- Gain exposure using self-retaining anal retractor (Lone Star)
				- Use cautery to mark out a 1-cm margin around lesion
				- Perform full thickness excision of the lesion with margin, orient the specimen
				- +/- closure of defect
				
				Low anterior resection (core):
				- Open vs MIS
				- Lithotomy, place ports
				- Retract the sigmoid colon to put mesentery on tension
				- Perform medial to lateral dissection in avascular plane
				- Identify left ureter, perform high ligation of IMA
				- Perform TME, find avascular plane behind the rectum starting at the sacral promontory, do rectal dissection posteriorly, then work laterally and then do anterior last
				- Transect rectum distally, need negative distal margin
				- Mobilize descending colon, transect colon at least 5 cm proximal to tumor
				- Reconstruct with EEA, end-to-side (Baker's type) anastomosis
				- Leak test +/- diverting loop ileostomy (DLI)
				  ◦ Typically divert if low anastomosis (<7 cm), received neoadjuvant chemoXRT, high-risk patient
				  ◦ DLI has not been shown to decrease anastomotic leak, but lessens the consequences associated with anastomotic leak
				
				Abdominoperineal resection (APR):
				- See anal cancer section
					Complications:
					- Anastomotic leak—5-10% risk with colorectal anastomosis
					  ◦ Risk factors for colorectal leak: malnutrition, chemoXRT, immunosuppression, smoking, male, obesity (BMI > 35)
					  ◦ Obtain CT with rectal contrast to evaluate for leak
					  ◦ If small, contained leak, and patient not sick, may be able to manage with IR drain and antibiotics but if large, uncontained leak and patient is sick, take patient back to OR
					- Sexual and urinary dysfunction common after pelvic dissection
					
					If diverting loop ileostomy was created, usually reverse ~6-10 wk later, get contrast enema pre-op to ensure anastomosis is healed
					
					Surveillance:
					- CEA q3mo x 2 y and then q6mo through 5 y
					- Annual CT C/A/P q6-12mo x 5 y
					- Colonoscopy at 1-y post-op
					  ◦ If adenomas found, repeat in 1 y
					  ◦ If normal, repeat in 3 y
						Benefits of neoadjuvant chemoXRT for local advanced rectal cancers:
						- Possibility for sphincter preservation
						- Shrink tumor
						- Decrease local recurrence
						- Higher rate of complete pathologic response seen with TNT than with the traditional approach (neoadjuvant chemoXRT, surgery, and adjuvant chemo)
						
						Watchful waiting for rectal cancer in patients with complete clinical response after TNT is being used for some patients, but would not answer it on boards at this point.
						
						Upper rectal cancers (above the peritoneal reflection) are treated like colon cancer. This is typically determined based on cross-sectional imaging.

Disease Process	Relevant H&P	Work-up/Staging	Treatment	Key Surgical Steps	Post-Op Care	Tips & Tidbits
Diverticulitis (core)	Number and frequency of prior episodes? Complicated (fistula, stricture, obstruction, large abscess) versus uncomplicated (microperforation, simple acute diverticulitis)? Most recent colonoscopy? Abdominal exam— evaluate for peritonitis	CBC, BMP CT with IV contrast Colonoscopy once acute episode resolves (~6 wk)	Stable, uncomplicated—consider outpatient PO antibiotics Stable with contained perforation/abscess—admission, IV antibiotics, bowel rest, IR drain as needed Unstable and/or frank perforation → OR for sigmoidectomy with end colostomy vs resection with primary anastomosis and DLI - Resection with anastomosis and DLI has become an increasingly utilized option, but Hartmann's is the safest answer on boards Recurrent diverticulitis—consider elective resection - Decision to operate depends on number and frequency of prior episodes, complicated vs uncomplicated, comorbidities, and discussion with patient - Elective resection for diverticulitis may be done open or minimally invasive with anastomosis vs ostomy depending on how the case goes	**Sigmoidectomy with end colostomy (Hartmann's) (core):** - Position in lithotomy, make lower midline laparotomy - Take down white line of Toldt and perform lateral to medial dissection of descending colon and sigmoid, identify ureter - Determine proximal transection point (take out frankly inflamed portion of colon but don't need to remove all diverticuli), transect - Mobilize rectosigmoid, divide at sacral promontory on the rectum (remove all sigmoid colon distally to decrease chance of recurrence), remove specimen - Create LLQ end colostomy **Laparoscopic sigmoidectomy:** - Position in lithotomy, place ports, sometimes hand-assist port needed - Mobilize sigmoid colon, determine proximal and distal transection points, identify and protect ureter - Divide mesentery, can stay close to the colon because not doing oncologic resection - Remove specimen via Pfannenstiel or periumbilical incision - Create end-to-side anastomosis using EEA stapler ○ Splenic flexure may need to be mobilized to decrease tension ○ Make sure bowel/mesentery isn't twisted or on significant tension prior to firing stapler - Perform flexible sigmoidoscopy with leak test **Colostomy creation (core):** - Pre-op stoma marking—stoma location should be visible to patient, lie within borders of rectus, not in skinfold - All stomas should be externalized through the rectus to prevent parastomal hernia formation - Circle of skin removed, incise the anterior fascia, split the rectus and then incise the posterior sheath, aperture should accommodate ~2 fingers - Pull bowel through, assess for reach and perfusion - Mature the colostomy	Complications: - Anastomotic leak - Recurrent diverticulitis after resection ~ 10% Typically wait at least 8wks after Hartmann's for reversal Colostomy reversal (core): - Position patient in lithotomy - Suture stoma closed to prevent spillage - Identify rectal stump, resect colon to get down to rectum, if needed - Separate stoma from surrounding skin at the mucocutaneous border, dissect colon circumferentially until it is free of the surrounding tissue - Insert anvil of EEA stapler into proximal colon and reduce it into the abdomen - Further mobilize the colon and take down splenic flexure, as needed for anastomosis without tension - Insert EEA stapler into rectum and connect with anvil, fire stapler to create anastomosis - Leak test - Close fascia at old colostomy site	While laparoscopic lavage for Hinchey grade III may be used by some, avoid answering this on the boards. Additional reading: Bridoux V, et al. Hartmann's procedure or primary anastomosis for generalized peritonitis due to perforated diverticulitis: a prospective multicenter randomized trial (DIVERTI). *J Am Coll Surg.* 2017 Dec;225(6):798-805.

Disease Process	Relevant H&P	Work-up/Staging	Treatment	Key Surgical Steps	Post-Op Care	Tips & Tidbits

Sigmoid volvulus (core)	Abdominal pain, distention, obstruction
	
	More common in patient with chronic constipation and/or neuropsychiatric disorders
		Abdominal XR (bent inner tube)
		
		CT scan—look for mesenteric swirling along with point of obstruction
		
		Contrast enema with bird's beak
			If no signs of intestinal ischemia or perforation, try endoscopic detorsion, if successful, leave rectal tube in place
			- 50-70% recurrence without operation → perform sigmoidectomy during same hospitalization, usually allow 24-72 h for the colon to decompress and administer bowel prep
			
			If peritonitis, free air, signs of perforation → OR immediately for sigmoid colectomy, possible Hartmann's
				Sigmoidectomy for volvulus:
				- Can approach laparoscopic versus open
				- Typically, minimal mobilization is needed due to excessive redundant sigmoid colon
				- Detorse colon if it has not already been endoscopically detorsed
				- Determine proximal and distal transection points—excise enough to reduce most of the sigmoid redundancy
				- Transect bowel and divide the mesentery of the specimen close to the bowel wall
				- Remove specimen
				- Create anastomosis vs colostomy
				  ○ In cases where colon has been detorsed endoscopically and bowel appears healthy, can typically create primary anastomosis
				  ○ If there is ischemic or questionable bowel or if there is significant size mismatch of the proximal and distal ends, colostomy may be preferred		

Cecal volvulus (core)	Abdominal pain, distention, obstruction	Abdominal XR (coffee bean sign) CT scan	Cecal volvulus—ileocecectomy or right hemicolectomy Do NOT attempt endoscopic treatment!	**Open ileocecectomy (core):** - Position patient supine with arms out - Make laparotomy and eviscerate volvulized bowel, detorse bowel - Determine proximal transection point on ileum and distal transection point on colon that appear healthy and well vascularized - Resect and perform primary anastomosis		Major missteps: - Attempting endoscopic detorsion of a cecal volvulus - Performing a cecopexy rather than resection—there is a very high rate of recurrence after cecopexy

Disease Process	Relevant H&P	Work-up/Staging	Treatment	Key Surgical Steps	Post-Op Care	Tips & Tidbits

Large bowel obstruction (core)	Family history? Most recent colonoscopy? Weight loss? Change in stools? Bloody stools?
	
	Abdominal exam and DRE
	
	Most common causes:
	• Diverticular disease
	• Cancer
	• Volvulus
		CBC, CMP
		
		CT abdomen/pelvis—Is there small bowel dilation? Do they have competent ileocecal valve? Where is the obstruction? Is there a mass?
			Diverticular stricture → will need resection
			
			Obstructing colon cancer → OR vs stenting
			- Stenting—carries risk of perforation or stent migration, difficult to stent if obstruction is proximal to splenic flexure, may be preferred for poor operative candidates
			- OR—diversion only vs resection
			  ○ Diverting stoma for distal obstruction → loop colostomy or end colostomy with mucus fistula
			Obstructing rectal cancer → diverting sigmoid colostomy
			- Rectal stenting not well tolerated due to pain, tenesmus, stent migration
			Cecal volvulus → OR for resection
			Sigmoid volvulus → endoscopic detorsion, sigmoidectomy
			
			If patient with large bowel obstruction has a competent ileocecal valve (no small bowel dilation), operative intervention is more urgent
				Hartmann's colectomy for obstructing sigmoid mass:
				- Laparotomy, explore the abdomen
				- Take down the white line of Toldt to free descending and sigmoid colon
				- Identify and protect the ureters
				- Divide colon proximally and distally to mass with at least 5cm margins
				- Perform an oncologic resection with high ligation of the IMA
				- Remove the specimen
				- Put Prolene sutures on rectal stump staple line for potential future reversal
				- Create an end colostomy
				  ○ Take out circle of skin in LLQ overlying rectus, make cruciate cut on the anterior sheath, split the muscle and then make cruciate cut on the posterior sheath, orifice should be large enough to fit 2 fingers
				- Pass colon through, be careful not to twist it
				- Remove staple line to open colon
				- Mature colostomy by taking full thickness bites of colon wall and suturing to dermis with interrupted 3-0 Vicryl +/- Brooking
					Complications:
					- Parastomal hernias
					  ○ Common with loop transverse colostomies (30-50%)
					
					Parastomal hernia management:
					• Asymptomatic/mildly symptomatic hernias should be treated with improving patient comfort and stoma care
					• Surgical repair or revision is indicated for symptomatic patients only, due to high recurrence rate
					• Reverse ostomy, if appropriate
						Major misstep: Creating a loop ileostomy for a patient with an obstructing sigmoid mass and competent ileocecal valve. An ileostomy does not decompress the colon if the patient has a competent ileocecal valve.

Lower GI bleed (core)	May present with varying severity of hematochezia or melena Differential diagnosis: - Diverticular bleed (MCC of LGIB) - Cancer - IBD - Colonic angiodysplasia Perform abdominal exam and anorectal exam with anoscopy to look for bleeding hemorrhoids	Large bore IVx2, resuscitation Full labs including type and screen Transfuse PRN NGT with lavage to rule out UGIB Localize: - Colonoscopy - CTA/angiogram (angiography can detect bleeding 1-1.5 mL/min) - Tagged RBC scan (can detect bleeding 0.1-0.4 mL/ min)	Try colonoscopy first, if patient is relatively stable If colonoscopy fails, IR angiography can be performed If colonoscopy and IR unsuccessful and/or patient is frankly unstable → OR for total abdominal colectomy (TAC) with end ileostomy - Important to localize bleeding as best as possible preoperatively—would obtain tagged RBC scan prior to taking patient for TAC - Can perform segmental resection if bleeding has been localized, otherwise patient needs TAC	**Total abdominal colectomy (core):** - Lithotomy position - Laparotomy - Mobilize entire colon, starting at terminal ileum and working distally, taking care to identify and protect the duodenum, stomach, pancreas, spleen, and ureters - Divide proximally at the ileum and distally across the upper rectum - Create end ileostomy		Do not be baited into doing primary anastomosis in unstable, hemorrhaging patient Most LGIB are successfully managed without surgery - Diverticular bleeding is self-limited in 80%

Disease Process	Relevant H&P	Work-up/Staging	Treatment	Key Surgical Steps	Post-Op Care	Tips & Tidbits
Anorectal abscess (core)	Perianal abscess—fluctuant, red area externally near anal canal, painful but patient usually not systemically ill Ischiorectal abscess—pain and erythema overlying area of ischiorectal fossa Intersphincteric abscess—not obvious externally but anal canal very tender on exam Neutropenic patients—can develop sepsis due to perianal abscess	Perianal and ischiorectal abscesses most common (>80%) Typically diagnosed based on exam (especially superficial abscesses) Get CT if diagnosis unclear based on physical exam Treatment of these abscesses requires a good understanding of the anatomy and the potential spaces for abscesses to develop (Figure 3.1)	Superficial abscesses (perianal, some ischiorectal)—incision and drainage in ED, no antibiotics unless significant cellulitis or immunocompromised Intersphincteric abscesses, deep post-anal abscesses → OR for EUA, I&D Supralevator abscess—transrectal drainage vs percutaneous transabdominal drainage Horseshoe abscess → modified Hanley procedure Neutropenic patients - ANC < 1000 → treat with antibiotics and majority will resolve (patient is so immunosuppressed they can't make pus to form an abscess) - ANC > 1000 → incision and drainage, antibiotics	**EUA with I&D:** - Perform an anoscopy, examine area for any other abnormalities, localize abscess - Drain collection, may need to remove section of skin so that it doesn't close and recur prematurely ○ Make the incision as close to the anus as possible so that if they fistulize, it's a short tract (higher success rates with closure of fistulas with short tract) - Packing not necessary **Modified Hanley procedure for horseshoe abscess:** - Make incision in the posterior midline, go through anococcygeal ligament to access deep post-anal space - Drain and curette the deep post-anal space - Look for internal opening in posterior midline, place seton looping through internal opening and incision into deep post-anal space, if found - Probe from deep post-anal space over to collections in the ischiorectal fossae and make counter incisions overlying collections, insert Penrose drains	Sitz baths 2-3x daily Antibiotics are not needed post-op unless cellulitis is present, systemic signs of infection, or in immunocompromised patient 50% of these patients will develop subsequent fistula, but this won't typically present until at least 1-mo post-op	Do not try to find fistula when patient initially presents with an abscess, just drain abscess and follow-up

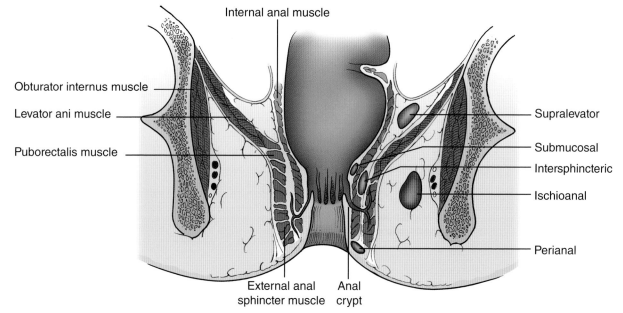

FIGURE 3.1: Potential spaces for anorectal abscesses to develop
- Perianal space—around the anal verge, from dentate line (medially) to the subcutaneous fat of buttocks (laterally), connected to the rectal wall via intersphincteric space
- Intersphincteric space—between the internal and external sphincters
- Ischiorectal fossa—pyramidal potential space between perineum and levator ani, bordered medially by levator ani and external sphincter and laterally by obturator internus muscle and ischium
- Supra-levator space—above levator ani, between pelvic wall and rectum, bilateral ischiorectal fossae are connected via the postanal space
- Deep post-anal space (not pictured)—posterior between the anococcygeal ligament and levator ani

Modified with permission from Minter RM, Doherty GM. *Current Procedures: Surgery*. New York, NY: McGraw Hill; 2010, Figure 26-4.

Labels on figure: Internal anal muscle; Obturator internus muscle; Levator ani muscle; Puborectalis muscle; Supralevator; Submucosal; Intersphincteric; Ischioanal; Perianal; External anal sphincter muscle; Anal crypt

Disease Process	Relevant H&P	Work-up/Staging	Treatment	Key Surgical Steps	Post-Op Care	Tips & Tidbits

Anorectal fistula (core)	May present with perianal drainage, history of anorectal abscess
	
	DRE, anoscopy
		Need to do EUA to determine location of fistula
		
		Normally don't need imaging but can get MRI if unable to determine tract on exam
		
		Fistulas classified based on relationship to the anal sphincter:
		- Intersphincteric fistula—does not penetrate the external sphincter
		- Trans-sphincteric fistula—penetrates the external sphincter below level of the puborectalis muscle and exits into ischiorectal fossa
		- Supra-sphincteric fistula—tract is over the top of the puborectalis, then downward again through the levators and ischiorectal fossa, to the skin
		- Extra-sphincteric fistula—from the perineal skin through the ischiorectal fat and levator muscles into the rectum, outside the sphincter complex
		- Submucosal fistula—tract just beneath the submucosa not involving the sphincter complex
			Choice of treatment depends on amount of sphincter involved in the fistula tract
			
			Fistula treatment options
			- Fistulotomy—preferred for simple fistulas with minimal sphincter involvement
			- Seton—can be placed for complex fistulas with too much sphincter involvement for fistulotomy, seton is usually a preliminary stage prior to a sphincter-preserving procedure
			- Endorectal or anal advancement flap—sphincter-preserving procedure for complex fistula
			- Ligation of intersphincteric fistula tract (LIFT) procedure— sphincter-preserving procedure for complex fistula
			- Fibrin glue, fistula plugs—typically have poor success rates
			
			In Crohn's patients with fistula, be more conservative
			- Place seton and optimize medical management of Crohn's rather than fistulotomy
			- For Crohn's patient with asymptomatic fistula, can just observe
				EUA, fistulotomy:
				- Identify internal and external openings of fistula, pass probe through, determine relationship of tract to sphincters and if it is appropriate for fistulotomy
				  ∘ If having issues identifying the internal opening, can use sparing amount of hydrogen peroxide and watch for bubbles internally
				  ∘ If still can't find the internal opening, abort and get MRI
				- If just internal sphincter is involved, okay to do fistulotomy
				- Can usually divide up to 1/3 of external sphincter
				  ∘ Should only be done in women if it is posterior, be more conservative dividing sphincter muscle in women due to risk of obstetric injury
				- If you can't do fistulotomy, then place seton
				
				Endorectal or anal advancement flap:
				- Patient may have had seton placed previously, remove seton
				- Debride area of external and internal openings, suture internal opening closed
				- Create flap—submucosal dissection, mobilization of vascularized, tension-free flap
				- Cover internal opening with flap that will extend at least 1 cm beyond the opening
				- Suture flap in place with absorbable suture
				
				LIFT procedure:
				- Patient should have had a seton in place to allow fistula tract to mature
				- Pass a fistula probe through the tract and remove the seton
				- Make curvilinear incision in intersphincteric plane at site of fistula
				- Dissect around intersphincteric portion of fistula tract being careful not to disrupt the tract
				- Ligate intersphincteric tract close to the internal and external sphincters with 2-0 Vicryl and transect it between the sutures
				- Test with hydrogen peroxide from external or internal opening to ensure closure
				- Curette external portion of the fistula tract
				- Reapproximate intersphincteric incision
						In a patient with recurrent anorectal fistulas, consider diagnosis of perianal Crohn's, obtain colonoscopy with biopsy
						
						Cutting setons have fallen out of favor and are now rarely used

Disease Process	Relevant H&P	Work-up/Staging	Treatment	Key Surgical Steps	Post-Op Care	Tips & Tidbits

Anal fissure (core)	Sharp pain during a bowel movement with burning and bleeding afterward
	
	Exam: examine perianal area, patient may not tolerate DRE or anoscopy due to pain
	- May have associated skin tag/sentinel pile (chronic fissure)
	- Majority of fissures are midline (posterior more common than anterior)
	- Suspect other process (IBD, TB, HIV, syphilis) if patient has lateral fissure
		Clinical diagnosis	Initial medical management: fiber, sitz baths, hydration, topical sphincter relaxing agents (nifedipine, nitroglycerin, or diltiazem), topical lidocaine, follow-up in 6 wk to assess healing
			- 50% will heal with medical management alone
			
			Botox injection—50% recurrence, can try in patients at high risk of incontinence
			
			Lateral internal anal sphincterotomy—95% fissure healing rate
				Lateral internal sphincterotomy (LIS) (core):
				- Position in prone jackknife
				- Perform perianal block
				- Anoscopy to look for any other abnormalities, inspect fissure
				- Locate intersphincteric groove in lateral position
				- Can do closed vs open sphincterotomy:
				  ◦ Closed: insert scalpel into intersphincteric groove parallel to muscle, turn 90° until blade is pointing inward and apply pressure to break internal muscle fibers but leave mucosa intact
				  ◦ Open: radial skin incision distal to dentate line, expose the intersphincteric groove, elevate internal sphincter fibers and divide, reapproximate the epidermis
				- Open and closed have similar outcomes
				- Can do tailored (sphincterotomy extends the length of the fissure) vs traditional (sphincterotomy extends to dentate line) sphincterotomy
					Risk of incontinence after LIS ~5%	

Disease Process	Relevant H&P	Work-up/Staging	Treatment	Key Surgical Steps	Post-Op Care	Tips & Tidbits

Hemorrhoids (core)	May present with bloody bowel movements, blood on tissue paper, anal itching, and/or perianal pain
	
	Constipation?
	
	Family history of colorectal cancer?
	
	Exam
	- Inspection
	- External palpation
	- DRE
	- Anoscopy
		Internal vs external hemorrhoid
		- Internal—above the dentate line, covered by mucosa, insensate
		- External—below the dentate, covered with keratinized tissue, sensate
		Grades of internal hemorrhoids:
		  I. Nonprolapsing
		  II. Prolapse and spontaneously reduce
		  III. Prolapse and have to manually reduce
		  IV. Chronic prolapse, can't reduce
			Grade I/II internal hemorrhoids → conservative treatment with fluid, fiber, avoid constipation and diarrhea
			Grade II/III internal hemorrhoids → can try RBL in the office, make sure hemorrhoid is above dentate line, do not want to band external hemorrhoid
			Grade III/IV internal hemorrhoids or combined internal/external → excisional hemorrhoidectomy
			Thrombosed external hemorrhoid—if patient presents early (<48-72 h) can do excision, otherwise leave them be and treat with supportive care
			Hemorrhoids in pregnancy—leave them alone, most will go away after delivery
			Hemorrhoids in patients with portal HTN—medical management, suture ligation, TIPS, avoid formal hemorrhoidectomy because these are more likely varicosities than true hemorrhoids, high risk of bleeding issues
				Excisional hemorrhoidectomy (core):
				- Anoscopy, identify hemorrhoidal cushions
				- Excise hemorrhoidal tissue starting externally and moving proximally, taking care to avoid the underlying sphincter muscle
				- Suture ligate hemorrhoidal pedicle proximally
				- If excising multiple columns, make sure you leave at least 1 fingerbreadth of normal mucosa between areas of excision to prevent anal stenosis
				- Leave hemorrhoid open (Milligan-Morgan) vs close (Ferguson)
					Complications:
					- Delayed post-hemorrhoidectomy bleeding usually happens ~2 wk out
					- Postoperative pelvic sepsis (very rare)—increasing pain, fever, urinary retention	

Disease Process	Relevant H&P	Work-up/Staging	Treatment	Key Surgical Steps	Post-Op Care	Tips & Tidbits

Anal squamous cell carcinoma (core)	Risk factors: HPV-16/18, AIN, anoreceptive intercourse, multiple partners, HIV, immunocompromised
	
	Presentation: asymptomatic, bleeding, pain, pruritis
	
	Exam: DRE, anoscopy, examine inguinal nodes, perform gynecologic exam in women
		Biopsy mass—squamous cell carcinoma (SCC) is most common type of anal cancer
		
		Staging of anal SCC:
		- CT C/A → rule out metastatic disease
		- CT pelvis or MRI pelvis to evaluate inguinal nodes
		  ○ FNA any abnormal inguinal LN
		- HIV testing
		- +/- colonoscopy
		- +/- PET— indicated for N+ and ≥ T2 anal canal and anal margin cancers
			Anal intra-epithelial neoplasia (AIN)
			- Premalignant lesion
			- Treat AIN with topical therapy (imiquimod, fluorouracil, trichloroacetic acid, or cidofovir) or EUA with excision and fulguration of any visible lesions
			- Recurrence rates high, require ongoing surveillance
			Anal SCC
			- ChemoXRT (Nigro protocol) is the primary treatment for localized disease
			- Mitomycin C + 5-FU + XRT → re-evaluate every ~8-12 wk, can wait up to 6 mo for complete remission
			  ○ Radiate the groin if inguinal nodes positive
			- If progressive disease, persistent disease at 6 mo, or recurrence → salvage APR
			  ○ ~10–30% of patients have persistent or recurrent disease after Nigro protocol
			  ○ Always re-biopsy and restage prior to performing salvage APR
			  ○ Patient should have inguinal node dissection along with APR if groin nodes are positive
			- Patients with metastatic disease are treated with systemic chemotherapy (5-FU/cisplatin)
				Abdominoperineal resection (APR) (advanced):
				- Lithotomy, place ports
				- Retract the sigmoid colon to put mesentery on tension
				- Perform medial to lateral dissection in avascular plane
				- Identify ureters, perform high ligation of IMA
				- Dissect down in TME plane all the way to the levators, once posterior dissection has been done, dissect laterally, then anteriorly
				- Identify and protect hypogastric nerves, ureters, and iliac vessels
				- Mobilize descending colon and divide colon with adequate proximal margin
				- Create an end colostomy
				- Perform perineal dissection, this can be done with patient in lithotomy or prone
				- Start dissection from perineal side in diamond configuration around the anus from the ischial tuberosities, coccyx, and midpoint of the perineum and dissect through the levator ani musculature to meet with previously performed pelvic dissection
				- Close perineal wound in layers
					Perineal wound dehiscence is common after APR
					
					Surveillance after complete remission with Nigro protocol → DRE, anoscopy, and exam of groin q3-6mo x 5 y, CT C/A/P, or PET/CT annually x 3 y
						Don't waste time memorizing the TNM staging of anal SCC, it does not play a significant role in determining treatment strategy.
						
						Additional reading:
						Stewart DB, et al. The American Society of Colon and Rectal Surgeons clinical practice guidelines for anal squamous cell cancers (Revised 2018). *Dis Colon Rectum.* 2018 Jul;61(7):755-774.
						
						Other types of anal cancer:
						Perianal SCC—cancer within 5-cm radius of anal verge
						- If T1-2N0, no sphincter involvement, mod-well differentiated → can try local excision if able to get negative margins without compromising the sphincters
						- T3-4, N+, poorly differentiated, or sphincter involvement → Nigro protocol
						
						Anal melanoma—may present as pigmented lesion, S-100+
						- Very aggressive, typically treated with local excision
						- Most patients with anal melanoma die of distant metastasis, APR does not offer a survival advantage
						
						Anal adenocarcinoma—treated like distal rectal cancer (ie, chemoXRT, APR)

Disease Process	Relevant H&P	Work-up/Staging	Treatment	Key Surgical Steps	Post-Op Care	Tips & Tidbits
Perianal condyloma, STDs (core)	Perianal condyloma usually asymptomatic, but can also cause pain, bleeding, and pruritus RF: HPV, HIV Exam should include visual inspection of anus and perianal area, DRE, and anoscopy Differential diagnosis for external anal lesion: HPV-associated anal condyloma, herpes (HSV), or syphilis Proctitis is most commonly due to gonorrhea, chlamydia, syphilis, or HSV	Condyloma diagnosed based on exam Patients with proctitis should have rectal swabs for gonorrhea, chlamydia, and HSV, as well as serologic STD/STI testing	Anal condyloma treatment: - Just a few condylomas ⟶ at home topical therapy (podofilox or imiquimod, for external condyloma only) or in office podophyllin, trichloroacetic (TCA), or cryotherapy - Lots of condylomas ⟶ surgical excision and fulguration	**Treatment of anal condyloma (core):** - Wear appropriate PPE - Position patient prone, tape buttocks apart - Perform perianal nerve block - Vaginal speculum examination in females - Anoscopy to inspect anal canal for lesions - Excise large, raised lesions and fulgurate or ablate small flat lesions - This is an epithelial disease, excision deeper than dermis and wide margins are not necessary - In patients with extensive disease, avoid creating a circumferential perianal wound, which can lead to stricture, can treat in staged fashion, if needed	One-third of patients will have recurrence of lesions after anal condyloma excision/fulguration	
C. diff colitis (core)	Watery diarrhea, abdominal pain, AKI Often have a history of recent antibiotic use	Infectious stool panel, C. diff stool toxin and PCR test CBC, BMP, lactate	Nonsevere ⟶ PO vancomycin or fidoxamicin x 10 d Severe ⟶ same Fulminant ⟶ PO vancomycin, vancomycin enemas, IV flagyl Peritonitis, perforation, or decompensation ⟶ TAC with end ileostomy Stool transplant for recurrent cases	See total abdominal colectomy with end ileostomy in lower GIB section	Some will do post-op vancomycin enemas to treat residual C. diff in the rectal stump	In practice, some surgeons will create a DLI and treat the patient with antegrade vancomycin enemas if there is no perforation or full thickness ischemia; however, it would be best to avoid this answer on boards.

Disease Process	Relevant H&P	Work-up/Staging	Treatment	Key Surgical Steps	Post-Op Care	Tips & Tidbits
Ischemic colitis (core)	May present with abdominal pain, distention, bloody stools, N/V, diarrhea Evaluate for peritonitis, perform DRE Colitis differential diagnosis: infectious, inflammatory, ischemic, diverticulitis, neutropenic enterocolitis	CBC, CMP, lactate, C. diff, stool panel/culture CT A/P with contrast— watershed areas (splenic flexure, rectosigmoid junction) most commonly affected by ischemic colitis Flexible sigmoidoscopy can be used to confirm diagnosis and assess extent of disease - Do not perform in unstable patient or patient with signs of perforation or full thickness ischemia	Supportive care with bowel rest, IVF, IV antibiotics, serial exams If patient develops signs of perforation or full thickness ischemia, take to OR for TAC	See total abdominal colectomy with end ileostomy in lower GIB section	Can develop strictures later on from ischemic colitis	If you end up taking a patient with ischemic colitis to the OR, do not create an anastomosis

Disease Process	Relevant H&P	Work-up/Staging	Treatment	Key Surgical Steps	Post-Op Care	Tips & Tidbits

Ulcerative colitis (core)	May present with abdominal pain, diarrhea, weight loss, bloody stools
	
	Extra-intestinal manifestations: primary sclerosing cholangitis, pyoderma gangrenosum, arthritis, uveitis
	
	Perform abdominal exam, DRE/anoscopy
		CBC, BMP, LFTs, CRP
		
		Infectious stool panel, C. diff—must rule out infectious etiology prior to starting immunosuppression
		
		Quantiferon Gold—ensure patient doesn't have tuberculosis prior to starting immunosuppression
		
		Colonoscopy with biopsy—do not do colonoscopy if patient has fulminant colitis
		- Involvement will be continuous from the rectum, extending proximally
		- Histologic: crypt abscesses
		- Take biopsy to check for CMV
		  ○ Can cause severe colitis
		  ○ Tx: ganciclovir
		
		Fulminant colitis presentation → 10 BM/d, rectal bleeding, fever, tachycardia, ESR > 30, "thumbprinting," pneumatosis, peritonitis
		
		Toxic megacolon—colonic dilation and systemic toxicity
			Medical management is first line:
			- GI consult
			- Many options for maintenance meds (TNF-alpha antagonists, mesalamine, 5-ASA, immunosuppressants [azathioprine, 6-MP, methotrexate])
			- Steroids for flares
			
			Indications for surgery:
			- Fulminant colitis/toxic megacolon
			  ○ If patient is stable and has no sign of perforation, can initially try rescue therapies (steroids, infliximab), resuscitation, antibiotics, bowel rest with close observation
			  ○ If patient worsens or fails to improve after several days → OR
			- Medically refractory disease, malnutrition, growth retardation
			- High-grade dysplasia
			
			Surgical options:
			- Total proctocolectomy with end ileostomy (TPC w/EI)
			- TPC with ileal pouch anal anastomosis (IPAA) with temporary DLI
			  ○ Two stage vs three stage approach
			- In the urgent setting (ie, fulminant colitis) perform TAC with end ileostomy, can remove rectum down the road, preserve option for IPAA in the future
				Emergent total abdominal colectomy with end ileostomy:
				- Laparotomy
				- Mobilize colon from lateral attachments starting at the cecum and working clockwise all the way to sigmoid
				- Take mesentery close to bowel—avoid high ligation of ileocolic or superior rectal vessels
				  ○ Taking the ileocolic vessels can ruin chances for a pouch in the future
				  ○ Taking superior rectal vessels violates presacral surgical plane for future proctectomy
				- Leave long rectal stump if emergent, can do completion proctectomy at a later date
				
				Ileal pouch anal anastomosis creation:
				- Total proctocolectomy either in same stage or already done during previous stage
				- Oversew the distal ileal staple line
				- Make sure vascular pedicle is not twisted
				- Mobilize ileum until there is no tension when reaching down to the anal canal
				  ○ Options to obtain additional length if having issues with reach:
				    ▪ Small bowel mobilization to root of mesentery
				    ▪ Lengthen mesentery with transverse mesenteric relaxing incisions
				    ▪ High ligation of the ileocolic vessels
				    ▪ Can leave pouch in the pelvis and come back in the future if absolutely unable to reach
				- Line up two 15-cm limbs of the small bowel and place a suture to approximate the bowel ends
				- Make an enterotomy in the apex of the pouch and place stapler through, fire to create pouch
				- Make purse string at the apex of the pouch around the anvil of EEA stapler
				- Place the EEA stapler into the anus and carefully advance under direct vision through the anal canal to engage with the anvil
				- Once the stapler is appropriately coupled, fire it
				- Create upstream loop ileostomy
					Complications:
					- Anastomotic leak rate for J pouch is ~20%
					- Cuffitis → mesalamine suppositories
					- Pouchitis—evaluate for stenosis, treat with cipro/flagyl, mesalamine, steroid enemas
					- Infertility—due to pelvic dissection, may be preferable to wait to do IPAA until patient is done with childbearing
					
					Surveillance for UC patients post TPC with IPAA:
					- Pouchoscopy with visualization and biopsies every 1-3 y
					- Anal transition zone dysplasia → transanal mucosectomy and pouch advancement to dentate line
						Patients with IBD on chronic steroids may need stress dose steroids in perioperative period
						- Stress dose steroids for major procedure → 100-mg IV hydrocortisone pre-op, then 50 mg q8h x 24 h, then taper dose by 1/2 per day down to home dose
						
						Do not do IPAA in patient with incontinence or with Crohn's, obesity is also a relative contraindication
						
						IBD screening colonoscopy should begin 8y after symptom onset, q1-3y with 4 quad bx every 10 cm

Disease Process	Relevant H&P	Work-up/Staging	Treatment	Key Surgical Steps	Post-Op Care	Tips & Tidbits

Crohn's disease (core)	Abdominal pain, diarrhea, weight loss, bloody stools, recurrent peri-anal abscess/fistula
	
	Terminal ileum most commonly affected, perianal disease fairly common
	
	Extra-intestinal manifestations: erythema nodosum, pyoderma gangrenosum, arthritis, uveitis, hepatitis
	
	Do abdominal exam, DRE/anoscopy
		CBC, CMP, CRP, ESR, P-ANCA
		
		Infectious stool panel to rule out infectious cause
		
		Quantiferon gold—rule out tuberculosis infection prior to starting immunosuppression
		
		CT vs MRI—MRI may be better at differentiating acute inflammatory stricture vs fibrostenotic stricture
		
		Colonoscopy with biopsy
		- Crohn's features: cobble stoning, segmental, skip lesions, non-caseating granulomas on histology
		- Biopsy any strictures to evaluate for malignancy
			Medical management is first line
			- GI should be involved early
			- "Top down" vs "step-up approach"—mesalamine, 5ASA, TNF-alpha antagonists (infliximab), immunosuppressants (tacro, azathioprine, 6-MP, methotrexate)
			- Steroids for flares
			Surgery only for complications
			Management of Crohn's stricture—CRP, endoscopy, CT enterography vs MRE → determine if it is from acute inflammation or fibrostenotic disease
			- Small bowel stricture
			  ○ For stricture related to acute inflammation - try NPO, TPN, steroids
			  ○ For chronic stricture - will need dilation vs stricturoplasty vs resection
			- Large bowel stricture—can try endoscopic dilation if it is an anastomotic stricture, otherwise should resect, do not treat with stricturoplasty (7% risk of malignancy in colon stricture)
				Tips for operating on Crohn's patients:
				- May require stress dose steroids when undergoing surgery
				- Perform segmental small bowel resection as needed, only remove grossly inflamed tissue, avoid resecting large amounts of small bowel
				- The Kono-S anastomosis is gaining popularity but would not recommend talking about it on boards, unless you have experience with it
				- Can do stricturoplasty if concerned for length of remaining small bowel
				Stricturoplasties:
				- Heineke-Mikulicz stricturoplasty—ideal for short strictures <10 cm in length
				  ○ Open bowel longitudinally and suture closed transversely
				- Jaboulay or Finney for intermediate strictures (10-25 cm)
				  ○ Jaboulay—bowel fold in U shape so that strictured bowel is at the apex and normal afferent and efferent limbs of bowel are side-by-side, open both limbs of bowel longitudinally and suture together, so that strictured segment is bypassed
				  ○ Finney—longitudinal enterotomy made on strictured segment, segment folded on itself in a U-shape and then sutured together like a diverticulum
				- Michelassi stricturoplasty—for strictures >20-25 cm
				  ○ Divide strictured bowel and its mesentery at the center of the stricture, advance one limb of bowel over the other end so they are overlapping in isoperistaltic orientation, longitudinal enterotomy over the length of the stricture on both limbs of bowel, limbs sutured together in sided-to-side orientation to create wider common channel
					IBD → screening colonoscopy beginning 8 y after onset of symptoms, q1-3 y with 4 quadrant bx every 10 cm
					- HGD in colon → colectomy
						Management of other Crohn's issues:
						Perianal disease—drain abscesses, if patient goes on to develop fistula place seton as needed, avoid fistulotomies and minimize tissue loss to preserve sphincter function, optimize medical management
						
						Bowel fistulas—try medical management and if no improvement perform segmental resection
						
						Perforation/abscess—take to OR if perforation uncontained and/or patient unstable, treat with antibiotics and IR drain if stable and contained, consider resection in 4-6 wk

Disease Process	Relevant H&P	Work-up/Staging	Treatment	Key Surgical Steps	Post-Op Care	Tips & Tidbits
Rectal prolapse (advanced)	Most common in older women, multiparous, history of constipation Typically, full thickness Don't be tricked by prominent, prolapsing hemorrhoids—prolapse will appear like concentric rings of mucosa Have patient strain on the toilet if not initially obvious on exam	Usually diagnosed based on exam Fluoroscopic defecography if needed	Initial management: fiber, fluid, minimize straining If patient remains symptomatic, should have surgical repair Transabdominal vs perineal approaches - Perineal approach preferred for older sicker patients, has lower risk of anastomotic leak but higher risk of recurrence	**Transabdominal rectopexy (advanced):** - Open vs MIS - Rectal mobilization anteriorly and posteriorly +/- preservation of lateral stalks - Consider sigmoid resection in patients with constipation - Pull rectum up out of pelvis and fix it to the sacral promontory with mesh or nonabsorbable suture - Watch out for presacral bleeding—manage with pressure, tacs, and/or hemostatic agents, if needed **Delorme—perineal approach for 1-3 cm of mucosal prolapse:** - Position patient in lithotomy or prone jackknife, Lone Star retractor can help with exposure - Grasp the prolapsing rectal tissue and pull it out, make a circumferential mucosal incision ~2 cm above the dentate line - Mucosal stripping—dissect the mucosa off of the muscularis by dissecting in the submucosal plane, excise the redundant mucosa - Plicate muscular layer - Close the mucosa over the plicated area **Altemeier (perineal proctectomy) - perineal approach for >3 cm prolapse:** - Position patient in prone jackknife or lithotomy, Lone Star retractor can help with exposure - Grasp redundant tissue with an Allis clamp - Make a full thickness circumferential excision 1-2 cm proximal to the dentate line - Dissect around the rectum, detaching it from mesorectum until peritoneal cavity is entered - Transect bowel at the level of rectosigmoid junction - Create handsewn coloanal anastomosis	Minimize straining, need a good bowel regimen Can have post-op urinary retention due to pelvic dissection	Ventral mesh rectopexy is an alternative to posterior rectopexy

Disease Process	Relevant H&P	Work-up/Staging	Treatment	Key Surgical Steps	Post-Op Care	Tips & Tidbits
Fecal incontinence (advanced)	Symptoms range from occasional involuntary passage of flatus to involuntary passage of stool Risk factors: increasing age, female, obstetric injury, pelvic XRT Underlying disorders may include prolapsing hemorrhoids, rectal prolapse, rectal mass, fecal impaction with overflow incontinence, or neuropathy Perform anorectal exam - Scar in perineum or thin perineal body may indicate old obstetric injury - DRE—assess sphincter tone	Try medical management first, if no improvement, get further tests Endoanal U/S or MRI can be used to look at sphincters and determine presence of tears, atrophy +/- anal manometry, defecography	Medical treatments: - Fiber to bulk stools - Antidiarrheal agents - Treat fecal impaction if present - Biofeedback physical therapy Fecal incontinence is a quality-of-life problem, intervention dictated by patient's desire to have invasive interventions Operative options for patients with incontinence refractory to medical treatment: - Sacral nerve stimulator - Overlapping sphincteroplasty—indicated in patients with anatomic sphincter injury, poor long-term durability - Colostomy			

Disease Process	Relevant H&P	Work-up/Staging	Treatment	Key Surgical Steps	Post-Op Care	Tips & Tidbits
Polyposis syndromes	Family history of colon cancer, history of polyps, GI bleeding, weight loss, abdominal pain May have known familial mutation or present with cancer Mucocutaneous pigmentation seen with Peutz-Jeghers	Refer for genetic testing if mutation is suspected Familial adenomatous polyposis (FAP) - APC gene mutation - Increased risk of colorectal cancer and duodenal cancer - Annual colonoscopy starting at 12 yo - EGD starting at 25 yo and repeat q1-5y depending on findings, looking for adenomatous duodenal polyps Juvenile polyposis—increased risk of colon and gastric cancer - Yearly colonoscopy and EGD starting at 12 yo and repeated q1-3y depending on findings HNPCC (Lynch syndrome)—increased risk of colon, endometrial, ureteral, bladder, and stomach cancer (among others) - MMR gene mutation—obtain mismatch repair testing looking for absence of MLH1, PMS2, MSH2, or MSH6 (ie, microsatellite instability) - Amsterdam criteria used to help identify families that may have HNPCC - Colonoscopy q1-2y beginning at 20-25 yo, yearly after 40 yo - Women should undergo annual endometrial biopsy and transvaginal U/S beginning at 35 yo to screen for endometrial and ovarian cancer - Prophylactic TAH/BSO recommended by age 40 or when childbearing complete - Annual U/A starting at 30-35 yo screen for urinary tract cancer Peutz-Jeghers—increased risk of gastric, colon, small bowel, pancreas, and breast cancer • Colonoscopy q2-3y beginning in adulthood	FAP—prophylactic colectomy recommended in early adulthood - Surgical options: TPC with end ileostomy vs TPC with IPAA vs TAC with ileorectal anastomosis - Can preserve rectum if patient has rectal sparing but have 12-29% risk of developing rectal cancer, need flex sig q6-12mo for surveillance Patient with Lynch syndrome and colorectal cancer - Colon cancer ⟶ TAC with ileorectal anastomosis - Rectal cancer ⟶ TPC with end ileostomy vs proctectomy with end colostomy and yearly colon surveillance			Additional reading: Rafferty JF, Feingold D, Steele SR. Clinical practice guidelines for the surgical treatment of patients with Lynch syndrome. *Dis Colon Rectum*. 2017 Feb;60(2):137-143.

4

Pancreas, Hepatobiliary, and Spleen

Mohamed Alassas, MD, FACS

DISEASES AND CONDITIONS

- Pancreatic adenocarcinoma (c), pancreaticoduodenectomy (a), distal pancreatectomy with splenectomy (c)
- Cystic pancreatic lesions including IPMN (c), spleen-sparing distal pancreatectomy
- Pancreatic neuroendocrine tumors (c)
- Pancreatitis (c), pancreatic debridement (c)
- Pancreatic pseudocyst, drainage of pancreatic pseudocyst (c)

- Chronic pancreatitis (a), operative management of chronic pancreatitis (a), total pancreatectomy (a)
- Peri-ampullary tumors, ampullary resection for tumor (a)
- Pancreas divisum (a), transduodenal sphincteroplasty
- Bile duct injury (c), choledochoenteric anastomosis (a)
- Choledochal cyst (c)
- Gallbladder polyps and cancer (c), gallbladder cancer operation (a)

- Cholangiocarcinoma, hepatic segmentectomy/lobectomy (a)
- Liver lesions (c), hepatic biopsy (c)
- Hepatic abscess (c), hepatic abscess drainage (c)
- Primary sclerosing cholangitis (a)
- Hematologic diseases of the spleen (c), splenectomy (c)
- Splenic abscess, cysts, and neoplasms (c)

GENERAL HEPATOBILIARY SURGERY TIPS

- Don't forget to stage in the cancer scenarios.

- Always mention that you will discuss cancer patients at a multidisciplinary tumor board.

(c) = **core topic**   (a) = **advanced topic**

Disease Process	Relevant H&P	Work-up/Staging	Treatment	Key Surgical Steps	Post-Op Care	Tips & Tidbits

Pancreatic adenocarcinoma (core)	Risk factors: cigarette smoking, EtOH, obesity, chronic pancreatitis
	
	May present with painless jaundice, new onset diabetes, weight loss, light stools, dark urine, itching
	
	Examine abdomen, look for jaundice and scleral icterus
		CBC, CMP, lipase, coagulation panel
		
		RUQ U/S in patients who present with jaundice
		
		CT pancreas protocol—look at lymph nodes, look for involvement of portal vein, SMA/SMV, common or proper hepatic artery, celiac artery
		
		CT C/A/P to rule out metastases
		
		CA 19-9—can be falsely elevated if total bilirubin >2.5
		- CA 19-9 > 130 concerning for occult metastatic disease
		
		+/- EUS with FNA biopsy
		
		+/- ERCP with stent, brushings—routine pre-op biliary drainage not recommended, but should be considered in patients with significant hyperbilirubinemia
			Discuss at multidisciplinary tumor board
			
			Tissue diagnosis is needed prior to starting chemo, but not required prior to surgery
			
			Criteria for Resectability:
			- Resectable: no arterial contact, <180° contact w/ SMV/PV
			- Borderline: <180° contact with SMA or celiac artery, reconstructable SMV/PV involvement
			- Unresectable: >180° contact with celiac or SMA, unreconstructable SMV/PV involvement, M1 disease, invading other unresectable structures
			
			All patients will get systemic therapy at some point in their treatment course
			- If borderline resectable, consider neoadjuvant chemo and then restage to determine if patient is a surgical candidate
			
			Preferred chemo regimen: FOLFIRINOX
			
			Head of pancreas mass → Whipple
			
			Body or tail of pancreas mass → distal pancreatectomy with splenectomy
				Whipple (Pancreaticoduodenectomy) (advanced) (Figure 4.1):
				- Consider diagnostic laparoscopy to rule out metastatic disease, convert to open if no mets seen
				- Take down hepatic flexure of colon, open gastrocolic ligament, gain access into lesser sac
				- Kocherize the duodenum, ensure no invasion into SMA
				- Dissect out inferior border of pancreas and start retropancreatic tunnel between SMV and neck of pancreas
				- Perform cholecystectomy
				- Dissect out portal structures, portal lymphadenectomy
				- Test clamp and divide GDA
				- Complete retropancreatic tunnel
				- Divide stomach, proximal jejunum 10 cm distal to LOT, CBD/CHD, and pancreatic neck
				  ◦ Free pancreatic head and uncinate from any remaining attachments
				  ◦ Send the pancreatic margin for frozen section
				- Reconstruct:
				  ◦ Pancreaticojejunostomy (PJ)—2-layer end-to-side duct-to-mucosa anastomosis, +/- stent
				  ◦ Hepaticojejunostomy—single layer end-to-side anastomosis
				  ◦ Gastrojejunostomy—antecolic loop of jejunum, 2-layer end-to-side anastomosis
				- Leave NGT in afferent limb of GJ
				- Leave drain posterior to PJ and drain near hepaticojejunostomy
				- Place J-tube if high risk for leak
				
				Distal pancreatectomy with splenectomy (core):
				- Consider diagnostic laparoscopy to rule out mets
				- Left subcostal vs midline incision
				- Divide gastrocolic ligament to enter lesser sac, take down splenocolic ligament
				- Divide short gastrics and then retract spleen medially and divide lateral attachments so that spleen and tail of pancreas can be rotated medially and mobilized off the retroperitoneum
				- Ligate and divide IMV if it drains into splenic vein
				- Mobilize spleen and pancreas medially to identify origin of splenic artery and vein at SMV-splenic vein junction
				- Ligate and divide splenic vessels
				- Divide neck of pancreas with GIA stapler, send frozen margin
				- Ensure hemostasis, leave drain in LUQ, close
					Complications:
					- Gastroparesis—common after Whipple, managed with dietary modification, glycemic control, motility agents
					- Pancreatic leak/fistula—check drain amylase on POD 3 to eval for leak
					  ◦ Treat with drainage, antibiotics, supportive care, make NPO and start TPN if output is high
					  ◦ Risk factors for leak—small pancreatic duct, soft pancreas
					
					Adjuvant chemo once recovered from surgery
					
					Surveillance:
					- H&P, CA 19-9, and CT C/A/P q3-6mo x 2 y, then q6-12mo
					
					5-y survival for patients with resectable pancreatic adenocarcinoma is 15-20%
						Acinar cell carcinoma—treat like pancreatic adenocarcinoma, better prognosis

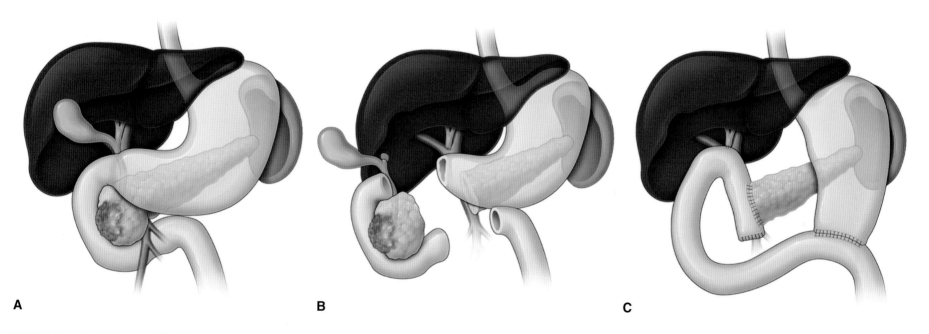

A   **B**   **C**

FIGURE 4.1: Pancreaticoduodenectomy. **A:** Head of pancreas mass. **B:** Resection of duodenum, proximal jejunum, head of the pancreas, gallbladder, and distal CBD. **C:** Reconstruction with pancreaticojejunosetomy, hepaticojejunostomy, and gastrojejunostomy. (Reproduced with permission from Zinner MJ, Ashley SW, Hines OJ. *Maingot's Abdominal Operations,* 13th ed. New York, NY: McGraw Hill; 2019, Figure 73-7.)

Disease Process	Relevant H&P	Work-up/Staging	Treatment	Key Surgical Steps	Post-Op Care	Tips & Tidbits

Cystic pancreatic lesions (core)	May have vague symptoms but often asymptomatic and identified incidentally on imaging
	
	Ask about history of pancreatitis and diabetes
		Differential diagnosis for pancreatic cystic lesion:
		- Simple pancreatic cyst
		- Pseudocyst
		- Mucinous cystic neoplasm (MCN)
		- Serous cystadenoma (SCA)
		- Intraductal papillary mucinous neoplasm (IPMN)
		- Solid pseudopapillary neoplasm (SPN)
		- Pancreatic neuroendocrine tumor (PNET)
		Labs—CBC, CMP, lipase, CA 19-9
		CT pancreas protocol
		+/- MRCP
		EUS with FNA and fluid studies (mucin, CEA, amylase, cytology)
		- SCA—low CEA, low amylase, (-) mucin
		- MCN—high CEA, low amylase, (+) mucin
		- IPMN—high CEA, high amylase, (+) mucin
			Indications for surgery for IPMN (simplified from Fukuoka guidelines):
			- Confirmed or suspected HGD or malignancy
			- Main duct IPMN
			- Branch duct IMPN > 3 cm
			- Symptomatic
			- Enhancing mural nodule > 5 mm
			- Main pancreatic duct > 10 mm
			If branch duct IPMN < 3 cm and no concerning features → surveillance MRI/EUS q3-12 mon (depending on size, characteristics)
			SCA—malignant transformation rare, resection not recommended
			MCN—significant malignant potential → resect
			SPN—10:1 female to male, young patients, good prognosis with resection (95% at 5 y)
			Head of pancreas mass → Whipple
			Body or tail of pancreas mass → distal pancreatectomy +/- splenectomy
			- Can preserve spleen if no known malignancy
				Laparoscopic spleen-preserving distal pancreatectomy:
				- Place ports triangulating LUQ
				- Enter lesser sac through gastrocolic ligament, confirm location of pancreatic pathology (can use U/S if needed)
				- Open plane along inferior border of pancreas
				- Dissect splenic vein from overlying pancreas, clipping any small branches
				- Dissect splenic artery away from superior border of pancreas, clipping any small branches
				- Divide pancreas with adequate margin
				- Send frozen section of proximal margin to ensure no HGD at margin
				- Leave drain and close
				- Alternatively, could do spleen-preserving distal pancreatectomy with ligation of splenic vessels and preservation of short gastrics (Warshaw technique)
				
				See pancreatic adenocarcinoma section for Whipple procedure
					Complications:
					- Pancreatic fistula—treat with drainage, supportive care, if persistent consider ERCP with sphincterotomy
					- Splenic artery pseudoaneurysm— usually occurs in setting of pancreatic leak, which erodes into vessels and causes hemorrhage
					  ○ May have herald bleed, new bloody drain output
					  ○ Treat with IR embolization
					Patients with IPMN with HGD s/p resection are at risk of recurrence, should have ongoing surveillance with MRI/EUS and tumor markers q6mo
						Main duct IPMN → 30-50% malignant
						Branch duct IPMN → 10-15% malignant
						Additional reading:
						Tanaka M, et al. Revisions of international consensus Fukuoka guidelines for the management of IPMN of the pancreas. *Pancreatology*. 2017 Sep-Oct;17(5): 738-753.

Disease Process	Relevant H&P	Work-up/Staging	Treatment	Key Surgical Steps	Post-Op Care	Tips & Tidbits

Pancreatic neuroendocrine tumors (PNET) (core)	Symptoms of functional PNET:
	- Insulinoma—hypoglycemia symptoms, relief of symptoms with administration of glucose
	- Gastrinoma—refractory peptic ulcer disease
	- Glucagonoma—dermatitis, diabetes, DVT
	- Somatostatinoma—diabetes, gallstones, steatorrhea, hypochlorhydria
	- VIPoma—watery diarrhea, low K+, achlorhydria
	
	Nonfunctional PNET may be found incidentally on imaging or due to obstructive symptoms
	
	Ask about family history
	- MEN I—pancreas (PNET), pituitary, parathyroid
		Biochemical testing to evaluate for functional PNET:
		- Chromogranin A, pancreatic polypeptide
		- Insulinoma
		  ○ Obtain pro-insulin, serum insulin, c-peptide (all will be elevated)
		- Gastrinoma
		  ○ Serum gastrin > 1000
		  ○ Secretin stim test—if gastrin is increased after secretin test (by more than 120), then positive
		- Glucagonoma
		  ○ Fasting glucagon > 1000
		- Somatostatinoma
		  ○ Somatostatin > 160
		- VIPoma
		  ○ Serum VIP >75
		+/- EUS with FNA for tissue biopsy—determine grade, differentiation, Ki67
		Consider DOTATATE scan—can help localize PNET and detect metastatic disease
		Localization of PNET can be difficult in certain cases and may require additional tests:
		1. Cross-sectional imaging (CT or MRI)—PNET will appear hyperdense on arterial phase
		2. EUS, DOTATATE scan, somatostatin receptor scintigraphy (doesn't work for insulinoma), venous sampling
		3. Intra-op U/S, palpation
		PNET graded and staged based on Ki67, mitotic rate, behavior (invasion, mets)
		Typical location of PNET (Figure 4.2)
			All functional and/or symptomatic PNET should be resected
			Nonfunctional:
			- < 1-cm nonfunctional, asymptomatic PNET can be observed, repeat imaging in 6 mo
			- 1- to 2-cm nonfunctional, asymptomatic PNET → observation vs resection
			  ○ consider enucleation vs traditional resection
			- >2 cm → resection with Whipple vs distal pancreatectomy +/- splenectomy
			
			Functional:
			- Insulinoma—rarely malignant
			  ○ If <2 cm, can perform enucleation
			  ○ If >2 cm, do traditional resection
			  ○ Can give diazoxide to treat hyperinsulinemia
			- Gastrinoma—give patient high dose PPI
			  ○ Treat with traditional resection (ie, Whipple)
			- Glucagonoma—commonly malignant and metastatic at presentation
			  ○ Perform traditional resection, if resectable
			- Somatostatinoma—commonly malignant
			  ○ Treat with Whipple, if resectable
			- VIPoma—distal pancreatectomy, if localized
			- If metastatic, can treat medically or debulk if you can get most of the disease (resection, RFA, etc) → symptomatic relief
			  ○ Chemo and polypeptide receptor radionuclide therapy
				See surgical steps for Whipple and distal pancreatectomy in preceding sections
				Intra-op U/S may be used to localize tumor, if not obvious
				- Open or laparoscopic
				- Use intra-op U/S to determine location of tumor relative to pancreatic duct and nearby vascular structures, which can help guide surgical resection
					Surveillance: H&P, biochemical testing, CT q3-12mo x 10 y depending on tumor aggressiveness	**Overall approach to PNET:**
						- Localize
						- Treat symptoms, start on somatostatin analog (except insulinoma)
						- Resect, if able—Whipple vs distal pancreatectomy vs enucleation, depending on tumor type, size, and location
						  ○ Don't enucleate if near pancreatic duct, high risk of leak
						Nonfunctional PNET—most common type overall
						Insulinoma—most common functional PNET
						Gastrinoma—most common PNET associated with MEN syndrome

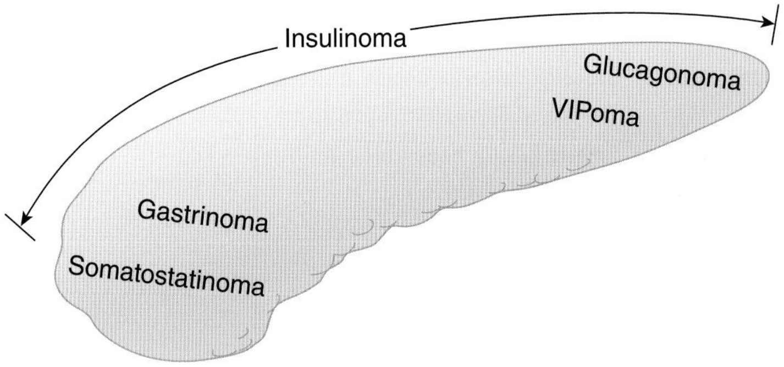

FIGURE 4.2: Location of pancreatic neuroendocrine tumors throughout the pancreas:
Insulinoma—evenly distributed throughout the pancreas
Gastrinoma—head of pancreas/Passaro's triangle
Glucagonoma—tail of pancreas
Somatostatinoma—head of pancreas
VIPoma—body/tail of pancreas

Disease Process	Relevant H&P	Work-up/Staging	Treatment	Key Surgical Steps	Post-Op Care	Tips & Tidbits
Pancreatitis (core)	Epigastric pain, abdominal distention, N/V May be related to EtOH use, gallstone disease, hereditary pancreatitis (PRSS1), autoimmune pancreatitis (IgG4)	CBC, CMP, lipase, amylase, lactate CT—Atlanta classification to describe fluid collections associated with pancreatitis: - <4 wk, no necrosis = peripancreatic fluid collection - <4 wk, + necrosis = acute necrotic collection - >4 wk, no necrosis = pseudocyst - >4 wk, + necrosis = walled-off necrosis Peripancreatic collections with gas concerning for infected necrosis Patients with severe pancreatitis may require repeat CT during their course due to change in clinical status (ie, new fevers, rising WBC, etc) RUQ U/S—look for gallstones	Supportive care, resuscitation, early enteral nutrition Antibiotics only if concerned for infected pancreatic necrosis Infected pancreatic necrosis → antibiotics, source control with percutaneous drain - If patient fails to improve, upsize drain - If deteriorates despite drainage, then VARDS or open necrosectomy - Avoid surgery until at least 4 wk, if possible Gallstone pancreatitis: lap chole prior to discharge to prevent recurrence, +/- ERCP	**Video assisted retroperitoneal debridement (VARDS):** - Incision is placed overlying percutaneous drain site - Use drain as a guide to access retroperitoneal collection - Laparoscope is placed through this opening - Collection is debrided with grasping forceps and suction - Additional drains placed within the cavity **Open pancreatic necrosectomy (core):** - Laparotomy, open lesser sac - Drain purulent material, debride (only remove pancreatic tissue that comes out with ring forceps) - Consider placing J-tube - Leave JP drains	Pseudocyst formation can occur Can develop diabetes if large amount of pancreas removed	Major misstep: Patients with pancreatitis can get very sick and have significant abdominal pain; however, do not get tricked into operating on a pancreatitis patient unnecessarily. Patients with severe pancreatitis are at risk of developing abdominal compartment syndrome. Additional reading: van Santvoort HC, et al; Dutch Pancreatitis Study Group. A step-up approach or open necrosectomy for necrotizing pancreatitis. *N Engl J Med*. 2010 Apr 22; 362(16):1491-1502.

Disease Process	Relevant H&P	Work-up/Staging	Treatment	Key Surgical Steps	Post-Op Care	Tips & Tidbits
Pancreatic pseudocyst	Epigastric pain, early satiety, gastric outlet obstruction History of pancreatitis	CT scan EGD/EUS with fluid sampling if diagnosis unclear - FNA fluid analysis: nonmucinous, low CEA, high amylase, negative cytology	Do not intervene on pseudocyst unless it is symptomatic Most will get better with time; however, pseudocysts >6 cm unlikely to resolve spontaneously Pseudocyst must be at least 4- to 6-weeks old prior to intervention to give time for cyst wall to mature Can do endoscopic decompression with cyst gastrostomy/cyst duodenostomy Surgical intervention only if endoscopic intervention fails Cyst-gastrostomy is most common, but can also perform cyst-duodenostomy if cyst is opposed to duodenum or create cyst-jejunostomy if cyst is not in opposition with stomach or duodenum	**Surgical cyst-gastrostomy (core):** - Upper midline laparotomy - Make anterior gastrotomy on stomach overlying the pseudocyst - Open the posterior wall of the stomach over area of cyst (can use U/S if needed) - Send a portion of the cyst wall to rule out malignancy - Suture cyst wall to posterior stomach wall with permanent sutures to keep it open - Close anterior gastrostomy - Remove gallbladder if patient has history of gallstone pancreatitis		Major misstep: performing endoscopic intervention on pancreatic pseudocyst prior to 4-6 wk, can result in free perforation

Disease Process	Relevant H&P	Work-up/Staging	Treatment	Key Surgical Steps	Post-Op Care	Tips & Tidbits
Chronic pancreatitis (advanced)	Abdominal pain is most common symptom, usually in epigastric area radiating to the back Steatorrhea, weight loss, diabetes History of prior pancreatitis episodes Ask about ETOH and tobacco use	Diagnosed on cross-sectional imaging—CT pancreas protocol or MRCP - Findings include calcifications, pancreatic duct dilatation, pseudocyst, and/or parenchymal atrophy ERCP can help delineate anatomy, treat strictures	Nonoperative management: • ETOH and tobacco cessation • Small low-fat meals • Pancreatic enzyme supplementation • Pain control • Manage diabetes ERCP with stenting, if pancreaticoduodenectomy (PD) dilated Celiac plexus block for pain control Consider surgical intervention in patients who fail medical management Many options for surgical treatment of chronic pancreatitis—choice of operation depends on pancreatic duct diameter and location of disease in pancreas (Figure 4.3): • Lateral pancreaticojejunostomy (PJ) • Duodenal sparing pancreatic head resection • Lateral PJ with localized pancreatic head resection • Pancreaticoduodenectomy • Distal pancreatectomy • Total pancreatectomy— indicated if other procedures fail	**Lateral pancreaticojejunostomy (advanced) (Figure 4.4):** - Must have PD > 7 mm in diameter - Midline laparotomy - Enter lesser sac and retract stomach upwards - Identify dilated PD, can aspirate with syringe or use U/S to localize - Make longitudinal incision along anterior pancreas, opening PD from tail to within ~2 cm of duodenum - Remove debris, ensure hemostasis - Divide jejunum ~20 cm distal to LOT and bring up a Roux limb through the transverse mesocolon - Open antimesenteric border of jejunum and create side-to-side PJ - Create JJ anastomosis ~50 cm distal to PJ **Total pancreatectomy (advanced):** - Midline laparotomy or bilateral subcostal incisions - Open lesser sac, take down hepatic flexure - Kocher maneuver - Dissect out inferior border of pancreas and begin tunnel between pancreas and SMV - Cholecystectomy, dissect out CBD - Test clamp GDA and divide - Complete retropancreatic tunnel from above - Mobilize the spleen, take down short gastrics, medially reflect spleen and distal pancreas up off the retroperitoneum, divide splenic vessels - Transect the stomach, CBD, and jejunum just distal to LOT, finish separating pancreas from retroperitoneum and pass specimen off the field - Bring jejunum up through transverse mesocolon - Create gastrojejunostomy and hepaticojejunostomy, leave drain	Patients require close glucose monitoring post-op	

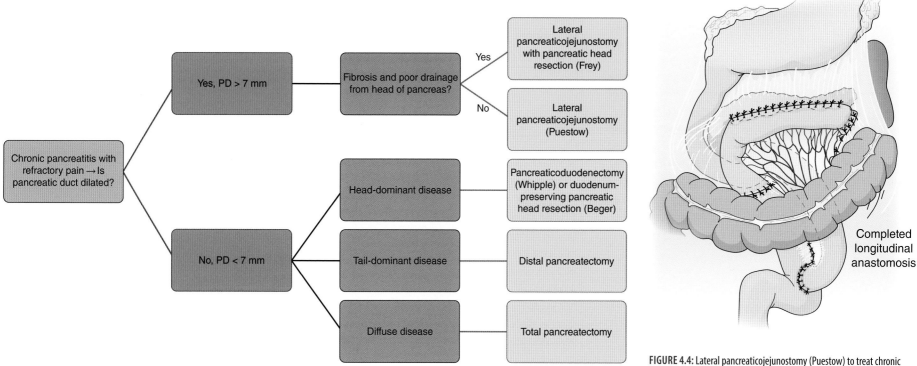

FIGURE 4.3: Surgical options for management of chronic pancreatitis.

FIGURE 4.4: Lateral pancreaticojejunostomy (Puestow) to treat chronic pancreatitis. (Modified with permission from Minter RM, Doherty GM. *Current Procedures: Surgery*. New York, NY: McGraw Hill; 2010, Figure 17-6.)

Disease Process	Relevant H&P	Work-up/Staging	Treatment	Key Surgical Steps	Post-Op Care	Tips & Tidbits
Periampullary tumor	May present with painless jaundice, weight loss	Full labs including LFTs, coagulation panel, tumor markers RUQ U/S CT/MRCP EGD/ERCP +/- stent/EUS with biopsy Potential etiologies include: • Pancreatic adenocarcinoma • Ampullary carcinoma • Duodenal polyp or carcinoma • Distal cholangiocarcinoma If diagnosis of malignancy confirmed, need to stage the patient	Adenoma—endoscopic resection, consider transduodenal resection if endoscopically unresectable Adenoma with HGD → usually treat with Whipple because most harbor occult malignancy Malignant mass → Whipple M1 disease → chemo	**Transduodenal local resection of periampullary mass (advanced):** - Upper midline laparotomy - Kocherize the duodenum - Make ~3-cm longitudinal duodenotomy along antimesenteric border of D2 - Dissect out the neoplasm, resect ampulla including division of CBD and pancreatic duct within head of pancreas, if needed - Reapproximate pancreatic duct and bile duct to duodenal mucosa with absorbable sutures - Leave stents in bile duct and pancreatic duct - Close duodenotomy transversely	Likely need chemo for malignant etiologies Endoscopic surveillance after local resection	
Pancreas divisum (advanced)	Most common congenital pancreatic anomaly, occurs in ~7% of population Most are asymptomatic May have epigastric pain, can develop pancreatitis	MRCP is best diagnostic test No further work-up needed if incidentally noted on imaging in asymptomatic patient	No treatment needed if asymptomatic Mild symptoms → low-fat diet, pain control Consider treatment in patients with severe pancreatitis ERCP with sphincterotomy of minor papilla Can consider transduodenal sphincteroplasty if endoscopic options exhausted	**Transduodenal sphincteroplasty:** - Kocher maneuver - Make longitudinal duodenotomy on lateral duodenal wall at the junction of the upper 2/3 and lower 1/3 of the duodenum - Identify the papilla - Cut the ampullary sphincter in the 11 o'clock position - Extend this to include the entire common tract of the sphincter of Oddi, pancreatic duct is typically located at the 5 o'clock position - Suture wall of CBD to the duodenal mucosa using interrupted fine absorbable sutures - Close the duodenotomy, +/- drain	NPO with NGT initially, consider UGI prior to starting diet	

Disease Process	Relevant H&P	Work-up/Staging	Treatment	Key Surgical Steps	Post-Op Care	Tips & Tidbits

Bile duct injury (core)	Important to determine the timing of the injury—injury may be noted at the time of surgery or patient may present in delayed fashion
	
	Determine if thermal injury was involved
		Full labs
		
		RUQ U/S—look for fluid collection or ductal dilation
		
		IR drain for any fluid collections—determine if fluid is bilious
		
		HIDA scan can be helpful if unclear diagnosis
		
		ERCP/MRCP to determine anatomy and level of injury
		
		CTA, MRA, or hepatic duplex to evaluate for associated vascular injury
		- May need vascular repair if patient has concomitant vascular injury
		
		Bile duct injuries are classified by the Strasberg classification
			Control sepsis and provide biliary drainage—antibiotics, may need IR drain and/or PTC
			
			Define the injury with ERCP or MRCP
			- ERCP can be use to treat minor biliary injury (eg. cystic duct leak)
			
			Evaluate for concomitant vascular injury with CTA, MRA or duplex
			
			Reconstruction
			- Roux-en-Y hepaticojejunostomy vs choledochoduodenostomy
			- Early (<72 h) vs delayed (6-8 wk) repair
			  ∘ Immediate repair in injury noted at time of surgery or detected within 72 h
			  ∘ Delay repair if patient presents >72 h after injury
			  ∘ If it is a thermal injury, delayed repair is preferred to allow for demarcation
				Roux-en-Y hepaticojejunostomy (advanced):
				- Right subcostal incision
				- Take down hepatic flexure
				- Kocherize the duodenum
				- Perform the portal dissection—use "anterior only" dissection on hepatic ducts to spare the vessels, expose the duct you will be sewing to
				- Bring up retrocolic Roux limb of jejunum
				- Create end-to-side biliary enteric anastomosis using 4-0 PDS
				- Create JJ anastomosis
				- Leave drain
					Biliary stricture formation is common	

Disease Process	Relevant H&P	Work-up/Staging	Treatment	Key Surgical Steps	Post-Op Care	Tips & Tidbits
Choledochal Cysts (core)	May present with obstructive jaundice and/or cholangitis due to debris collecting in the cysts May be found incidentally on imaging, sometimes seen on prenatal imaging Increased risk of malignancy throughout the biliary tree Can develop primary choledocholithiasis in cysts	RUQ U/S, LFT MRCP is best test to delineate biliary anatomy Can get ERCP to relieve obstruction and define anatomy Types of choledochal cysts: - Type I: fusiform dilation of the CBD (most common) - Type II: diverticulum off of the CBD, malignant potential low - Type III: cystic dilation of the CBD within the wall of the duodenum, aka choledochocele - Type IVa: extrahepatic and intrahepatic cysts - Type IVb: multiple extrahepatic cysts - Type V: only intrahepatic cysts (Caroli disease)	Treatment recommended due to risk of recurrent cholangitis and malignancy Type I: cyst excision with Roux-en-Y hepaticojejunostomy or hepaticoduodenostomy Type II: resection of diverticulum off the CBD Type III: endoscopic sphincterotomy versus transduodenal excision and sphincteroplasty Type IVa: cyst excision followed by Roux-en-Y hepaticojejunostomy or hepaticoduodenostomy, consider partial hepatectomy if cysts are limited to one lobe Type IVb: cyst excision followed by Roux-en-Y hepaticojejunostomy or hepaticoduodenostomy Type V: partial hepatectomy (if cysts limited to one lobe) vs liver transplant	See hepaticojejunostomy in bile duct injury section	Anastomotic stricture is common Lifetime risk of developing biliary malignancy remains elevated despite resection, but is thought to be reduced - Consider annual LFTs and cross-sectional imaging to monitor for malignancy	

Disease Process	Relevant H&P	Work-up/Staging	Treatment	Key Surgical Steps	Post-Op Care	Tips & Tidbits

Gallbladder polyps, gallbladder cancer (core)	Risk factors for gallbladder cancer: cholelithiasis, increased age, gallbladder polyps, choledochal cysts, PSC
	
	Gallbladder polyps after noted on imaging or found incidentally at time of cholecystectomy
	
	Gallbladder cancer may be found incidentally at time of cholecystectomy or present with symptoms, if advanced
		Gallbladde cancer staging work-up:
		• CT C/A/P
		• CA 19-9, CEA
		• +/- staging laparoscopy
		T staging—important to be familiar with T staging for treatment purposes
		- Tis—Carcinoma in situ
		- T1a—Invades lamina propria
		- T1b—Invades muscular layer
		- T2a—Invades perimuscular connective tissue on the peritoneal side
		- T2b—Invades perimuscular connective tissue on the hepatic side
		- T3—Perforates serosa, invades adjacent structures
		- T4—Invades portal vein, hepatic artery or 2+ extra-hepatic structures
			Management of gallbladder polyps seen on imaging:
			- Polyp < 5 mm ⟶ no further intervention
			- Polyp 6-9 mm ⟶ 6 mo follow-up U/S
			- Polyp 1-2 cm ⟶ laparoscopic cholecystectomy
			- Polyp > 2 cm ⟶ treat like gallbladder cancer, stage and then do radical cholecystectomy if no signs of metastatic disease
			Gallbladder cancer
			- If resectable, do radical cholecystectomy with portal lymphadenectomy (need at least 6 LN)
			  ○ Consider adjuvant chemo (capecitabine)
			- If unresectable/M1, patient gets palliative chemo (gemcitabine + cisplatin)
			GB cancer incidentally found on pathology after laparoscopic cholecystectomy (0.2% incidence):
			- T1a ⟶ perform staging and ongoing surveillance
			- T1b or greater ⟶ staging with CT C/A/P, CEA, CA19-9
			  ○ If resectable ⟶ do 4b/5 segment resection and portal LN dissection
			  ○ Unresectable ⟶ chemo
			Surgery is best chance for long-term survival
			No strong evidence for XRT
				Radical cholecystectomy (advanced):
				- Diagnostic laparoscopy
				- Right subcostal incision
				- Open cholecystectomy including at least a 2-cm rim of liver tissue around gallbladder fossa (segments 4b/5, nonanatomic)
				- Perform portal lymphadenectomy
				- Obtain frozen section on cystic duct margin, if positive should do CBD resection with hepaticojejunostomy
				- Consider intraoperative hepatic U/S
					For all comers, median overall survival is only 12 mo	Polyps > 1 cm have > 40% risk of malignancy
						
						Polyps > 2 cm have nearly 100% risk of malignancy

Disease Process	Relevant H&P	Work-up/Staging	Treatment	Key Surgical Steps	Post-Op Care	Tips & Tidbits

Cholangiocarcinoma	May present with jaundice, pruritis
	
	Often presents late, especially if intrahepatic
	
	Risk factors: PSC, hepatitis, liver fluke infection
		Staging: MRI/CT, LFTs, tumor markers, +/- ERCP/ EUS with brushings and/ or FNA
		
		Can diagnose based on imaging alone, don't need biopsy prior to surgery
			ERCP with stent for biliary decompression, if needed
			
			Surgery indicated when cholangiocarcinoma is localized and R0 resection is possible
			- Contraindications to resection: invasion of main portal vein or hepatic artery or their branches bilaterally, metastatic disease
			- Can still resect if portal LN are positive, but not if the disease has spread to other LN groups
			
			Surgery depends on location of cholangiocarcinoma:
			- Intrahepatic tumor → partial hepatectomy, possible liver transplant, liver-directed therapy (TACE, RFA, etc)
			- Hilar (Klatskin) tumor → partial hepatectomy, possible liver transplant
			- Distal tumor → Whipple
			
			Adjuvant chemo—capecitabine
			
			Unresectable disease managed with chemo, XRT, and/or liver-directed therapies (TACE, RFA, etc)
				Partial hepatectomy (advanced):
				- Ranges from simple wedge resection to extended right hepatectomy, can be anatomic versus nonanatomic
				- Begin with diagnostic laparoscopy to rule out peritoneal metastasis
				  ○ If metastatic disease is found, consider palliative bypass (hepaticojejunostomy) versus aborting and getting ERCP with metal stent
				- Incision—upper midline, subcostal, or Chevron
				- Mobilize the liver
				- Use intra-op U/S to localize the lesion and major vascular and biliary structures, mark out planned line of transection
				- Get vessel loop around hepatoduodenal ligament in case Pringle maneuver is needed
				- Portal lymph node dissection
				- If performing formal right or left hepatectomy, isolate the inflow vessels to the associated hemi-liver in the hepatic hilum
				  ○ Will see demarcation in liver once inflow is taken
				- Isolate the associated proximal bile duct, perform cholecystectomy if needed
				- Isolate the outflow vessels
				- Transection of liver parenchyma
				  ○ Biliary and vascular structures may be divided before or after parenchymal transection
				- Examine cut liver edge for ongoing bleeding or bile leak, +/- drain
				
				General liver resection tips:
				- Familiarity with hepatic anatomy, including typical location of major vascular and biliary structures, is essential to safe resection (Figure 4.5)
				- Hepatic resections can be anatomic or nonanatomic (Figure 4.6)
				  ○ Anatomic resection generally preferred for malignant disease
				- Can use intra-op U/S to identify lesions, determine proximity to major vascular and biliary structures, and mark out line for parenchymal transection
				- Maintain a low CVP during parenchymal transection (ideally <5 cm H20) to minimize blood loss from hepatic veins
				- Have vessel loop with Rummel tourniquet around hepatoduodenal ligament so you can Pringle, as needed
				- Methods for parenchymal transection: finger-fracture technique, clamp-crushing method, cautery, LigaSure, stapler, CUSA, precoagulation with RFA or MWA
					Complications post liver resection:
					- Bile leak— diagnosed by drain bilirubin 3x serum, managed primarily with drainage, can do ERCP if persistent
					- Post-op portal vein and hepatic artery thrombosis— diagnosed on duplex, treat with anticoagulation
					- Post-hepatectomy liver failure—due to inadequate functional liver remnant, presents as rising INR and hyperbilirubinemia, managed with supportive care	

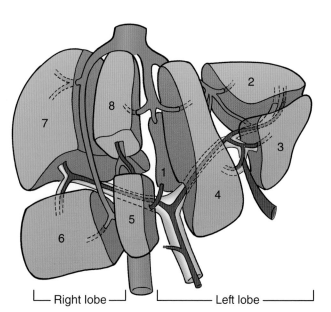

FIGURE 4.5: Segmental liver anatomy and course of the vascular and biliary structures. Right and left lobe are separated by Cantlie's line. Right lobe includes segments V-VIII. Left lobe includes segments II-IV. (Modified with permission from Minter RM, Doherty GM. *Current Procedures: Surgery.* New York, NY: McGraw Hill; 2010, Figure 14-1.)

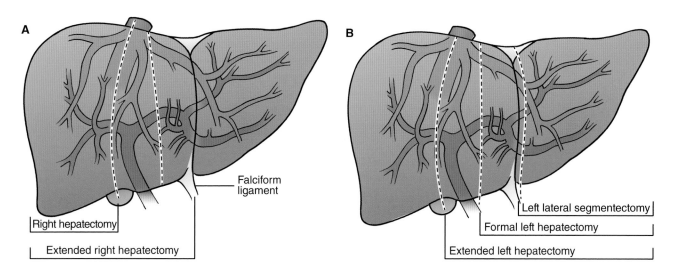

FIGURE 4.6: Types of major anatomic liver resections. **A:** Right lobectomy/hepatectomy (segments V-VIII), extended right hepatectomy (segments IV-VIII). **B:** Extended left hepatectomy (segments II-V, VIII), Formal left hepatectomy (segments II-IV), left lateral segmentectomy (segments II-III). (Modified with permission from Minter RM, Doherty GM. *Current Procedures: Surgery.* New York, NY: McGraw Hill; 2010, Figure 14-2 A-B.)

Disease Process	Relevant H&P	Work-up/Staging	Treatment	Key Surgical Steps	Post-Op Care	Tips & Tidbits

Liver lesions (core)	Often incidentally noted on imaging
	
	May have abdominal discomfort, fullness
	
	Ask about risk factors for liver disease—EtOH, IVDU, hepatitis, obesity, previous malignancy
	- OCP/steroid use associated with hepatic adenoma
	
	Look for any signs of liver disease on exam (ascites, caput medusae, etc)
		CBC, BMP, LFT, INR, hepatitis panel, tumor markers (AFP, CEA)
		
		Triphasic MRI/CT—avoid biopsy, liver lesions are typically diagnosed based on imaging
		
		Liver lesions and their characteristic imaging findings:
		- Hemangioma—most common benign liver lesion
		  ○ Peripheral, nodular enhancement on arterial phase, peripheral-to-central (centripetal) filling on portal venous and delayed phases
		- Follicular nodular hyperplasia (FNH)—bright arterial enhancement on arterial phase with central stellate scar, lights up on sulfur colloid scan
		- Hepatic adenoma—well demarcated, heterogenous mass, homogeneously enhances during arterial phase
		- Hepatocellular carcinoma (HCC)—heterogeneous, poorly circumscribed mass, enhances on late arterial phase and quickly washes out on venous phase, pseudocapsule on delayed phase
		  ○ If HCC diagnosed, obtain staging chest CT
		- Intrahepatic cholangiocarcinoma—low-attenuating mass with minor peripheral enhancement that becomes stronger in venous phases, proximal bile ducts may be dilated
		- Metastatic tumor—either high or low attenuating lesions depending on primary
		  ○ Colorectal cancer most common
		  ○ May require biopsy if primary unknown
		- Simple cyst—thin-walled fluid-filled structure
		
		If planning resection, need to determine if patient will have adequate future liver remnant (FLR)
			Hemangioma—no treatment, unless symptomatic
			
			FNH—no treatment, unless symptomatic
			
			Hepatic adenoma—stop OCP, resect if >5 cm due to risk of rupture or malignant transformation
			
			Intrahepatic cholangiocarcinoma—see cholangiocarcinoma section
			
			Hepatocellular carcinoma
			- Surgical resection with partial hepatectomy indicated if R0 resection possible
			  ○ Contraindications to resection: extrahepatic metastases, inadequate FLR, involvement of main bile duct, presence of portal thrombus in main portal vein or IVC
			- Liver-directed therapies may be used for unresectable tumors and as a bridge to transplant
			- Certain patients may qualify for liver transplant (Milan Criteria)
			
			Metastatic lesion—treatment depends on etiology and extent of disease
			- if primary site is unknown, can obtain biopsy for tissue diagnosis and molecular testing
				See partial hepatectomy in cholangiocarcinoma section
				
				Laparoscopic liver biopsy (core):
				- Place a camera port plus 1-2 additional ports
				- Identify target lesion, use intra-op U/S if needed
				- Biopsy with Tru-Cut needle
				- Can use pressure, cautery, argon, or hepatorrhaphy with #1 chromic and/or topical sealants to control post biopsy hemorrhage
					Complications:
					- Monitor for bile leak—may present with N/V, fevers, RUQ pain, jaundice, elevated LFTs, increasing bilious drain output
					- At risk for liver failure if inadequate liver remnant
						Spend some time getting familiar with the appearance of these more common liver lesions on CT scan (ie, FNH, hepatic adenoma, hemangioma), in case you are asked to identify one
						
						Milan criteria for liver transplant in patients with HCC:
						- One tumor < 5 cm
						- ≤ 3 tumors, all < 3 cm
						- No macrovascular invasion
						- No extracapsular spread
						
						Future liver remnant (FLR)—volume of liver parenchyma remaining after liver resection, inadequate FLR results in post-op hepatic insufficiency
						- FLR can be measured pre-op using volumetric CT or MRI
						- Need 20-30% FLR in a normal healthy patient
						- Need 30-40% FLR in a patient post chemo
						- Need 40-50% FLR in a cirrhotic patient
						- Portal vein embolization may be used to induce hypertrophy and increase FLR

Disease Process	Relevant H&P	Work-up/Staging	Treatment	Key Surgical Steps	Post-Op Care	Tips & Tidbits
Hepatic abscess (core)	May present with fever, chills, abdominal pain History of recent intra-abdominal infection? IVDU? HIV? Pyogenic abscess—often present with history of cholangitis, appendicitis, or diverticulitis, subsequently develop fever and abdominal pain Amoebic abscess—patient with recent travel history Echinococcus (hydatid cyst)—recent travel to Mediterranean, exposure to sheep, may have palpable liver mass with eosinophilia	CBC, CMP RUQ U/S CT scan Serum antibody test for Entamoeba histolytica and Echinococcus	If pyogenic: - Can try percutaneous drainage, upsize drain as needed - If patient is not improving, will need surgical intervention If amoebic: - Perform serum antibody test → if positive, administer metronidazole x 10 d If echinococcal cyst: - Pre-op albendazole, then surgical removal or PAIR technique (puncture, aspiration, injection of hypertonic saline, re-aspiration) - Requires 4 d of pre-op albendazole and 3 mo post-op	**Hepatic abscess drainage (core):** - Can do laparoscopic vs open - Superficial liver abscesses can be treated with simple fenestration and drainage - Deep abscesses may require intra-op U/S localization or limited hepatic resection for drainage - Leave a drain		

Disease Process	Relevant H&P	Work-up/Staging	Treatment	Key Surgical Steps	Post-Op Care	Tips & Tidbits

Primary sclerosing cholangitis (PSC) (advanced)	May be asymptomatic or present with fatigue, pruritis, jaundice
	Associated with UC
		Elevated alkaline phosphatase and bilirubin
		U/S—abnormal bile ducts with wall thickening and focal dilations
		MRCP—multifocal, short strictures
		ERCP—multifocal strictures and dilations, dilate and place stents as needed
		Screening:
		- U/S or MRI q6-12 mo due to increased risk of gallbladder cancer and cholangiocarcinoma
		  ◦ Focal liver masses seen on imaging should raise concern for cholangiocarcinoma
		- Appropriate colonoscopy surveillance if patient also has UC
			ERCP to treat strictures with dilation and stenting
			Surgical intervention
			- Biliary reconstruction—can be considered if there is dominant stricture at the hepatic bifurcation that could be resected and reconstructed
			- Liver transplantation recommended for patients with cirrhosis (MELD ≥ 15)
			  ◦ Survival post OLT up to 85% at 5 y
			  ◦ Recurrence in 14-20% of patients			

Hematologic diseases of the spleen (core)	Medically refractory ITP Hereditary spherocytosis with significant symptoms or transfusion dependent	CBC, coagulation panel CT scan	Splenectomy Patient should receive splenectomy vaccines at least 2-wk pre-op	**Open splenectomy (core):** - Upper midline laparotomy - Open the lesser sac - Take down splenic flexure of the colon - Take down short gastrics - Take down lateral attachments to spleen - Staple across the splenic hilum but be careful to avoid the tail of the pancreas **Laparoscopic splenectomy:** - Position patient supine with left side bumped, can break the bed to increase space between costal margin and ASIS - Place ports to triangulate the LUQ - Open lesser sac, take down splenic flexure - Divide the short gastrics - Dissect out and staple or clip the splenic artery and vein - Take down splenophrenic and splenorenal ligaments - Place spleen in bag and morcellate		Watch out for accessory spleens

Disease Process	Relevant H&P	Work-up/Staging	Treatment	Key Surgical Steps	Post-Op Care	Tips & Tidbits

Splenic masses (abscesses, cysts, neoplasms) (core)	Splenic cysts and masses often incidentally found on imaging
	
	Patient with abscess may present with LUQ pain and tenderness, fever, history of recent infection
	
	Can develop splenic cysts after trauma
		CT scan
		- Abscesses—hypodense lesions, may have peripheral enhancement and septations, usually polymicrobial
		- Benign cysts—simple low-density lesions
		- Echinococcal/cyst—parasitic
		- Neoplasms—irregular margins, heterogeneous, density of soft tissue, may have central necrosis, vascularity, or invasion into other structures
		  ◦ Primary splenic neoplasms are rare (angiosarcomas, lymphangiomas)
		  ◦ Can have splenic metastasis from breast, lung, melanoma, other sources
		  ◦ Lymphoproliferative lesions—lymphoma, leukemia
			Splenic abscess—antibiotics and IR drainage vs splenectomy
			
			Echinococcal cyst—splenectomy, avoid rupture, which can cause anaphylaxis
				For splenectomy see "Hematologic diseases of the spleen" section
				
				If doing splenectomy for malignancy, do not morcellate		

5

Breast Surgery

David White, MD, FACS

DISEASES AND OPERATIONS

- Radiographic abnormalities of the breast (c), excisional biopsy (c)
- Breast mass, invasive breast cancer (c), partial mastectomy (c), sentinel lymph node biopsy (c)
- Locally advanced breast cancer, simple mastectomy (c), axillary lymph node dissection (c)

- Inflammatory breast cancer (c), modified radical mastectomy (c)
- Breast cancer in pregnancy (c)
- Male breast disease (c)
- Hereditary breast cancer (c)
- Paget's disease of the breast

- Fibroadenoma, phyllodes tumors (c)
- Nipple discharge (c), duct excision (c)
- Infectious breast disease (c)
- Benign breast disease (c), breast cyst aspiration (c)

GENERAL TIPS FOR BREAST SCENARIOS

- There is a set of questions you should ask for essentially every patient with a breast complaint to evaluate for risk factors for breast cancer including:
  - Prior breast abnormalities/biopsies?
  - Age of menarche/menopause?
  - Number of pregnancies? Age at time of pregnancies?
  - Breast feeding history?
  - Estrogen exposure (ie, OCPs, hormone replacement therapy)?
  - Family history of cancer (including age of cancer diagnoses)?
  - History of radiation (XRT)?
- Discuss all patients with breast cancer at a multidisciplinary committee, which should include the medical oncology, radiation oncology, and surgery teams.
- Patients with breast cancer need axillary staging—in general, patients with a clinically negative axilla should have a sentinel lymph node biopsy (SLNB) while patients with a clinically positive axilla should undergo axillary lymph node dissection (ALND).
  - Caveat: There is potential to downstage a clinically positive axilla with neoadjuvant chemotherapy so that the patient can undergo SLNB.
- Make sure that you discuss all reasonable treatment options in a given scenario with the patient (breast conserving therapy, mastectomy, neoadjuvant chemo, etc), rather than choosing for the patient.
- You must remember that breast-conserving therapy (BCT) includes partial mastectomy and adjuvant whole breast radiation. Patients with a large tumor to breast ratio, widespread calcifications, or multicentric disease may not be candidates for breast-conserving therapy. Additionally, patients with a history of prior XRT and scleroderma are not able to receive XRT and, therefore, are not candidates for BCT.
  - Addition of adjuvant XRT reduces recurrence, but makes no difference in overall survival.
- When performing excision, The recommended margin for DCIS is 2 mm; however, the recommended margin for invasive cancer is no tumor on ink.
- The management of breast cancer is rapidly evolving and getting more nuanced all the time. Try to focus on the big picture and be well-versed in the management of the more common breast scenarios.

(c) = core topic   (a) = advanced topic

Disease Process	Relevant H&P	Work-up/Staging	Treatment	Key Surgical Steps	Post-Op Care	Tips & Tidbits

Radiographic abnormalities of the breast (core)	Ask patient the breast cancer risk factor questions (see general tips)
	
	Examine bilateral breasts, axilla, and other nodal basins
		Screening mammograms should start at age 40 yo for standard-risk patients
		
		Routine screening breast MRI recommended for patients with >20% lifetime risk of breast cancer
		
		For any abnormality picked up on screening mammogram, get a diagnostic mammogram (more views)
		
		BIRADS—used to classify mammography findings based on risk of malignancy
		- 0—insufficient → need more imaging
		- 1—negative → routine follow-up
		- 2—benign → routine follow-up
		- 3—likely benign → short interval follow-up
		- 4—suspicious → core needle biopsy (CNB)
		- 5—highly suspicious for malignancy → CNB
		- 6—biopsy proven malignancy → treat accordingly
			Excisional biopsy, if indicated based on CNB result
			Management of borderline and high-risk lesions:
			- Radial scar/complex sclerosing lesions—excision typically recommended
			  ○ May present as spiculated, suspicious mass on imaging or be identified incidentally on CNB
			  ○ Associated malignancy found in 10-25% when excised
			  ○ Some small, incidentally noted radial scars diagnosed with CNB and concordant with imaging can be observed
			- Flat epithelial atypia—typically excision is not recommended, unless there is imaging and pathology discordance
			  ○ Upstaging rate < 5%
			- Papillary lesions/intraductal papillomas—excision recommended if atypia present or symptomatic (nipple discharge), otherwise observe
			- Atypical lobular hyperplasia (ALH)—excision not recommended unless there is imaging and pathology discordance
			  ○ Relative risk of breast cancer 3-5x
			  ○ Upstaging ~5%
			  ○ Consider chemoprevention if ER/PR+
			- Lobular carcinoma in situ (LCIS)—observation vs surgical excision, can manage with close follow-up with imaging, as long as there is pathology and imaging concordance
			  ○ Risk factor for future breast cancer (1%/y), NOT premalignant
			  ○ Do not need to re-resect if positive margins after excision
			  ○ Pleomorphic or florid LCIS are a more aggressive subtype and should always be treated with excision, re-excise if margins positive
			  ○ Consider chemoprevention if ER/PR+
			- Atypical ductal hyperplasia (ADH)—surgical excision recommended
			  ○ 4-5x increased relative risk for breast cancer
				Excisional biopsy (core):
				- Wire localization or preop implanted radiographic marker—use imaging to help determine surgical approach
				- Incision options:
				  ○ Lesion above nipple—use transverse or curvilinear incisions
				  ○ Central lesion—can use peri-areolar incision
				  ○ Lesion below nipple—radial incision
				- Excise area of concern
				- Orient the specimen
				- Make sure biopsy clip is in the specimen (XR)
					Surveillance:
					- ALH, ADH, or LCIS → exam q6-12mo, annual mammography
					- DCIS post partial mastectomy → mammogram 6-mo post-op, then annually
					- DCIS post mastectomy → exam q6mo x 2 y, then annually
						Major misstep: Getting a fine needle aspiration (FNA) of a breast lesion, instead of a CNB.
						
						When working up a breast lesion, Imaging and biopsy results should be concordant! You need to pursue further work-up if they are not.
						
						Additional reading:
						The American Society of Breast Surgeons. (2018). *Consensus Guideline on Concordance Assessment of Image-Guided Breast Biopsies and Management of Borderline or High-Risk Lesions.* https://www.breastsurgeons.org/docs/statements/Consensus-Guideline-on-Concordance-Assessment-of-Image-Guided-Breast-Biopsies.pdf

Disease Process	Relevant H&P	Work-up/Staging	Treatment	Key Surgical Steps	Post-Op Care	Tips & Tidbits
Radiographic abnormalities of the breast (*Cont.*)			∘ 20% rate of upgrade to DCIS or IDC when excised ∘ Do not need to re-excise if margins positive for ADH ∘ Consider chemoprevention if ER/PR+ Ductal carcinoma in situ (DCIS)—a premalignant lesion, should be treated with surgical excision - Often presents as microcalcifications on mammogram - 10-15% risk of upstaging to IDC - Treat with BCT (lumpectomy + XRT) or mastectomy - Need 2-mm negative margins, re-excise if margins positive - Axillary staging for DCIS ∘ If performing mastectomy, do SLNB ∘ Do not need to routinely do SLNB when treating DCIS with BCT ▪ Consider SLNB for patients with DCIS > 4 cm or with aggressive features (comedo necrosis) ▪ DCIS with microinvasion (invasive cancer < 1 mm) have 6% risk of + SLN, so should do SLNB ▪ If DCIS is upgraded to invasive cancer after excision, then you must do SLNB - Chemoprevention if ER/PR+ - No role for chemo in treatment of DCIS Chemoprevention - Reduces the risk of breast cancer in patients with high risk lesions - Should be offered to patients diagnosed with hormone receptor positive ADH, ALH, DCIS, LCIS, and invasive cancer ∘ Premenopausal ⟶ tamoxifen ∘ Postmenopausal ⟶ tamoxifen, raloxifene, or anastrozole ∘ Risks associated with tamoxifen: thromboembolic events (CVA, PE, or DVT) and uterine cancer ▪ Women with history of DVT or stroke should not be offered tamoxifen - Give for 5 y			

Disease Process	Relevant H&P	Work-up/Staging	Treatment	Key Surgical Steps	Post-Op Care	Tips & Tidbits

Breast mass, Invasive breast cancer (core)	Patient may present with palpable breast mass or cancer detected on imaging
	
	Ask patient the breast cancer risk factor questions (see general tips)
	
	Is mass growing in size? How long has it been present? Nipple discharge?
	
	Obtain review of systems evaluating for any symptoms of metastatic disease
	
	Examine bilateral breasts, axilla, and other nodal basins
	- Mass size? Soft vs hard? Mobile vs fixed?
		Initial imaging evaluation of palpable breast mass depends on age:
		- Women < 30 yo → start with U/S
		  ◦ Mammogram less sensitive due to dense breast tissue
		- Women >30 yo → get diagnostic mammogram and U/S
		Core needle biopsy
		- Invasive ductal carcinoma (IDC) vs invasive lobular carcinoma (ILC)
		- Always ask hormone receptor and Her2 status if the examiner did not automatically tell you
		If suspicious axillary LN on exam, obtain axillary U/S with FNA or CNB of suspicious nodes
		- Some providers routinely get axillary U/S as part of the work-up for all breast cancers; however, it is recommended on an as needed basis by NCCN
		- Clip suspicious nodes at time of biopsy
		Pregnancy test if childbearing age
		TNM staging of breast cancer is quite complicated and you don't need to know all the details, just focus on the basics in Table 5.1
		Full staging (CT C/A/P, bone scan, brain MRI) reserved for locally advanced (T3+ or N2+) and inflammatory breast cancers, or those with symptoms concerning for metastatic disease
			Treatment of localized (M0) invasive breast cancer:
			- BCT vs mastectomy with axillary staging
			  ◦ BCT (lumpectomy + adjuvant XRT)
			    ▪ XRT can be omitted in patients >70 yo with ER+ T1-2 N0 IDC
			  ◦ Mastectomy +/- XRT
			    ▪ XRT can be omitted after mastectomy if SLNB is negative, tumor < 5 cm, and R0 resection
			- Axillary staging/treatment:
			  ◦ SLNB if clinically node negative
			  ◦ ALND if clinically node positive
			- Chemo can be given before or after surgery
			  ◦ Typical regimen is ACT—**A**driamycin, **C**yclophosphamide, pacli**T**axel
			  ◦ Candidates for neoadjuvant chemo
			    ▪ Inflammatory breast cancer
			    ▪ HER2+ or triple negative
			    ▪ ≥ cT2 or ≥ cN1
			    ▪ T4 invading chest wall
			    ▪ Bulky/matted axillary LNs (N2) or N3 nodal disease
			    ▪ Large tumor in patient who wants BCT
			    ▪ Attempting to downstage positive axilla to avoid ALND
				Partial mastectomy (core):
				- Wire localization or preop implanted radiographic marker, if not palpable—use imaging to help determine surgical approach
				- Incision options:
				  ◦ Lesion above nipple → use transverse or curvilinear incisions
				  ◦ Central lesion → use periareolar incision
				  ◦ Lesion below nipple → radial incision
				- Develop flaps, thickness depends on depth of the lesion
				- Excise lesion and orient it
				  ◦ If lesion is close to the skin, may need to include skin in specimen
				- X-ray specimen to ensure you have the biopsy clip
				- Take additional margins, if any appear close on the imaging
				- Check for hemostasis, place clips in the cavity, and close
				
				Sentinel lymph node biopsy (core):
				- Use radiotracer and/or dye (methylene or isosulfan blue)
				- Make incision just below hair-bearing area in axilla, overlying area with highest radiotracer signal
				- Dissect through clavipectoral fascia
				- Resect all abnormal nodes, blue nodes, and "hot" nodes until background count < 10% of "hottest" sentinel node
				  ◦ If you cannot find any sentinel nodes, you should perform ALND
					If margin is positive after partial mastectomy, take back for re-excision of margins
					Lymphedema:
					- SLNB → 3-5% risk of lymphedema
					- Ax dissection → 15-30% risk of lymphedema
					Surveillance for invasive breast cancer:
					- S/p partial mastectomy → mammogram 6-mo post-op, then annually
					- S/p mastectomy → exam q6mo x 2 y, then annually
					Reconstruction options post mastectomy:
					- Autologous flap reconstruction, free or pedicled—DIEP flap, TRAM flap, latissimus dorsi muscle flap
					- Implant based—direct to implant vs tissue expander to implant
					- Combo using flap reconstruction augmented with implant
						When to obtain genetic testing and counseling in patient with breast cancer:
						- triple negative cancers
						- patients < 45 yo
						- Male breast cancer
						- If concerned for hereditary breast cancer
						- Presence of increased risk mutation may influence decision making (ie, desire for prophylactic bilateral mastectomy)
						Additional reading:
						Giuliano AE, et al. Axillary dissection vs no axillary dissection in women with invasive breast cancer and sentinel node metastasis: a randomized clinical trial. *JAMA.* 2011 Feb 9; 305(6):569-575.
						Boughey JC, et al; Alliance for Clinical Trials in Oncology. Sentinel lymph node surgery after neoadjuvant chemotherapy in patients with node-positive breast cancer: the ACOSOG Z1071 (Alliance) clinical trial. *JAMA.* 2013 Oct 9;310(14):1455-1461.

Disease Process	Relevant H&P	Work-up/Staging	Treatment	Key Surgical Steps	Post-Op Care	Tips & Tidbits
Breast mass, Invasive breast cancer (*Cont.*)			○ Need for adjuvant chemo based on multiple factors including pathologic stage, tumor receptor status (ER, PR, Her2), patient age, etc - Gene assay tests (Oncotype DX, MammaPrint, etc) can be used for ER+ cancers to predict the benefit of adding adjuvant therapy - Endocrine therapy x 5 y if ER+ - Trastuzumab x 1yr if Her2+ and >5 mm 　○ If tumor <5 mm and LN (-) → +/- trastuzumab Refer to plastic surgery preoperatively to discuss reconstruction options if planning to do mastectomy	○ If you are doing targeted axillary sentinel node dissection in patient who previously had + axillary nodes and then underwent neoadjuvant chemo, you must use dual tracer (dye and radiotracer) remove the previously biopsied/clipped node in addition to any sentinel nodes, send LN for frozen, and if positive for tumor, proceed with ALND Previously, +SLNB would lead to ALND; however, now select patients with ≤2 +SLN can avoid axillary dissection based on the ACOSOG Z0011 trial: - Inclusion criteria: T1-2 tumor (<5 cm), clinically node negative, patient getting BCT (including XRT), did not get neoadjuvant chemo - If there are ≥ 3 LN+ or LN with gross extra-nodal extension, proceed with ALND		

Table 5.1: TNM staging of breast cancer	
T staging	Tis—DCIS T1— < 2 cm T2—2-5 cm T3— > 5 cm T4—invading skin or chest wall
N staging	$pN1_{mi}$ —micrometastases in LN (~200 cells, > 0.2 mm but < 2 mm) N1—clinical: movable ipsilateral level I/II axillary nodes, pathologic: 1-3 LN+ N2—clinical: fixed/matted ipsilateral level I/II axillary nodes, pathologic: 4-9 LN+ N3—clinical: ipsilateral level III axillary nodes, internal mammary LN and/or supraclavicular LN involved, pathologic: >10 LN+
M staging	M0 – no metastasis M1 - metastasis

Disease Process	Relevant H&P	Work-up/Staging	Treatment	Key Surgical Steps	Post-Op Care	Tips & Tidbits

Locally advanced breast cancer (core)	Ask patient the breast cancer risk factor questions (see general tips)
	
	Obtain thorough ROS evaluating for symptoms of metastatic disease
	
	Examine bilateral breasts, axilla, and other nodal basins
		Mammogram and U/S with CNB of mass
		
		Axillary U/S w/FNA or CNB of abnormal LNs
		
		Genetic testing and counselling if indicated
		
		Pregnancy test if childbearing age
		
		Full staging indicated for locally advanced (T3+ or N2+) breast cancers or those with signs/ symptoms concerning for metastatic disease:
		- CBC, CMP
		- CT C/A/P
		- Bone scan
		- +/- XR, brain MRI, or spine MRI, if concerning symptoms
		- PET can be obtained instead of CT and bone scan
			Treatment order can vary:
			Surgery + adjuvant chemoXRT vs neoadjuvant chemo + surgery + XRT
			
			Chemotherapy can be given before or after surgery, depending on patient and disease factors
			- Typical chemo regimen: **A**driamycin, **c**yclophosphamide, **p**aclitaxel (ACT)
			
			Surgery options—it may help to think of management of the breast and axilla separately
			- Management of breast: BCT (if amenable) vs mastectomy
			- Axillary staging: SLNB (if clinically LN- or downstaged with neoadjuvant chemo) vs ALND
			
			XRT for all BCT patients and some mastectomy patients (+margin, LN+, tumor > 5 cm)
			
			Adjuvant chemo and hormonal treatment as indicated
			
			Inoperable breast cancer, M1 disease → systemic therapy
			- If becomes operable, then progress to surgery
			- If still inoperable, then consider for additional chemo +/- XRT
				Simple mastectomy (core):
				- Elliptical incision
				- Raise skin flaps to free breast tissue from the skin
				- Take breast off chest wall
				  ∘ Borders of the breast:
				    ▪ Superior = clavicle
				    ▪ Inferior = inframammary fold/rectus
				    ▪ Lateral = latissimus
				    ▪ Medial = sternal border
				- Irrigate and ensure hemostasis
				- Leave drain
				
				Axillary lymph node dissection (core) (Figure 5.1):
				- Patient positioned supine with arm abducted ~90° on an arm board
				- Make oblique incision near inferior axillary hair line
				- Dissect through subcutaneous tissues and clavipectoral fascial into the area of axillary fat
				- Identify axillary vein and start dissection just inferior
				- Elevate pectoralis muscles to dissect out level II lymph nodes
				- Identify and avoid long thoracic and thoracodorsal neurovascular bundles
				- Eventually mobilize and remove axillary contents en bloc
				- Ensure hemostasis, leave drain, close
					XRT, hormonal therapy, and adjuvant chemo, as indicated
					
					Surveillance:
					- Post partial mastectomy → mammogram at 6-mo post-op, then annually
					- Post simple mastectomy → exam q6mo x 2 y, then annually
						Major misstep: Do not let examiners lead you down the road of operating on a patient with M1 disease.
						
						Radical mastectomy— pioneered by Halsted, en bloc resection of breast, overlying skin and nipple, underlying chest muscle (including pec major and minor), and axillary lymph nodes, no longer used unless patient has invasion into chest wall and positive axillary LN.
						
						Nipple-sparing mastectomy has equivalent rates of local control for breast cancer when compared with conventional mastectomy
						
						C/I to nipple-sparing mastectomy:
						∘ Nipple involvement, Paget's disease
						∘ Inflammatory breast cancer
						∘ Active smoker

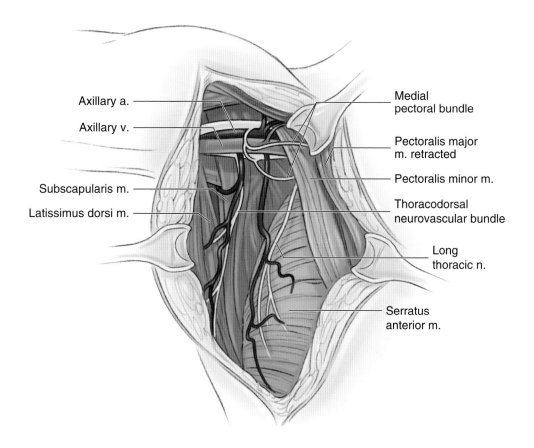

FIGURE 5.1: Axillary anatomy—the axillary vein, long thoracic nerve, and thoracodorsal nerve should be identified and protected. (Reproduced with permission from Kuerer HM. *Kuerer's Breast Surgical Oncology*. New York, NY: McGraw Hill; 2010, Figure 63-2.)

Disease Process	Relevant H&P	Work-up/Staging	Treatment	Key Surgical Steps	Post-Op Care	Tips & Tidbits

Inflammatory breast cancer (IBC) (core)	Ask patient the breast cancer risk factor questions (see general tips)
	
	Examine bilateral breasts, axillary nodes, and other LN basins
	
	May see breast erythema, edema, and peau d'orange
		CBC, CMP
		
		Bilateral diagnostic mammogram with CNB of any abnormalities seen
		
		Skin punch biopsy—pathologic diagnosis of IBC made if dermal lymphatic invasion seen, however dermal lymphatic invasion is only present in 50% and is not required for diagnosis of IBC!
		
		IBC can also be a clinical diagnosis in patient with invasive breast cancer and erythema/edema affecting at least 1/3 of breast, even if there is no dermal lymphatic invasion seen
		
		Determine ER/PR and Her2 status
		
		CT C/A/P, bone scan +/- PET
		
		Genetic counseling, if appropriate
		
		Inflammatory breast cancer = cT4d; Stage IIIB (at minimum)
		
		>50% have +LN and ~25% have distant metastasis at time of presentation
			Treat with neoadjuvant chemo, followed by modified radical mastectomy, then adjuvant XRT
			- Chemotherapy (ACT = Adriamycin, cyclophosphamide, paclitaxel) +/- trastuzumab
			  ○ If patient does not respond to initial chemo, consider XRT or additional chemo prior to surgery
			- Modified radical mastectomy = mastectomy with axillary dissection
			  ○ Not eligible for BCT, skin/nipple sparing mastectomy, or SLNB!
			- Adjuvant radiation
			- Hormonal therapy if ER/PR+
				Modified radical mastectomy (core):
				- Elliptical incision centered around nipple areolar complex
				- Raise flaps superiorly and inferiorly
				- Dissect breast off pectoralis, including pectoralis fascia with specimen
				- Make sure to include the axillary tail
				- Orient specimen
				- Perform axillary node dissection—can often be done via the mastectomy incision
				- Remove level I and II axillary LNs
				  ○ Include level III if there is gross disease in level II and/or III
				- Start by incising clavipectoral fascia along lateral edge of the pectoralis
				- Identify axillary vein and start dissection inferior to it, removing all the axillary nodal tissue between axillary vein, pectoralis muscle, serratus anterior muscle, and latissimus dorsi
				- Identify and preserve long thoracic nerve, thoracodorsal nerve, and axillary vein
				- Leave drain(s), close flaps
					Complications:
					- Long thoracic nerve injury → winged scapula
					- Thoracodorsal nerve injury → difficulty with arm extension/ adduction
					
					5-y survival for IBC is 40%
						It is reasonable to trial a course of antibiotics in a patient who presents with breast erythema, especially in a patient with risks factors for mastitis; however, if they fail to improve, this should immediately prompt concern for IBC.
						
						Major missteps: Do NOT be dissuaded from treating patient for IBC by a negative skin biopsy.
						
						Do not tricked into doing, BCT, SLNB, or nipple sparing mastectomy for a patient with IBC!

Disease Process	Relevant H&P	Work-up/Staging	Treatment	Key Surgical Steps	Post-Op Care	Tips & Tidbits

Breast cancer in pregnancy (core)	Ask patient the breast cancer risk factor questions (see general tips)
	
	What trimester of pregnancy is the patient in?
	
	Examine bilateral breasts, axilla, and other nodal basins
		U/S is initial imaging
		
		Bilateral mammogram with shielding
		
		CNB of mass
		
		Consider axillary U/S → FNA or CNB of any abnormal nodes
		
		Genetic testing, if indicated (ie, patient ≤45 yo)
		
		Complete staging for advanced breast cancer:
		- CXR with shielding
		- Liver U/S or MRI
		- CT, PET, and bone scan should be avoided in pregnancy
		
		Discuss with multidisciplinary team including surgery, medical oncology, radiation oncology, and maternal fetal medicine
			Treatment depends on trimester
			
			First Trimester:
			- Should have mastectomy
			- BCT not recommended because patient can't get XRT until after delivery
			- SLNB vs ALND—should have ALND if clinically LN+
			- No chemo in the first trimester!
			- Can give adjuvant chemo later in pregnancy, and XRT and hormonal therapy postpartum, if indicated
			
			Second Trimester/Early Third Trimester:
			- LN(-) → mastectomy vs BCT
			  ∘ SLNB to stage the axilla
			  ∘ XRT for BCT given after delivery
			- LN(+) → upfront surgery with ALND vs neoadjuvant chemo followed by surgery
			  ∘ Surgery = mastectomy or BCT (adjuvant XRT given after delivery)
			  ∘ Patients who want to shrink tumor size to permit BCT or to attempt to downstage the axilla should be offered neoadjuvant chemo
			- Chemo okay in second and third trimesters
			- Postpartum XRT and hormone therapy, if indicated
			
			Late Third Trimester:
			- Postpartum treatment per usual breast cancer guidelines
			
			Chemo regimen during pregnancy = Adriamycin, Cyclophosphamide, 5-FU (instead of paclitaxel)
				Partial mastectomy (see invasive breast cancer section)
				
				Sentinel lymph node biopsy (see invasive breast cancer section)
				
				Simple mastectomy (see locally advanced breast cancer section)
				
				Axillary lymph node dissection (see locally advanced breast cancer section)
					Adjuvant treatment as indicated	Treatments and medications to be avoided during pregnancy:
						- XRT
						- Trastuzumab
						- Hormonal therapy (ie, tamoxifen)
						- Avoid using methylene blue for SLNB, okay to give radiotracer
						- Chemo okay in second and third trimesters

Disease Process	Relevant H&P	Work-up/Staging	Treatment	Key Surgical Steps	Post-Op Care	Tips & Tidbits
Male breast disease (core)	Breast enlargement or breast mass in male patient Gynecomastia—mostly occurs in neonatal, pubertal, and elderly men - Causes: puberty, medications (antiandrogens, hormones, H2 blockers, PPI, psych meds, alcohol, marijuana), cirrhosis, malnutrition, idiopathic Pseudogynecomastia—fatty tissue, not fibroglandular tissue Male breast cancer <1% of breast cancers occur in men Risk factors for breast cancer in men: increased age, obesity, conditions with abnormal estrogen-to-androgen ratio (cirrhosis, Klinefelter syndrome, hormone use), BRCA2 (7% lifetime risk of breast cancer) Examine the bilateral breasts and axilla - Gynecomastia—usually bilateral, tissue primarily subareolar with rubbery consistency - Pseudogynecomastia—usually in obese patients, bilateral, soft, adipose tissue - Carcinoma—irregular, hard, nontender	Gynecomastia work-up: check testosterone, luteinizing hormone, estradiol, hCG, TSH, thyroxine For suspected breast cancer → mammogram and U/S with CNB All men with breast cancer should be referred for genetic testing	Gynecomastia—benign and self-limited - Pubertal gynecomastia— usually resolves spontaneously within 6-24 mo - Persistent gynecomastia → consider resection, if patient wishes Breast cancer → simple mastectomy - SLNB if clinically LN-, ALND if LN+ Same indications for endocrine therapy, chemo, and adjuvant XRT as in women - Adjuvant tamoxifen preferred over aromatase inhibitor for ER/PR+ cancers - Neoadjuvant chemo should be considered for men with T4 cancer, + LN and/or high-risk cancer (triple-negative or HER2+ cancers)	**Resection for gynecomastia:** - Start with periareolar incision, limit it to <1/2 circumference of the nipple-areolar complex to minimize risk of necrosis - Palpate and excise rubbery disk of subareolar tissue	Surveillance for male patients post mastectomy: exam q3-6mo x 5 y, then annually	BCT in men with breast cancer may be safe but would not advise answering that on boards because it is an ongoing area of study. Stage for stage, outcomes in men with breast cancer are similar to women, although men often present at a later stage than women.

Disease Process	Relevant H&P	Work-up/Staging	Treatment	Key Surgical Steps	Post-Op Care	Tips & Tidbits
Hereditary breast cancer (core)	Patient may have strong family history of breast, ovarian, and other cancers 5-10% of breast cancers are hereditary Genetic mutations associated with breast cancer - BRCA1 mutation: breast and ovarian cancer - BRCA2 mutation: breast, ovarian, prostate, and pancreatic cancer - CHEK2 mutation: breast, colorectal, and bladder cancer - PALB2 mutation: breast and pancreatic cancer - CDH1 mutation: breast and gastric cancer - p53 mutation (Li-Fraumeni): breast, brain, lung, hematologic malignancies, sarcoma, adrenal cortical carcinoma	Genetic testing should be done with a genetic counselor Consider BRCA mutation screening in asymptomatic women with personal or family history of breast, ovarian, or peritoneal cancer or who have known family history of BRCA1/2 gene mutation Indications for genetic testing in breast cancer patient: - Patient <45 yo - Triple negative breast cancer - 2+ primary breast cancers in same patient - Family member with breast cancer at <50 yo, known BRCA mutation, 2+ relatives on same side of family with breast, ovarian, or pancreatic cancer - Personal history of peritoneal, ovarian, or fallopian cancer - Male breast cancer Surveillance for known BRCA carriers: - Annual MRI starting at 25 yo and annual mammogram starting at 30 yo, staggered every 6 mo - Transvaginal U/S, CA-125, and annual pelvic exam starting at 30 yo	Bilateral prophylactic mastectomy recommended for BRCA carriers - Can be considered at any age - Reduces risk of breast cancer by >90% Consider prophylactic BSO once childbearing complete, BSO also significantly reduces the risk of breast cancer			Women with BRCA1: Risk of breast cancer ~60%, risk of ovarian cancer ~40% Women with BRCA2: Risk of breast cancer ~50%, risk of ovarian cancer ~15% BRCA2 associated with male breast cancer

Disease Process	Relevant H&P	Work-up/Staging	Treatment	Key Surgical Steps	Post-Op Care	Tips & Tidbits
Paget's disease of the breast	Ask patient the breast cancer risk factor questions (see general tips) Examine bilateral breasts, axilla, and other nodal basins - Chronic nipple ulceration and scaly/eczematous area near nipple	Patients with Paget's commonly have an underlying breast cancer Obtain U/S and diagnostic mammogram - CNB of any abnormality Full thickness skin biopsy of involved skin - Paget cells = intraepithelial adenocarcinoma cells	Biopsy negative for Paget's and malignancy → clinical follow-up, re-biopsy if not healing Skin biopsy with Paget's, no underlying cancer found → BCT (central lumpectomy/ excision nipple areolar complex with XRT) vs total mastectomy with SLNB Biopsy with DCIS or IDC → treatment per typical DCIS/IDC algorithm Even if imaging negative for abnormality, most patients with Paget's usually have underlying malignancy			

Fibroadenoma, Phyllodes tumor (core)	Ask patient the breast cancer risk factor questions (see general tips)
	
	Examine bilateral breasts, axilla, and other nodal basins
		Obtain U/S
		Obtain mammogram for patients >30 yo
		CNB vs clinical observation based on imaging findings and level of concern
		- Concerning findings—rapid rate of growth, size >3 cm, atypical imaging findings
		Consider chest staging (CXR vs chest CT) for patients with malignant phyllodes tumor
			Biopsy results:
			- Fibroadenoma → common benign breast mass, observe
			- Benign phyllodes → clinical follow-up x 3 y
			- Borderline or malignant phyllodes → wide excision
				Excision of phyllodes tumor:
				- Perform wide excision with 1-2 cm margin of normal breast tissue
				  ○ In cases of large tumors, a mastectomy may be required
				- Axillary staging is not required
				  ○ Phyllodes spread hematogenously, LN mets rare, similar to sarcoma		

Disease Process	Relevant H&P	Work-up/Staging	Treatment	Key Surgical Steps	Post-Op Care	Tips & Tidbits

Nipple discharge (core)	Ask patient the breast cancer risk factor questions (see general tips)
	
	Is discharge spontaneous vs express-able? Unilateral vs bilateral? Discharge from 1 duct or multiple ducts? Fluid characteristics? New meds?
	
	Examine bilateral breasts and axilla, try to express discharge
	
	Differential diagnosis:
	- Physiologic—bilateral and non-bloody discharge
	  ◦ Hyperprolactinemia
	  ◦ Pregnancy
	  ◦ Medication effect
	- Pathologic—unilateral, bloody, spontaneous
	  ◦ Intraductal papilloma (MCC)
	  ◦ Duct ectasia
	  ◦ Malignancy
	  ◦ Infection
		Guaiac test of bloody-appearing nipple discharge to confirm
		
		U/S, mammogram
		- May see intraductal mass if intraductal papilloma present
		
		CNB and clip placement for any radiographic abnormalities seen
		
		+/- ductography
			Suspicious lesion on imaging → excision
			
			No lesion on imaging → excision of discharging duct (subareolar duct excision)
			
			If malignant → cancer work-up and treatment
				Terminal duct excision (core):
				- Preoperative wire localization of mass, if applicable
				- Attempt to cannulate offending duct with lacrimal duct probe
				- Make circumareolar incision
				- Elevate areola
				- Leave subcutaneous fat on underside of nipple areola complex to preserve blood supply
				- Isolate and excise duct (~4 cm length of duct)—can excise single duct if able to localize versus doing terminal duct excision
				- Excise localized mass, if present
					Persistent discharge post excision can be expected for 4-6 wk after surgery from draining seroma	

Disease Process	Relevant H&P	Work-up/Staging	Treatment	Key Surgical Steps	Post-Op Care	Tips & Tidbits

Infectious breast disease (core)	Patient may present with breast pain, erythema, fever, malaise
	
	Ask about smoking, breastfeeding, trauma to the breast, diabetes, and nipple piercing
	
	Examine bilateral breasts and axilla
	- May have redness, pain, fluctuance, drainage
	- Granulomatous mastitis—can present with a single, solid, irregular mass or masses within the breast
		Ultrasound
		- Abscess—will appear hypoechoic, well circumscribed, may be loculated
		- Solid mass → get mammogram and CNB to rule out malignancy
		  ○ CNB of mass demonstrating granulomas = granulomatous mastitis
		    ■ Send tissue for AFB and fungal stains to rule out TB or sarcoid, send tissue culture to rule out Corynebacterium
		
		Biopsy should be performed on any "infection" that fails to respond to appropriate antibiotics and drainage to rule out underlying malignancy
			Uncomplicated case of mastitis or cellulitis without abscess—treat with antibiotics (cover for staph/strep), NSAIDs, and cold compresses
			- Lactating women—antibiotics + continue breastfeeding or pumping to promote drainage
			- If symptoms do not improve in 48-72 h, reevaluate with U/S to rule out abscess
			- Uncomplicated mastitis should resolve within 2 wk, if it does not, other possibilities should be considered, including resistant organism, abscess requiring surgery, or underlying malignancy
			
			Small abscess—Cephalexin 500 mg QID x 1 wk, if persistent then do needle aspiration
			
			Abscess—U/S-guided needle aspiration with 16-gauge needle + antibiotics
			- Can perform repeat aspirations as needed
			- Abscess s/p multiple failed aspirations → incision and drainage
			
			Lactational abscess—penicillin antibiotic x 10 d and aspiration + frequent pumping of the breast
			- Do not perform incision & drainage because milk fistula can form (often heal spontaneously, but mother may have to stop breast feeding until healed)
			
			Treatment of granulomatous mastitis—treat with observation (may take months to resolve), some treat with steroids
			- If fails to resolve, excision can be considered but often results in wound-healing issues
				Breast abscess aspiration (core):
				- Use U/S for localization
				- Use 16-gauge needle to aspirate fluid collection
				  ○ Avoid going through nipple areolar complex
				- Send fluid for gram stain, sensitivities +/- cytology (if worried about malignancy)
				- See patient back in clinic in several days to reevaluate, re-aspirate if needed
				
				Incision & drainage (core):
				- Incision over area of fluctuance
				- Drain fluid collection and break up any loculations
				- Send fluid for culture
				- Take sample of cavity wall to send for pathology to rule out malignancy
				- Irrigate cavity and pack
					Should get posttreatment mammogram, once everything is resolved, to rule out underlying malignancy
					
					Smoking cessation
						Mondor disease—thickened palpable cord in the subcutaneous breast tissue, or lateral chest wall, +/- associated erythema and tenderness
						- diagnosis made on exam, but get imaging if there is concern for malignancy
						- Treat with warm compresses, NSAIDs, should resolve within 4-6 wk

Disease Process	Relevant H&P	Work-up/Staging	Treatment	Key Surgical Steps	Post-Op Care	Tips & Tidbits

Benign breast disease (core)	Examine bilateral breasts and axilla
	
	Fat necrosis—may develop following trauma or breast surgery, often presents as mass or area of firmness
	
	Breast cysts/fibrocystic disease—can present as mass or be identified incidentally on imaging, cysts feel like smooth mobile mass, may fluctuate in size with menstrual cycle
	
	Fibroadenoma—feels like rubbery mobile mass, common benign tumor in young women
		U/S—preferred initial imaging for younger women (<30 yo) due to dense breast tissue
		- Simple cysts—anechoic, round/oval, thin-walled, smooth contour
		- May see Calcifications associated with fat necrosis
		
		Mammogram for older women or to further evaluate concerning finding
		
		CNB if concerning findings on imaging
			- Fat necrosis—benign, no specific follow-up necessary
			- Breast cyst
			  ○ Simple cyst does not require any treatment unless symptomatic
			  ○ Symptomatic cyst may be aspirated for symptom relief
			  ○ No cytology needed for cysts with non-bloody fluid that resolve after aspiration
			  ○ Recurrent cysts and cysts with bloody fluid should be sent for cytology
			  ○ Cysts with a solid component need to be biopsied
			- Fibroadenoma—typically no treatment required if diagnosis of fibroadenoma made on CNB
			  ○ Excise if symptomatic, >3 cm, rapid growth, or unable to exclude possibility of phyllodes tumor
				Breast cyst aspiration (core):
				- Localize cyst using ultrasound, advance 18-gauge needle into fluid collection and aspirate until cavity collapses
				- Bloody fluid should be sent for cytology
				- Green or straw-colored fluid with collapse of the cyst after aspiration is likely benign
				- If unable to fully aspirate fluid, obtain CNB
					Discordant pathology results should be managed with repeat CNB or excisional biopsy
					
					Post-biopsy hematoma can be managed with compression and ice, usually self-limited	

6

Vascular Surgery

Xuan-Binh Pham, MD

DISEASES AND CONDITIONS

- Acute limb ischemia (c), arterial embolectomy (c)
- Peripheral arterial disease (c), lower extremity bypass (a)
- Popliteal artery aneurysm (a)
- Diabetic foot infection (c)
- Nonhealing foot wound, lower extremity amputations (c)
- Cerebrovascular disease (c), carotid endarterectomy (a)

- Acute mesenteric ischemia (c), SMA embolectomy/thrombectomy (a)
- Chronic mesenteric ischemia, operations for mesenteric occlusive disease (a)
- Central venous access (c), port placement (c)
- Venous thromboembolism (c), IVC filter placement (a)
- Hemodialysis access (c), arteriovenous graft/fistula creation (a)
- Lower extremity swelling, venous disease (c)

- Aortoiliac occlusive disease, aortoiliac reconstruction for occlusive disease (a)
- Acute aortic dissection (a)
- Abdominal aortic aneurysm (a), abdominal aortic aneurysm repair (a)
- Splenic artery aneurysm (a)
- Thoracic outlet syndrome (a)
- Vascular graft infection and graft-enteric fistula (a), extra-anatomic bypass (a)
- Femoral artery pseudoaneurysm

GENERAL VASCULAR SURGERY TIPS

- Be familiar with common vascular exposures—these will help you get through many of the vascular scenarios. Descriptions of the most common vascular exposures are included in this chapter.
- You are also expected to be familiar with the basics of endovascular intervention and the use of ultrasound in the diagnosis and management of vascular disease.

- Work-up of vascular patients frequently includes duplex U/S because it is useful for rapidly identifying venous or arterial disease, so don't forget this as part of your work-up, if indicated.
- Don't forget to heparinize!
- Consider HIT if the examiners present you with a patient with a drop in platelets and thrombosis while on heparin—send HIT assay, stop heparin, start argatroban or bivalirudin.

- Be familiar with how and when to obtain an ankle brachial index (ABI).
- Have a low threshold to perform fasciotomy when patient has had limb ischemia >4-6 h.
- Consider obtaining cardiac work-up (ECG, ECHO, +/- stress test) in patients undergoing elective vascular operations as many of these patients will have underlying cardiac disease.

(c) = core topic   (a) = advanced topic

Disease Process	Relevant H&P	Work-up/Staging	Treatment	Key Surgical Steps	Post-Op Care	Tips & Tidbits

Acute limb ischemia (core)	Patient will present with a cold, painful leg
	
	History of atrial fibrillation? History of prior stenting or bypass?
	
	Neurovascular exam—check pulses/doppler signals, motor and sensory function
	
	Assess for 6Ps: pain, paralysis, paresthesia, pulselessness, pallor, poikilothermia
		Labs, ECG
		
		Duplex U/S—will help determine location of occlusion
		
		Rutherford classification for acute limb ischemia used to classify acutely ischemic limbs based on exam findings (table 6.1)
			Heparinize ASAP, want ACT >250
			
			Patient with Rutherford I/IIA ischemia for <14 d may be candidates for catheter-directed thrombolysis
			
			If Rutherford IIb → emergent OR for thrombectomy vs bypass
			
			If Rutherford III → amputation
			
			In patient with likely embolic acute limb ischemia (ie, history of afib), take for embolectomy
			
			Patients with significant preexisting peripheral arterial disease are more likely to need bypass
				Femoral embolectomy (core):
				- Make longitudinal groin incision overlying femoral artery
				- Identify inguinal ligament, then dissect down onto common femoral artery (CFA), get control of CFA, profunda, and superficial femoral artery (SFA)
				- Heparinize
				- Open CFA transversely
				- Perform proximal and distal embolectomy with 4-5 Fr Fogarty
				- Once you have 2 clean passes, check to see if you have back bleeding, if you do then patch/close the artery
				- Check distal pulses/signals
				  ∘ If present, then close
				  ∘ If still absent, move distally and do popliteal cutdown and embolectomy
				- Can do angiogram if having issues
				- May need to do endarterectomy/bypass if embolectomy unsuccessful
				- Do fasciotomies if >4-6 h of ischemia time (see lower extremity compartment syndrome section in trauma chapter)
					Frequent neurovascular checks during immediate post-op period
					
					Continue therapeutic anticoagulation and antiplatelet
						Additional reading: Rutherford RB. Clinical staging of acute limb ischemia as the basis for choice of revascularization method: when and how to intervene. *Semin Vasc Surg.* 2009 Mar;22(1):5-9.

Table 6.1: Rutherford classification of acute limb ischemia					
Classification	**Prognosis**	**Sensory loss**	**Motor deficit**	**Arterial doppler**	**Venous doppler**
I: viable	No immediate threat	None	None	+	+
IIA: marginally threatened	Salvageable if promptly treated	None or just toes	None	-	+
IIB: immediately threatened	Salvageable if immediately revascularized	More than toes, rest pain	Mild/mod	-	+
III: irreversible	Major tissue loss, permanent damage	Anesthetic	Profound, paralysis	-	-

Source: Modified with permission from Rutherford RB, Baker JD, Ernst C, et al. Recommended standards for reports dealing with lower extremity ischemia: revised version. *J Vasc Surg.* 1997;26(3):517-538.

Disease Process	Relevant H&P	Work-up/Staging	Treatment	Key Surgical Steps	Post-Op Care	Tips & Tidbits

Peripheral arterial disease (core)	Lifestyle-limiting claudication vs critical limb-threatening ischemia (CLTI)
	- Claudication—lower extremity pain with activity, relieved by rest
	- CLTI—tissue loss and/or rest pain
	
	Ask about cardiovascular risk factors (HTN, HLD, DM, smoking)
	
	Full pulse exam, check doppler signals, look for skin changes or wounds
		ABI:
		• <0.9 abnormal
		• 0.4-0.9 mild to mod PAD
		• <0.4 typically have CLTI
		
		Duplex U/S
		
		CTA vs angiogram
		
		Obtain vein mapping if planning to do bypass, need vein > 3 mm and of adequate length
		
		Pre-op cardiac work-up if planning to undergo surgery—ECG, ECHO, +/- stress test
			Claudication → start with medical management
			
			Optimal medical treatment: ASA, statin, DM control, smoking cessation, walking program, cilostazol (PDE inhibitor, avoid in patients with CHF)
			
			CLTI—skip medical management and go straight to intervention
			
			Revascularization:
			- Endovascular—TASC system used to classify arterial disease based on severity and how amenable it would be to endovascular intervention
			- Surgery—need inflow, outflow, conduit
			
			CFA disease → not typically amenable to endovascular intervention, need femoral endarterectomy with patch angioplasty
				General principles of bypass (advanced):
				- Harvest GSV or use prosthetic (PTFE, Dacron), if needed
				- Obtain proximal and distal exposure
				- Pass tunneler with conduit, heparinize, then clamp vessels, and set up for anastomoses
				- Proximal anastomosis before distal
				- Suture choice:
				  ◦ Femoral anastomosis → 5-0 Prolene
				  ◦ Tibial/popliteal → 6-0 Prolene
				  ◦ Pedal/tibial → 7-0 Prolene
				Exposure of CFA:
				- Longitudinal incision in groin overlying femoral artery
				- Dissect down and identify CFA as it passes under inguinal ligament
				- Dissect out and get loops around CFA, SFA, and profunda
				Exposure of below knee popliteal artery:
				- Longitudinal incision made 1 cm posterior to medial border of tibia
				- Open fascia of superficial posterior compartment, retract gastroc posteriorly
				- Dissect soleus off of the tibia to expose the popliteal artery, which is running with popliteal vein and tibial nerve
					Continue aspirin
					
					Follow-up U/S 1 mo post-op
					
					Complications:
					- Graft thrombosis
					  ◦ Patient loses pulse in PACU → return to OR
					  ◦ Early graft failure (within 30 d)—typically due to technical failure
					  ◦ Late graft failure (> 6 mo)—typically due to intimal hyperplasia or progression of vascular disease
					- Lymphatic leak—serous fluid leaking from groin wound, take back for washout and ligation of lymphatics, +/- Sartorius flap
					- Graft infection—excise infected prosthetic graft, extra-anatomic bypass
						CLTI → 25% risk of amputation in 1 y, 50% risk of death in 5 y

Disease Process	Relevant H&P	Work-up/Staging	Treatment	Key Surgical Steps	Post-Op Care	Tips & Tidbits
Popliteal artery aneurysm (advanced)	Popliteal artery aneurysms are the most common type of peripheral aneurysm May be asymptomatic or present with symptoms (thrombosis and distal embolization, claudication) RF: connective tissue disorder	Duplex CTA Vein mapping to look for suitable conduit, if planning to repair Screen for other aneurysms - 30-60% have AAA - 50% have contralateral popliteal artery aneurysm	Repair if >2 cm or symptomatic Exclusion and bypass - Preferably use GSV - In patients who present with acute ischemia due to popliteal aneurysm thrombosis, consider thrombolysis to restore patency prior to open repair Can stent in poor operative candidates	**Exclusion and bypass of popliteal artery aneurysm:** - Supine positioning - Flex knee slightly with bump under distal thigh - Harvest GSV - Expose distal SFA with incision on distal medial thigh along posterior border of the femur, push sartorius posteriorly (Figure 6.1) - Expose below knee popliteal artery or proximal tibial artery with incision on upper medial calf along posterior border of tibia, divide pes anserinus if needed - Tunnel conduit from proximal exposure to distal exposure, then heparinize and clamp - Perform bypass from SFA to below knee popliteal artery with reversed GSV or PTFE, do proximal anastomosis first with 5-0 Prolene, then popliteal anastomosis with 6-0 Prolene - Ligate native popliteal artery segment proximally and distally to prevent subsequent embolization - Unclamp, check signals - Alternatively, can expose popliteal artery from posterior approach with lazy S incision	Follow-up in clinic at 1, 6, and 12 mo with ABI and duplex of graft Popliteal aneurysm sac may continue to grow due to geniculate branches → embolize if needed	CFA aneurysms are the second most common type of peripheral artery aneurysm - Cut-off for repair of femoral artery aneurysm is > 2.5 cm - Typically require open surgery, with aneurysm resection and interposition prosthetic bypass Cut-off for repair of common iliac artery aneurysm is >3.5 cm, and >3 cm for internal iliac artery aneurysms - Iliac artery aneurysms may be amenable to stenting, depending on characteristics

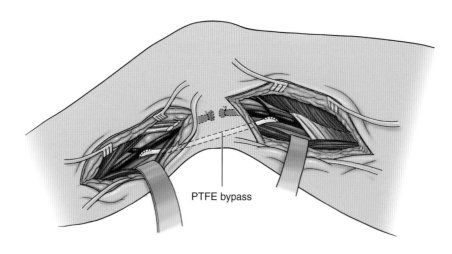

PTFE bypass

FIGURE 6.1: Exposure of above and below knee popliteal artery for popliteal artery bypass. (Reproduced with permission from Feliciano DV, Mattox KL, Moore EE. *Trauma*, 9th ed. New York, NY: McGraw Hill; 2021, Figure 77B.)

Disease Process	Relevant H&P	Work-up/Staging	Treatment	Key Surgical Steps	Post-Op Care	Tips & Tidbits
Diabetic foot infection (core)	History of diabetes, neuropathy, smoking, PVD Perform pulse exam, look for ulcers on foot, location and appearance of infection Differentiate between wet vs dry gangrene	CBC, BMP, HgA1C XR of foot ABI, duplex, +/- toe pressures to assess arterial supply TcPO$_2$ can be helpful to assess potential for healing	Ulcer/dry gangrene—manage initially with offloading, excellent foot care, wound care If does not show signs of improvement within 3-4 wk, then consider revascularization (endovascular vs bypass) If wet gangrene is present, patient needs debridement, consider guillotine amputation if infection is making patient systemically ill	**Guillotine lower extremity amputation:** - Place tourniquet, typically set at ~200 mm Hg - Select level for transection, go as distal as possible to preserve soft tissue for eventual closure but must remove all grossly infected tissue - Transect soft tissue - Divide bone with saw - Ligate major vessels, release tourniquet, establish hemostasis	Return to OR for formal BKA when patient stabilized and wound looks healthy	

Nonhealing foot wound, lower extremity amputation (core)	Patient will present with lower extremity wound or trauma
	
	Vascular process? Infection? Diabetes? Ambulatory status?
	
	Extremity and pulse exam
		CBC, BMP
		
		Obtain wound culture and blood cultures for patient with infected wound
		
		If it is a vascular issue, should get ABI and arterial duplex to assess blood supply
		- +/- angiogram
		- Typically need open popliteal artery to heal BKA and open CFA or profunda to heal AKA
		
		TcPO$_2$ can help determine level to amputate
		- TcPO$_2$ > 40 associated with better amputation healing rates, TcPO$_2$ < 20 associated with failure
			Antibiotics if patient has infected wound
			
			BKA vs AKA depending on ambulatory status, infection, blood supply
			- AKA easier to heal but less chance of being ambulatory
			
			If patient is sick from infected limb, may need to do guillotine amputation and formally close later
				Below-knee amputation (core) (Figure 6.2):
				- Apply tourniquet
				- Mark out skin incisions:
				  ○ Anterior skin incision should be 12 cm distal to tibial tuberosity
				  ○ Posterior skin incision should be 15 cm distal to the anterior flap
				  ○ The anterior flap should encompass 2/3 of the circumference of the leg and posterior flap length should be 1/3 the circumference
				  ○ Create flaps in a "fish mouth" fashion
				- Tibia should be cut 1 cm proximal to anterior skin incision
				- Fibula should be cut 1 cm proximal to tibial bone cut
				- Bevel bone edges
				- Fold posterior muscle flap forward, close the incision in layers
				
				Above-knee amputation (core) (Figure 6.2):
				- Apply tourniquet
				- Make skin incision 4 fingerbreadths above patella (fish mouth incision)
				- Cut femur 2 fingerbreadths above skin incision
				- Ligate femoral vessels
				- Can do myodesis with adductor longus tendon to prevent abduction contracture
				- Close fascia over bone, close incision in layers
					Stump shrinker, work with PT/OT, do exercises to minimize risk of contracture, eventually fitted for prosthetic	

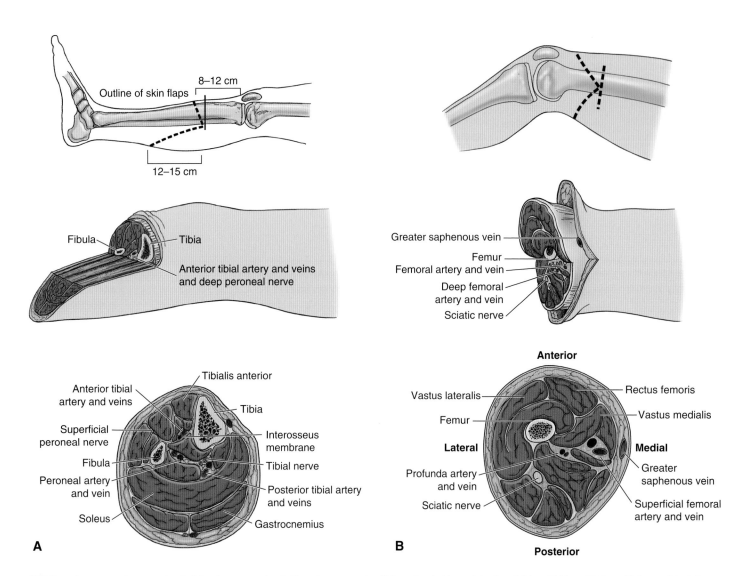

FIGURE 6.2: Lower extremity amputation. **A.** Below-knee amputation. **B.** Above-knee amputation. (A: Reproduced with permission from Feliciano DV, Mattox KL, Moore EE. *Trauma*, 9th ed. New York, NY: McGraw Hill; 2021. Figure 86. B: Reproduced with permission from Feliciano DV, Mattox KL, Moore EE. *Trauma*, 9th ed. New York, NY: McGraw Hill; 2021. Figure 85.)

Disease Process	Relevant H&P	Work-up/Staging	Treatment	Key Surgical Steps	Post-Op Care	Tips & Tidbits

Cerebrovascular disease (core)	Asymptomatic? TIA? CVA?
	
	Amaurosis fugax?
	
	Risk factors: HTN, DMII, smoking, HLD, CAD
	
	Prior neck radiation or surgery?
		Duplex U/S—peak systolic velocity corresponds to degree of stenosis
		• <125 cm/s = < 50% stenosis
		• 125-230 cm/s = 50-69% stenosis
		• >230 cm/s = 70-99% stenosis
		• Undetectable flow = occlusion
		CTA neck
		
		Pre-op cardiac work-up— ECG, ECHO, +/- stress test
			Medical management—HTN, HLD, DM control, smoking cessation, aspirin
			
			Symptomatic with > 50% stenosis → CEA
			
			Asymptomatic with > 80% stenosis → consider CEA
			
			Timing of CEA after stroke— ideally wait at least 48 h but perform within 1-2 wk of stroke
			
			Carotid artery stenting (CAS) may be preferred in patients with history of prior neck surgery or XRT
			- CAS associated with higher risk of perioperative stroke than CEA
				Carotid endarterectomy (CEA) (advanced):
				- Awake vs under general anesthesia +/- intra-op EEG, can do routine shunting vs measure carotid stump pressures for selective shunting (shunt for pressure <40 mm Hg)
				- Incision along anterior border of sternocleidomastoid (SCM), dissect down through platysma
				- Retract SCM laterally to reveal carotid sheath
				- Ligate facial vein and open carotid sheath
				- Identify and preserve vagus and hypoglossal nerves
				- Encircle common carotid artery (CCA), external carotid artery (ECA), and internal carotid artery (ICA)
				- Heparinize with 100 U/kg
				- Clamp ICA, CCA, then ECA
				- Longitudinal arteriotomy from CCA on to ICA
				- +/- shunting
				- Perform endarterectomy
				- Close with bovine pericardial patch
				- Unclamp in reverse order ECA, CCA, then ICA
				- Close neck +/- drain
				- Wake patient up and check neuro status before going to PACU
					ICU post-op for BP monitoring
					Goal SBP 100-140 mm Hg
					Complications:
					- Post-op stroke → get STAT U/S to look for thrombosis, if thrombosed take back to OR
					- Reperfusion syndrome—HTN, headache, seizure, hemorrhagic stroke
					  ○ Tx: control BP and obtain STAT head CT to eval for stroke
					- Neck hematoma—intubate to protect airway, wait until in OR to open incision because if it is a patch blowout the patient may have significant hemorrhage
					- Nerve palsy:
					  ○ Vagus nerve injury → hoarseness, airway issues (RLN deficit)
					  ○ Glossopharyngeal nerve injury → ipsilateral tongue deviation
					Duplex 3-mo post-op
						Transcarotid arterial revascularization (TCAR) is an alternative to CEA that is increasingly being used for patients with carotid disease, but we would not advise doing TCAR on the boards at this time
						Additional reading:
						Brott TG, et al; CREST Investigators. Stenting versus endarterectomy for treatment of carotid-artery stenosis. *N Engl J Med*. 2010 Jul 1;363(1):11-23.

Disease Process	Relevant H&P	Work-up/Staging	Treatment	Key Surgical Steps	Post-Op Care	Tips & Tidbits
Acute mesenteric ischemia (AMI) (core)	Abdominal pain out of proportion to exam Common in older patients with vascular disease Embolic AMI—common in patients with afib Nonocclusive mesenteric ischemia (NOMI)—sick, elderly patients with CHF, recent cardiac/vascular surgery, hypotension Mesenteric vein thrombosis—patients in hypercoagulable state	CBC, CMP, lipase, coagulants, lactate ECG—if examiner tells you the patient is in afib, this may be a clue they have embolic AMI CTA Four types: - Embolic AMI—embolus typically lodges more distally after takeoff of first jejunal branches, resulting in proximal jejunal sparing - Thrombotic AMI—usually at the ostia of the SMA, resulting in ischemia from distal duodenum to splenic flexure - NOMI - Mesenteric venous thrombosis (MVT) In case of embolic AMI, will eventually need to do embolic work-up (ECHO, ECG, CTA) to look for source	Anticoagulation (except for NOMI) Resuscitation, correction of hypovolemia and metabolic acidosis, antibiotics Take patients with embolic and thrombotic AMI to the OR ASAP NOMI—improve cardiac output as much as possible, consider intraluminal papaverine MVT—anticoagulation, bowel rest, supportive care Indications for urgent laparotomy in patients with NOMI or MVT: - Peritonitis - Evidence of transmural necrosis or perforation - Worsening abdominal exam - Abdominal compartment syndrome - Worsening metabolic acidosis or sepsis	**SMA embolectomy/bypass (advanced):** - Laparotomy - Elevate the transverse colon and locate middle colic artery at the base of the transverse mesocolon, which can be followed to locate the SMA - Get proximal and distal control of the SMA and then make transverse arteriotomy - Perform proximal and distal embolectomy with Fogarty balloon, if flow improves, close arteriotomy - If flow remains poor and/or patient has more chronic vascular disease changes, may require aortomesenteric bypass to SMA or retrograde ilio-SMA bypass - Resect any bowel that appears non-viable after reperfusion - If bowel viability is questionable, temporarily close the abdomen and return for second look	Perioperative mortality is high (30-60%) Need for ongoing anticoagulation depending on etiology Patients with arterial disease need lifelong statin and antiplatelet	
Chronic mesenteric ischemia	Abdominal pain, food fear, weight loss, diarrhea Abdominal exam, pulse exam Same risk factors as PAD/CAD (*HTN, DMII, smoking, HLD*)	Rule out other potential causes of postprandial pain (PUD, biliary colic, etc) Mesenteric duplex U/S or CTA Mesenteric angiogram—can be diagnostic and therapeutic, reveals extent of disease	Endovascular angioplasty and stenting If endo fails, then surgery—aortomesenteric endarterectomy vs bypass If doing bypass, can go to celiac artery and/or SMA	**Antegrade aortomesenteric bypass (advanced) (Figure 6.3A):** - Midline laparotomy - Expose the supraceliac aorta via lesser sac with mobilization of left lobe of liver and left crus - Follow the anterior surface of the aortic inferiorly to locate the celiac artery within the lesser sac - Take down LOT and isolate SMA at the base of small bowel mesentery - Heparinize (80-100 U/kg), then clamp proximally and distally - Use GSV, PTFE, or Dacron as conduit (no prosthetic if bowel spillage) - Create proximal anastomosis to supraceliac aorta - Create distal anastomosis to celiac/common hepatic artery and/or SMA - Check intestinal and extremity viability Can also do retrograde bypass with distal aorta or iliacs as inflow (Figure 6.3B)	Patient should be kept on an antiplatelet	

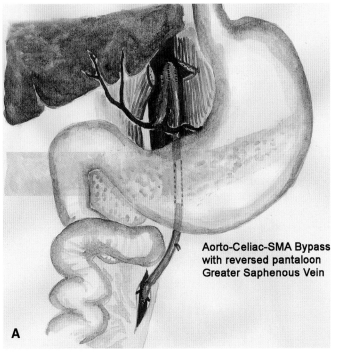

Aorto-Celiac-SMA Bypass
with reversed pantaloon
Greater Saphenous Vein

A

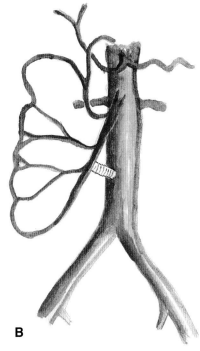

B

FIGURE 6.3: Surgical management of chronic mesenteric vascular disease. **A.** Antegrade bypass from supra-celiac aorta to celiac artery and SMA with GSV. B. Retrograde bypass from infrarenal aorta to SMA with prosthetic graft. (Reproduced with permission from Dean SM, Satiani B, Abraham WT. *Color Atlas and Synopsis of Vascular Diseases.* New York, NY: McGraw Hill; 2014, Figure 47-8 A and Figure 47-9 A.)

Disease Process	Relevant H&P	Work-up/Staging	Treatment	Key Surgical Steps	Post-Op Care	Tips & Tidbits
Central venous access (core)	Patient may need central access for a variety of reasons—sick ICU patient, need for dialysis, port for chemo, etc	Typically none needed	Potential sites for central venous access—IJ, subclavian, femoral Typically use IJ, rather than subclavian, for temporary dialysis access because it has lower rates of central venous stenosis and easier to do U/S guided	**Port placement (core):** - Obtain venous access with needle and wire using U/S - Confirm wire placement in the SVC using fluoro - Make pocket for port to sit in - Tunnel device tubing from the pocket to venous access site - Dilate access point with dilator sheath over the wire - Remove the wire and stylet and Thread catheter into SVC through the access sheath, catheter tip should sit of the SVC-right atrial junction - Secure device to the pectoralis fascia, aspirate and flush the device with heparinized saline - Close the wound	Get post-op CXR to eval placement and rule out pneumothorax Complications: - Carotid stick with needle—can typically remove needle and hold pressure - Central line in carotid—confirm by attaching to transducer and looking at wave form and/or sending blood gas, will likely need to heparinize and take patient to OR for cutdown and primary repair of arteriotomy	Additional reading: Parienti JJ, et al; 3SITES Study Group. Intravascular complications of central venous catheterization by insertion site. *N Engl J Med.* 2015 Sep 24; 373(13):1220-1229.

Disease Process	Relevant H&P	Work-up/Staging	Treatment	Key Surgical Steps	Post-Op Care	Tips & Tidbits
Venous thromboembolism (VTE) (core)	DVT—pain and swelling in leg - Phlegmasia cerulea dolens: severe presentation of DVT, blue discoloration of limb, limb threatening PE—SOB, chest pain, tachycardia, hypoxia RF for VTE: post-op period, prior VTE, malignancy, hypercoagulable disorder, critically ill, immobility Differential diagnosis for a swollen leg: - DVT - Chronic venous insufficiency - Arterial occlusion - Infection	CBC, BMP, ABG, ECG Venous duplex to look for DVT CT PE if concerned for pulmonary embolism ECHO in patient with PE and concern for right heart strain	Initiate anticoagulation (AC) immediately - First episode of VTE → AC for at least 3mon - Consider indefinite AC if patient has active malignancy - Patient with VTE but contraindication to therapeutic AC or recurrent VTE while on AC → IVC filter DVT treatment: - Typically, do not treat asymptomatic below knee DVTs, just follow-up with weekly U/S x 2 wk to ensure no progression - Consider endovascular intervention (thrombolysis, thrombectomy) for phlegmasia +/- iliofemoral DVT to reduce risk of chronic venous insufficiency PE treatment: - Anticoagulation - Large embolus with right heart strain or hemodynamic instability → consider percutaneous pulmonary artery thrombolysis or thrombectomy	**IVC filter placement (advanced):** - Place patient supine, in slight Trendelenburg with head rotated away from site of access - Access right IJ with 18-gauge needle - Place guidewire in IVC under fluoroscopic guidance - Advance sheath over wire, then place catheter through sheath - Pull wire and shoot venogram, mark the renal veins (renal veins usually at L1) - Place the filter through sheath and position inferior to renal veins, deploy filter - Completion venogram	Post-thrombotic syndrome—extremity pain, swelling, heaviness, skin pigmentation, ulceration - Tx: limb elevation and compression IVC filter complications: pneumothorax, access site thrombosis, filter fracture, migration, perforation, IVC thrombosis Post IVC filter placement: Follow-up to see when anticoagulation can be restarted and filter removed	Recurrent LLE DVT → rule out May Thurner, may need venogram, IVUS, venoplasty, and stenting Avoid using warfarin in pregnant patients Additional reading: Stevens SM, et al. Antithrombotic therapy for VTE disease: second update of the CHEST Guideline and Expert Panel Report. *Chest.* 2021 Dec; 160(6):e545-e608.

Disease Process	Relevant H&P	Work-up/Staging	Treatment	Key Surgical Steps	Post-Op Care	Tips & Tidbits
Hemodialysis access (core)	CKD4 (GFR < 30) → refer for dialysis access (fistula first initiative) When is patient anticipated to initiate dialysis? ○ Want arteriovenous fistula (AVF) 6 mo prior and arteriovenous graft (AVG) 6 wk prior to starting dialysis, gives time for access to mature Handedness? Location of prior access, lines? ○ More likely to have significant central stenosis after subclavian line than IJ Pulse exam, Allen's test	Duplex U/S of upper extremities—need vein >3 mm and artery > 2 mm Make sure there is no proximal stenosis	Acute renal failure → hemodialysis via catheter in IJ opposite arm for future dialysis access is best option if immediate access needed, create AVF/ AVG once stable (if needed) ○ Nontunneled line—can be used for days to weeks (inpatient only) ○ Tunneled line—can be used for weeks to months Long term dialysis options—hemodialysis, peritoneal dialysis, kidney transplant Selecting site of AVF/AVG: ○ Create AVG/AVF in nondominant arm and as distal as possible ○ Preference order—radiocephalic, radiobasilic, brachiocephalic, brachiobasilic, AVG	**Brachiocephalic arteriovenous fistula creation (advanced):** - Check K+ pre-op - Can be done with MAC and local - Use U/S to look at possible targets - Make transverse incision in antecubital fossa - Dissect out ~3 cm cephalic vein by creating skin flaps - Incise bicep aponeurosis to expose brachial artery for 2-3 cm - Heparinize with 5000 U IV heparin - Clamp vessels - Make ~0.75-1 cm arteriotomy with 11 blade and Potts - End to side anastomosis with 6-0 Prolene - Check for thrill and distal pulses	- Get duplex in 4-6 wk - Rule of 6s—AVF ready for dialysis when: ~6 wk post-op, >6 mm in diameter, <6 mm from skin, >600 mL/min flow - If you do brachiobasilic, will need transposition in ~ 6 wk Complications: - Ischemic monomelic neuropathy—severe hand pain but good pulse in PACU ○ Tx: ligate access - Steal syndrome—ischemic hand with poor pulse that improves with access compression ○ Tx: consider access ligation, banding, or distal revascularization interval ligation (DRIL) - Failure to mature - Graft stenosis and/or thrombosis ○ Evaluate with duplex of fistula ○ Tx: fistulagram, thrombectomy, balloon dilation as needed	

Disease Process	Relevant H&P	Work-up/Staging	Treatment	Key Surgical Steps	Post-Op Care	Tips & Tidbits
Lower extremity swelling, venous disease (core)	Leg swelling May complain of leg pain, fatigue and/or heaviness History of DVT? Chronic venous insufficiency is often the result of prior DVT Examine patient for pulses/signals, telangiectasias, varicose veins, leg edema, pain, wounds, skin changes, and skin ulceration Venous stasis ulcers classically appear in area of medial malleolus	Venous duplex U/S—rule out DVT, look for venous reflux (reflux > 500 ms for superficial or perforator veins; >1000 ms for deep veins) CEAP classification used to categorize venous disorders	Most patients with venous reflux should start with trial of compression stockings and leg elevation x 6 wk - Skip trial of compression and offer intervention if patient has wound associated with venous insufficiency, manage wound with compression/unna boot Intervention warranted if they fail trial of compression Symptomatic venous disease with documented superficial venous reflux → can treat with GSV ablation or vein stripping Varicose veins can be treated with microphlebectomy or sclerotherapy at same time as ablation Telangiectasias—treated with sclerotherapy and surface laser therapy	**Greater saphenous vein ablation:** - Leg sterilely prepped and draped - Access GSV just below the knee using U/S and micropuncture, place sheath - Advance ablation catheter until tip is ~3 cm distal to saphenofemoral junction - Inject tumescent fluid +bicarb+lidocaine) along course of GSV (provides pain control and buffer from ablation for surrounding tissues) - Begin ablating and withdrawing the catheter - Small branch varicosities can be treated at the same time with microphlebectomy or sclerotherapy	Risk of post-op DVT formation (EHIT—endothermal heat-induced thrombosis) - Obtain U/S 3-4 d after GSV ablation to rule out formation of DVT - If patient develops DVT, usually treat with several weeks of anticoagulation and then repeat duplex to make sure it has resolved	
Aortoiliac occlusive disease (advanced)	May present with claudication, impotence and/or absent femoral pulses (Leriche syndrome) Ask about smoking, other risk factors for vascular disease	Basic labs, ECG ABI, Duplex CTA	Medical optimization (exercise, smoking cessation, statin, BP and DM control, etc) Some cases may be amenable to endovascular intervention Surgical bypass required for more advanced disease not amenable to endovascular treatment	**Aortobifemoral bypass (advanced):** - Bilateral femoral artery exposure - Laparotomy - Retract transverse colon up and small bowel to the right - Incise the retroperitoneum overlying the aorta - Identify the left renal vein, dissect the aorta at the level of the left renal vein and prepare it for clamping - Create a tunnel from the aorta to each femoral artery, staying posterior to the ureters - Give 100 U/kg of heparin (goal ACT 250-300) - Clamp the aorta proximally below the renal arteries and distally at the level of the IMA - Make aortic arteriotomy ~3 cm - Create proximal anastomosis with PTFE or Dacron conduit - Bring conduit through tunnel to femoral artery - Clamp CFA, SFA, and profunda - Make arteriotomy on CFA, perform endarterectomy if needed - Create distal anastomosis to CFA - Repeat bypass to the contra-lateral femoral artery - Release clamps - Check bowel viability, distal pulses, and hemostasis	Close monitoring, frequent neurovascular checks on POD 0	

Disease Process	Relevant H&P	Work-up/Staging	Treatment	Key Surgical Steps	Post-Op Care	Tips & Tidbits
Aortic dissection (advanced)	RF: HTN, connective tissue disorders Sudden onset severe chest/back pain, different blood pressures in the arms, new aortic regurgitation, cardiac tamponade (type A) Look for evidence of malperfusion	ECG, CBC, CMP, lipase, troponin, lactate CXR (widened mediastinum), CTA, TEE Determine if Type A vs B - A—involves ascending aorta or arch - B—distal to left subclavian	Beta-blocker for impulse control (keep HR < 60, SBP < 120) Type A → CT surgery consult, emergent repair Type B → Determine if complicated (malperfusion, aneurysmal, rupture, progression, refractory HTN, or refractory pain) - Type B, uncomplicated—medical management (impulse control, serial labs to evaluate renal or intestinal malperfusion), surveillance, repeat CTA to determine stability at 24 h, transition to PO anti-HTN meds if stable - Type B, complicated → Initially treat same as uncomplicated, with impulse control, but need endovascular (TEVAR) or open repair	**Thoracic endovascular aortic repair (TEVAR):** - Review 3D recon of CTA, need 2-cm landing zone above intimal tear, can usually cover left subclavian if needed - If placing long segment graft, have anesthesia place spinal drain - Drape neck to knees - Obtain bilateral percutaneous CFA access with ultrasound ○ CFA should be punctured in area overlying the femoral head, so that it can be compressed - Confirm placement of guidewire into true lumen with IVUS, place catheter, perform aortogram - Insert and deploy stent to cover proximal intimal tear - Evaluate mesenteric vessels and stent if needed - Perform completion angiogram - Close arteriotomies, check pulses	Complications s/p TEVAR: - LUE ischemia after covering left subclavian → subclavian-carotid bypass - Paraplegia after covering artery of Adamkiewicz → lumbar drain Uncomplicated dissection: follow-up CTA at 24 h, 7 d, then 6 wk to assess stability Post TEVAR: Follow-up CTA at 1, 6, and 12 mo, then annually	

Disease Process	Relevant H&P	Work-up/Staging	Treatment	Key Surgical Steps	Post-Op Care	Tips & Tidbits

Abdominal aortic aneurysm (AAA) (advanced)	Screening recommendations: one-time U/S screening for AAA in all patients 65-75 yo with history of tobacco use, men >55 yo with family history of AAA, and women > 65 yo who have smoked or have family history of AAA.
	
	Signs of rupture: sudden severe abdominal or back pain, hypotension, pulsating abdominal mass
	
	Rupture may be intra-abdominal vs retroperitoneal
		Normal abdominal aorta 2-2.5 cm
		
		Surveil known AAA with U/S at 6 mo, and then annually if stable
		
		Get CTA with 3D recon if planning to fix AAA electively
		
		If ruptured, permissive hypotension (allow SBP 70-80s if mentating appropriately), type and cross
		- U/S or CTA if stable vs straight to OR if unstable
		- Put up aortic balloon, if needed
			Criteria for elective repair: > 5.5 cm in men, > 5.0 cm in woman, or expanding > 0.5 cm/6 mo
			
			Endovascular aneurysm repair (EVAR) criteria:
			- Aneurysm neck at least 1-cm long, < 32-mm wide, and angulation < 60%
			- Iliacs must be > 6-8 mm in diameter and without significant tortuosity
			
			If unable to repair endovascularly, repair open
			
			Ruptured AAA may be approached endovascularly vs open depending on aneurysm characteristics
				Endovascular aortic repair (EVAR):
				- Look at CTA and choose appropriate graft
				- Access bilateral CFA, heparinize, perform aortogram
				- Mark out renal arteries
				- Insert main body of graft, taking care not to cover the renal arteries
				- Get wire access to the contralateral side gate and place contralateral limb
				- Balloon angioplasty to seal
				- Obtain completion angiogram and access for endoleaks, fix if needed
				- Close groins, check distal pulses
				
				Open AAA repair (advanced):
				- Midline laparotomy
				- Retract small bowel to the right and transverse colon up
				- Dissect duodenum off of aorta and define proximal clamping site
				- Dissect distal aorta/iliacs, get distal control
				- Choose appropriate graft size
				- Heparinize, clamp proximal aorta and iliacs
				- Open sac, oversew back bleeding (lumbar arteries)
				- Sew in graft
				- Reimplant IMA if needed (do not need to reimplant if completely occluded or if has very profuse flow, consider reimplantation if <35 mm Hg)
				- Close sac and retroperitoneum over graft
					Endoleaks:
					• Ia—proximal seal issue
					• Ib—distal seal issue
					• II—continued flow into sac from side branch
					• III—leak at junction
					• IV—pressure in sac from tiny holes in graft
					• V—mysterious "endotension"
					
					Complications:
					- Ischemic colitis after AAA repair
					  ○ More common after open AAA repair but can also happen after EVAR
					  ○ Presents as bloody diarrhea, and pain, and/or distention after AAA repair
					  ○ Endoscopy can be used to confirm diagnosis, evaluate severity
					  ○ Treat with supportive care (IV hydration, antibiotics, bowel rest, etc) unless there are signs of perforation/full thickness ischemia, in which case patient should go to OR
					
					CTA at 1 and 12 mo, then aortic duplex or CTA annually
						Annual risk of rupture based on AAA size:
						• 5-6 cm AAA → 2-5%
						• 6-7 cm → 3-10%
						• 7 cm → > 10%
						
						Risk of rupture is higher in female patients

Disease Process	Relevant H&P	Work-up/Staging	Treatment	Key Surgical Steps	Post-Op Care	Tips & Tidbits
Splenic artery aneurysm (SAA) (advanced)	Usually incidentally found, may have vague epigastric or LUQ pain Associated with pregnancy, portal HTN, post liver transplant Determine if patient is pregnant or planning on becoming pregnant When presenting with rupture, will often have "double rupture phenomenon" due to rupture into lesser sac, then free rupture into abdominal cavity	CTA Splenic artery arteriogram—can be diagnostic and therapeutic	Criteria for treatment: - Symptomatic SAAs - SAA > 2 cm - All SAA in pregnant women and women of childbearing age due to risk of rupture while pregnant Typically send to IR, but if patient is too unstable or unable to do it endovascularly, then they need to go to OR for ligation of SAA	**Endovascular SAA treatment:** - Retrograde puncture of right CFA - Catheterize celiac artery and get wire into splenic artery - Perform splenic artery arteriogram to identify aneurysm - Place covered stent to exclude aneurysm/embolize - Post-stent arteriogram for confirmation **Open ligation of splenic artery aneurysm:** - Left subcostal incision - Access lesser sac through the gastrohepatic ligament - Expose celiac artery and its branches, including the splenic artery - Get proximal and distal control of splenic artery and ligate - Assess viability of the spleen, perform splenectomy if it does not look viable	Splenectomy vaccines 2 wk pre- or post-op: • Strep pneumoniae • H. influenzae • Neisseria meningitidis	Visceral artery pseudoaneurysms—can develop after pancreatitis, trauma, or instrumentation Indications for intervention for other types of visceral aneurysms: - Celiac, SMA and hepatic artery aneurysms >2 cm - Symptomatic aneurysms - Visceral artery pseudoaneurysms
Thoracic outlet syndrome (TOS) (advanced)	Arm swelling, numbness, and pain More common in patients with repetitive arm movement (painters, pitchers, swimmers) Neurogenic TOS (nTOS)—compression of brachial plexus leads to upper extremity numbness and weakness, aggravated by repeated overhead movement, accounts for 95% of cases of TOS Venous TOS (vTOS, Paget-Schroetter syndrome)—venous compression causes DVT, extremity swelling, accounts for 3% of TOS Arterial TOS (aTOS)—arterial compression leads to thrombosis, distal thromboembolism, and arm pain with exertion ("claudication")	Duplex to evaluate for vTOS and aTOS CXR—look for cervical rib CTA—better delineate anatomy Electrophysiological evaluation indicated if nTOS suspected, poor sensitivity Thoracic outlet anatomy (Figure 6.4)	nTOS—4-6 wk of physical therapy, can also try scalene Botox injections vTOS—anticoagulation, thrombolysis to reestablish venous patency, surgery to decompress thoracic outlet and prevent reocclusion aTOS—anticoagulation, thrombolysis/thrombectomy, thoracic outlet decompression, fasciotomy if needed for compartment syndrome Surgery for thoracic outlet decompression is indicated for patients with aTOS and vTOS, as well as patients with significant nTOS refractory to nonoperative management	**Thoracic outlet decompression:** - Multiple approaches including transaxillary, supraclavicular, and infraclavicular - Choice of approach depends on type of decompression and surgeon preference - Decompression may entail first/extra rib resection, scalenectomy, vascular reconstruction and/or brachial plexus neurolysis		

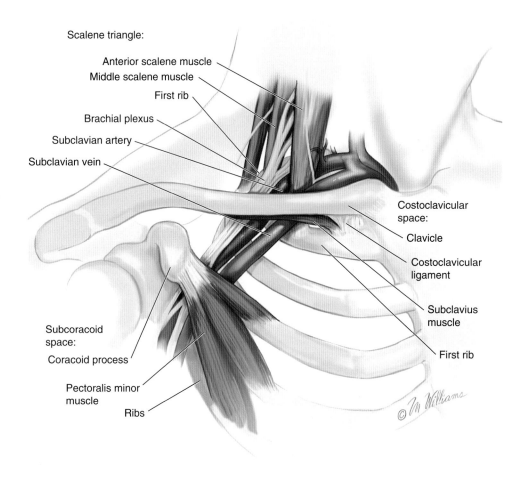

FIGURE 6.4: Anatomy of the thoracic outlet. (Reproduced with permission from Sugarbaker DJ, Bueno R, Burt BM, et al. *Sugarbaker's Adult Chest Surgery*, 3rd ed. New York, NY: McGraw Hill; 2020, Figure 144-2.)

Disease Process	Relevant H&P	Work-up/Staging	Treatment	Key Surgical Steps	Post-Op Care	Tips & Tidbits
Graft infection, graft-enteric fistula (advanced)	Patient with history of vascular graft presents with unexplained sepsis, failure to thrive, malaise, erythema/cellulitis in the area, anastomotic pseudoaneurysm, or draining sinus near incision Patient with history of AAA repair and GIB → concern for aorto-enteric fistula Infection may happen due to direct contamination, graft erosion, or seeding when patient is bacteremic Graft infection may lead to systemic infection, anastomotic disruption, graft thrombosis, or graft bleeding issues	Full labs, blood cultures U/S of the area CTA—may see perigraft fluid and/or gas, loss of tissue planes, pseudoaneurysm If able, get tissue sample and cultures to confirm diagnosis - CT-guided aspiration of perigraft fluid collection - Most infections involve Staph but can also be due to GNR - Fungal graft infections less common, typically in immunosuppressed patients Urgent EGD if concern for aortoenteric fistula, usually involves third or fourth part of duodenum	Broad spectrum antibiotics +/- antifungal Debridement for source control Staged graft excision and extra-anatomic revascularization (ie, axillofemoral bypass, bifemoral bypass) is the conventional treatment of graft infections, especially in cases with extensive contamination - Patient with aortoenteric fistula will need axillofemoral bypass, then graft excision Graft excision and in situ reconstruction using autologous femoral vein, antibiotic impregnated graft or cryopreserved graft may be acceptable in cases with minimal contamination Endovascular temporizing measures can be used to delay open repair, especially in acutely unstable patients Graft preservation/local therapy can be performed in patients without sepsis or anastomotic involvement Some patients with chronic graft infections require lifelong suppressive therapy	**Axillo-bifemoral bypass (advanced):** - Expose axillary artery from infraclavicular approach - Make transverse incision 1-2 cm inferior to clavicle from just lateral to the sternal head of the clavicle extending to upper deltopectoral groove - Clavipectoral fascia incised transversely and pec major muscle fibers are split, separating sternal and clavicular heads - Axillary artery should be exposed and controlled for 3-5 cm - Expose femoral arteries bilaterally - Select conduit material, usually 8-mm ringed PTFE - Tunnel from axillary artery to ipsilateral femoral artery along anterior axillary line, then from ipsilateral femoral artery to contralateral femoral artery - Heparinize - Create axillary anastomosis in end to side fashion as medial as possible (where artery does not move as much with arm abduction) - Create femoral anastomoses - Unclamp and check signals **Sartorius flap:** - Use a sartorius flap for soft tissue coverage in cases of groin infection - Sartorius muscle exposed lateral to the femoral vessels - Divide sartorius proximally from its attachment to the ASIS - Mobilize medially without tension and suture in place overlying femoral vessels (Figure 6.5)	Graft surveillance is important to assess patency and ensure there is no evidence of recurrent graft infection - ABI and bypass duplex should be obtained q3-4mo during first year, then q6-12mo - Axillo-bifemoral primary patency is 60-70% at 5 y	

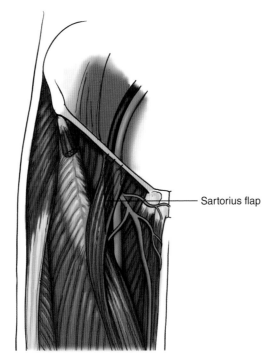

Sartorius flap

FIGURE 6.5: Sartorius flap. (Reproduced with permission from Feliciano DV, Mattox KL, Moore EE. *Trauma*, 9th ed. New York, NY: McGraw Hill; 2021, Figure 74.)

Disease Process	Relevant H&P	Work-up/Staging	Treatment	Key Surgical Steps	Post-Op Care	Tips & Tidbits
Femoral artery pseudoaneurysm (PSA)	Pulsatile groin mass, recent groin access/operation, skin changes, limb ischemia Rupture can lead to hemodynamic instability Assess peripheral pulses, examine recent access sites and incisions	Typically diagnosed with groin duplex U/S CTA if diagnosis unclear	U/S-guided compression may be attempted if PSA is <2 cm, less successful if patient is anticoagulated U/S-guided thrombin injection is an option if PSA has a fairly long, narrow neck Can treat endovascularly with coil embolization and/or stent Surgical repair indicated if: - Extensive skin necrosis requiring debridement - Infection suspected - Arteriovenous fistula - Hemodynamic instability - Limb ischemia - Failed less invasive options	**Repair of femoral artery pseudoaneurysm:** - Cut down on CFA, be ready to apply digit pressure for hemorrhage control, if needed - Get proximal and distal control on the femoral artery ○ For large PSA and difficulty getting proximal control, can make retroperitoneal incision to get control of external iliac - Evacuate hematoma and define vessel wall, debride aneurysmal and nonviable tissue back to normal appearing vessel wall - Can close primarily or use a patch, if needed - If infected, treat with extra-anatomic bypass or autogenous patch with sartorius or gracilis muscle flap		Peripheral artery pseudoaneurysms can form after vascular access, IV drug injection, vasculitis, infection, or trauma

7

Trauma Surgery

Shelby Reiter, MD, and Danielle Hayes, MD

DISEASES AND CONDITIONS

- Initial assessment and management of a trauma patient (c)
- Penetrating neck injury (c)
- Penetrating chest injury (c)
- Subclavian artery injury
- Hollow viscus injury (c)
- Solid organ injury (c)
- Duodenal and pancreatic injuries (c)

- Diaphragmatic injury (c)
- Pelvic fracture, retroperitoneal hematoma (c)
- Upper urinary tract injuries (c)
- Lower urinary tract injuries (c)
- Extremity injury (a)
- Lower extremity compartment syndrome (c), fasciotomy (c)
- Traumatic brain injury (c)

- Burns (c), skin grafting (c)
- Frostbite and hypothermia (c)
- Geriatric trauma (c)
- Pediatric trauma (c)
- Trauma in pregnancy (c)

GENERAL TIPS FOR TRAUMA SCENARIOS

- In trauma cases, you MUST be able to efficiently and effectively go through the ATLS protocol.

- Practice talking succinctly through the primary survey until it rolls off your tongue.

- Do not send an unstable patient to the CT scanner.

(c) = core topic   (a) = advanced topic

Disease Process	Relevant H&P	Work-up/Staging	Treatment	Key Surgical Steps	Post-Op Care	Tips & Tidbits

Initial assessment and management of a trauma patient (core)	Mechanism? Penetrating vs blunt
	
	Primary survey—ABCDE—the starting point for every trauma patient
	
	Airway—Confirm patent airway
	- Early intubation in patients with unstable airway
	- If unable to establish an orotracheal or nasotracheal airway, perform a cricothyroidotomy
	
	Breathing—Confirm presence of bilateral, equal, breath sounds
	
	Circulation—Evaluate central pulses, BP, and HR
	- Ensure patient has appropriate access for resuscitation
	- Start initial resuscitation for hypotension, if indicated
	- Gain temporary hemorrhage control with manual compression, packing, or tourniquet, if needed
	
	Disability—Calculate GCS, evaluate for neuro deficits, maintain spine immobilization
	
	Exposure—Remove all clothing so that entire body can be evaluated
	
	Adjuncts to primary survey:
	- CXR
	- Pelvic XR
	- FAST—initial use was in blunt, hypotensive trauma patients, also helpful in penetrating trauma for cavitary triage
	  ○ eFAST includes pleural views to look for lung sliding and presence of PTX
	  ○ Need ~200 mL of abdominal free fluid for FAST to be positive
		Trauma labs: CBC, CMP, lipase/amylase, ABG, lactate, type and screen, coagulants, UDS
		
		Adjuncts to primary survey: CXR, pelvic XR, FAST
		
		Stable patients often go for a "trauma pan scan" which includes:
		- Noncontrast head CT
		- Noncontrast cervical spine CT
		  ○ Get CTA of the neck if concerned about BCVI
		- Chest CT with contrast (arterial phase)
		- Abdomen and pelvis CT with contrast (portal venous phase)
		
		You must be effective in identifying and treating these life-threatening diagnoses:
		- Obstructed airway
		- Tension pneumothorax (PTX)—may have hypotension, decreased breath sounds, tracheal deviation, JVD
		  ○ Diagnosis is based on clinical exam and you should not delay treatment to obtain imaging if clinical signs are present
		- Massive hemothorax (HTX)—hypotension, decreased breath sounds and opacification of hemithorax on CXR
		- Hemorrhagic shock—hypotension, tachycardia, and large amount of blood loss
		  ○ Large amount of blood loss may come from bleeding into abdomen, thoracic cavity, pelvis, retroperitoneum, thigh, and/or externally
		  ○ Localize and control source of hemorrhage
		  ○ Initiate resuscitation with early use of blood products
			In a hypotensive trauma patient, initiate resuscitation immediately
			- In some situations, starting with 1L of crystalloid may be acceptable; however, often times, early use of blood products is appropriate
			- Use balanced transfusion ratio with FFP, pRBC, and platelets in a 1:1:1 ratio (or whole blood)
			- Initiate massive transfusion protocol (MTP), if needed, for quick preparation and transfusion of uncrossed blood products
			- Give TXA within 3 h of injury in patient requiring large blood resuscitation
			- In some cases, allow for permissive hypotension, titrating based on mental status and presence of radial pulse, until definitive hemorrhage control obtained
			
			Resuscitative thoracotomy (RT) indicated for select group of trauma patients—consider mechanism, location of injury, duration of cardiac arrest, and presence of signs of life:
			- Penetrating trauma: Pulseless patient or patient with profound shock with signs of life and/or CPR < 15 min, can consider RT*
			- Blunt trauma: Pulseless patient or patient with profound shock with signs of life in the ED and/or < 10 min CPR, can consider RT*
			- In patients with blunt trauma, if no signs of life are present and CPR has been ongoing for >10 min, successful ROSC unlikely, RT should not be performed
				Resuscitative thoracotomy:
				- Patient supine, left arm over the head
				- Incision is made in fourth or fifth ICS immediately below nipple or in inframammary fold, extending from midline all the way to the bed
				- Sharp dissection (scissors or scalpel) used to get through soft tissue and muscle into the thoracic cavity
				- Rib spreader (Finochietto retractor) placed with handle pointed down toward the left axilla to allow access to vital structures
				- Mobilize lung by dividing inferior pulmonary ligament
				- Pericardium opened vertically anterior to phrenic nerve to decompress hemopericardium and allow for control of cardiac injury and cardiac massage
				- Cross clamp the thoracic aorta to improve perfusion to heart and brain in cases of abdominal/pelvic hemorrhage
				- Incision can be extended to the right chest for improved exposure
				
				Damage control laparotomy (DCL):
				- Goals of DCL are to (1) control hemorrhage and (2) control contamination
				- Overarching goal is quick operation to allow for transfer to the ICU for ongoing resuscitation and correction of acidosis, hypothermia, and coagulopathy
				- Indications for use of damage control strategy include acidosis, hypothermia, and coagulopathy
				- Efficiently enter the abdomen, pack all quadrants and systematically explore the zones of the retroperitoneum and quadrants of the abdomen, control bleeding and bowel spillage
				- Abdomen is packed as needed for hemorrhage control and left open with negative pressure dressing
						Major misstep: waiting to get a CXR when a patient is exhibiting signs of a tension pneumothorax
						
						Additional reading:
						
						Western Trauma Association guidelines regarding RT: Moore EE, WTA Study Group. Defining the limits of resuscitative emergency department thoracotomy: a contemporary Western Trauma Association perspective. *J Trauma.* 2011 Feb;70(2):334-339.
						
						Eastern Association for the Surgery of Trauma guidelines regarding RT: Seamon MJ, et al. An evidence-based approach to patient selection for emergency department thoracotomy: a practice management guideline from the Eastern Association for the Surgery of Trauma. *J Trauma Acute Care Surg.* 2015 Jul;79(1):159-173.

Disease Process	Relevant H&P	Work-up/Staging	Treatment	Key Surgical Steps	Post-Op Care	Tips & Tidbits

Initial assessment and management of a trauma patient (core) (*Cont.*)	If at any time you do an intervention during the primary survey (ie, place chest tube, intubate patient, etc), restart the primary survey from the top
	Secondary exam—once primary survey complete and any immediately life-threatening issues are dealt with, do a full head-to-toe exam, including rolling the patient, to make a full inventory of the patient's injuries
		- Pericardial tamponade—hypotension, muffled heart sounds, JVD
		  ∘ Hemopericardium can be identified on FAST, however, may not be apparent if blood is decompressing into the pleural space
		- High cervical spinal cord injury—patient with hypotension and bradycardia
		  ∘ Diagnosed on exam with absent distal motor function and sensation
		- Severe TBI—patient may present with labile BP and HR
		  ∘ Diagnosed by exam, and CT scan
			- Patients most likely to benefit from RT are those who present after penetrating thoracic trauma with signs of life and <15 min CPR
			*Per Western Trauma Association guidelines
			REBOA is an alternative to RT, can decrease hemorrhage in noncompressible cavities, especially the pelvis, and act as a bridge to OR or IR
			Unstable patient's with abdominal trauma are taken for damage control laparotomy			

Penetrating neck injury (core)	Initial evaluation per ATLS - High likelihood a patient with significant neck injury will need to be intubated "Hard signs" of vascular or aerodigestive injury mandate operative exploration - Pulsatile bleeding - Expanding hematoma - Hypotension - Audible bruit or palpable thrill - Loss of distal pulse - Neurologic deficit - Air bubbling from wound - Significant subcutaneous emphysema - Stridor, airway compromise - Hoarseness, difficulty swallowing On exam, determine whether the wound violates the platysma Control hemorrhage—use digital pressure, can also place a Foley balloon in wound tract and inflate for hemorrhage coming from area not amenable to digital pressure	Cervical XR, CXR Hard signs of vascular or aerodigestive injury → OR for operative exploration If no hard signs, but violates the platysma → CTA of the neck, then EGD/esophagogram and bronchoscopy/laryngoscopy, as needed Neck zones - Zone I—sternal notch to cricoid cartilage - Zone II—cricoid cartilage to angle of the mandible - Zone III—angle of the mandible to the base of the skull	If wound doesn't violate platysma → washout and close Neck exploration, if indicated	**Neck exploration:** - Extend neck and turn head to contralateral side - Incision along anterior border of SCM (line from ear lobe to sternal notch) - Dissect down through subcutaneous tissue and platysma, posterolateral retraction of the SCM → expose carotid sheath - Ligate and divide middle thyroid vein and facial vein - Open carotid sheath and evaluate for injury - If concerned for esophageal injury, dissect around esophagus, encircle with Penrose drain to retract and examine, avoid injury the RLN		Patients with penetrating neck injury do not need a C collar unless there is clinical suspicion of SCI injury as it tends to get in the way Blunt cerebrovascular injury (BVCI)—patients with the following findings should be screened for BCVI with a CTA of the neck: - C spine or basilar skull fractures - High-energy mechanism - Near-hanging - Direct blow to the neck - Significant neck soft tissue injury - Horner syndrome - Le Fort II/III fractures - Diffuse axonal injury

Disease Process	Relevant H&P	Work-up/Staging	Treatment	Key Surgical Steps	Post-Op Care	Tips & Tidbits

Penetrating chest trauma (core)	Stab wound or GSW to the chest
	
	Initial evaluation per ATLS
	
	"The cardiac box"—bordered by sternal notch superiorly, xiphoid process inferiorly, and nipples laterally
	- High risk for cardiac injury in patients with wound in "the box"
	- Cardiac injury can still occur with wounds outside the box
		CXR—PTX? HTX? Mediastinal widening?
		FAST—subxiphoid view to look for pericardial effusion, can also do lung windows to look for PTX
		Transmediastinal GSW:
		- CXR, pericardial U/S
		- Place chest tube if needed
		- CTA, if stable
		- Bronchoscopy, EGD/esophagram, thoracotomy/sternotomy, pericardial window PRN
		Stab to "the box"—rule out cardiac injury
		- Pericardial view with U/S
		  ○ If equivocal, proceed with pericardial window
		  ○ Pericardial U/S may be falsely negative in setting of cardiac injury if blood is decompressing into pleural space
		  ○ RV is most anterior portion of heart, most likely to be injured with an anterior stab
		Injury to the thoracic vessels—CTA chest is useful screening test for stable patients with concern for thoracic vessel injury
		- Aortic injury may present with hypotension, unequal arm BP, widened mediastinum and/or indistinct aortic notch on CXR
			Resuscitation
			Profound shock/loss of vitals in the trauma bay → resuscitative thoracotomy
			Cardiac injury—OR ASAP for repair
			- Pericardiocentesis can be used as a temporizing measure if immediate surgical intervention not possible
			- Complex cardiac injuries involving cardiac valves or atrial/ventricular septa usually require cardiopulmonary bypass for repair
			Injury to the thoracic vessels
			- Patients with penetrating thoracic vessel injury typically present unstable and require operative repair via left anterolateral thoracotomy, clamshell, or median sternotomy
			Hemothorax/Pneumothorax—place chest tube first, thoracotomy indicated if:
			- >1.5 L blood out initially
			- >250 mL bloody drainage/h x 3-4 h
			- >2 L bloody drainage/24 h
			- Hemodynamic instability, signs of ongoing surgical bleeding
			- Massive air leak
			- Drainage of esophageal contents from the chest tube
			Lung injury—may present as HTX or PTX
			- Many parenchyma lung injuries do not require any intervention other than a chest tube
				Thoracotomy incisions and exposures:
				- Left anterolateral thoracotomy → exposure of pericardium, left lung, descending aorta
				  ○ Preferred incision for exploring hemodynamically unstable patient
				  ○ Excellent exposure to left pleural space and anterior mediastinum but poor exposure of posterior structures
				  ○ Can be extended as a clamshell for access to contralateral side
				- Clamshell thoracotomy → access to both sides of the chest
				- Median sternotomy → excellent exposure of heart, great vessels, good for isolated cardiac injuries
				- Left posterolateral → exposure left pulmonary hilum, descending aorta
				- Right posterolateral → exposes right lung hilum, esophagus
				
				Subxiphoid pericardial window, repair of cardiac injury:
				- Avoid intubation until you are prepped and ready, as patient can code on induction
				- Make upper midline incision adjacent to the xyphoid
				- Incise the linea alba, entering the preperitoneal space, but do not enter the abdomen
				- Xyphoid excised and sternum retracted upward so that cardiophrenic fat pad can be visualized
				- Bluntly dissect the fat pad away and grab the pericardium with 2 graspers
				- Suction the field to ensure it is dry prior to entering the pericardium
				- Make incision into the pericardium
				  ○ If the fluid that comes from the pericardium is clear, this is negative
				  ○ If fluid that comes from the pericardium is bloody, this is considered positive, proceed with median sternotomy
				- Median sternotomy
				- Open the pericardium vertically, avoid injury to phrenic nerves
					Retained HTX—persistent HTX despite chest tube placement
					- Get CT if concerned for retained HTX based on CXR
					- If still within first 24 h, placing a second chest tube can help drain significant retained hemothorax can lead to posttraumatic empyema and fibrothorax with trapped lung
					- Small HTX (<300 mL) can typically be observed, but if >300 mL, likely needs VATS for evacuation of retained HTX
					
					Persistent air leak, bronchopleural/alveolar-pleural fistula
					- Leak that continues beyond 5-7 d
					- Perform bronchoscopy if concerned for major airway injury
					- Challenging to manage
					  ○ Ventilated patient—may have significant loss of tidal volumes, minimize airway pressures
					  ○ Can try autologous blood pleurodesis, endobronchial one-way valves, Heimlich valves
					  ○ Operative intervention may be needed
						CXR has low sensitivity in the diagnosis of a pneumothorax, missing up to 50%, whereas eFAST has 86-100% sensitivity
						
						Rib fractures—significant rib fractures more common with blunt trauma
						- Often have underlying pulmonary contusion
						- Flail chest: 2+ contiguous rib fractures with 2+ fractures per rib
						- At risk for pneumonia, respiratory failure, need for intubation
						- Require multimodal pain control, good pulmonary hygiene
						- Some patients with significant fractures may benefit from operative fixation

Disease Process	Relevant H&P	Work-up/Staging	Treatment	Key Surgical Steps	Post-Op Care	Tips & Tidbits
Penetrating chest trauma (core) (*Cont.*)		Tracheobronchial injury—classic presentation of a distal tracheal/proximal bronchial injury is large PTX and significant air leak/persistent PTX after placing chest tube - May require direct laryngoscopy, bronchoscopic-guided intubation, or surgical airway to establish secure airway	- More extensive injuries require surgical intervention: ◦ Simple primary repair (pneumorrhaphy)—generally used to treat superficial pulmonary lacerations ◦ Wedge resection—peripheral lacerations not amenable to simple repair can be treated by wedge resection with stapler ◦ Pulmonary tractotomy—used to address through and through injuries, stapler inserted into tract and fired to open the tract so that bleeding vessels and damaged airways can be oversewn ◦ Nonanatomic and formal anatomic resections may be needed for more extensive injuries ◦ Hilar injuries—patient typically in hemorrhagic shock ▪ Rarely amenable to direct repair, may require pneumonectomy—in a trauma patient, this is a last resort, very high mortality rate	- Can typically repair cardiac injury with 3-0 Prolene horizontal mattress sutures with pledgets - Injury adjacent to coronary artery is repaired with deep mattress sutures passing underneath the vessel to avoid ligation of the coronary artery - Alternatively, pericardial window can be done through the transdiaphragmatic approach if you are already in the abdomen **Surgical management of tracheobronchial injury:** - Bronchoscopy can be used to help localize injury - Distal half of the trachea, right mainstem bronchus, and proximal left mainstem bronchus are best approached through right posterolateral thoracotomy - Distal left mainstem bronchus accessed via left posterolateral thoracotomy - Place ETT in contralateral mainstem bronchus during repair of mainstem bronchus - Repair tracheal injury with interrupted absorbable sutures, cover with tissue flap		

Disease Process	Relevant H&P	Work-up/Staging	Treatment	Key Surgical Steps	Post-Op Care	Tips & Tidbits

Subclavian artery injury	Penetrating or blunt injury
	
	Initial evaluation per ATLS
	
	Evaluate for hard signs of vascular injury in upper extremity
	
	Check brachial-brachial index (BBI)
	
	Hemorrhage control—difficult area to control hemorrhage due to inability to put direct pressure
		Full trauma labs
		
		CXR
		
		CTA neck/chest if stable and concerned for subclavian or other major vessel injury
		- CTA indicated in stable patient with abnormal BBI
		- Make sure contrast is given in side contralateral to injury
		
		Can perform on table angiogram to further characterize injury if in hybrid OR
			Transfuse as needed
			
			Immediate operative intervention for unstable patients with subclavian injury
			
			Can consider endovascular intervention in stable patient with contained injury
			- Blunt injury is typically more amenable to endovascular repair
				Subclavian artery repair:
				- Prep neck to knees, may need to harvest GSV
				- Exposure—subclavian artery exposure can be difficult!
				  ◦ Proximal subclavian artery exposure via median sternotomy (tends to be best) or anterolateral thoracotomy (if patient is unstable)
				  ◦ Make infra-clavicular extension and resect part of the clavicle for additional exposure of subclavian artery and distal control
				    ▪ Exposure of most distal part of the subclavian does not require clavicle resection
				  ◦ Trap door—anterolateral thoracotomy + median sternotomy + clavicular incision
				    ▪ This incision is time-consuming and morbid
				- Once you have proximal and distal control, define the injury, debride nonviable tissue
				- Primary repair vs vein patch vs interposition graft with ringed PTFE
				- Can usually ligate concomitant venous injury
				- Replace clavicle fragment at end of case or freeze it for later if patient unstable
					If subclavian vein was ligated, monitor for forearm compartment syndrome	

Disease Process	Relevant H&P	Work-up/Staging	Treatment	Key Surgical Steps	Post-Op Care	Tips & Tidbits

Hollow viscus injuries (core)	Initial evaluation per ATLS
	
	Signs that should raise concern for hollow viscus injury
	- Peritonitis—may be minimal to absent for the first several hours
	- Seatbelt sign
	- Handlebar marks
	- Bloody NGT output
	- Blood on DRE
	
	Colorectal injury may be intra or extraperitoneal
	- Intraperitoneal injuries more likely to present with peritonitis
	- Extra/retroperitoneal injuries more likely to present with abscess and/or sepsis if not identified early
		Full trauma labs, CXR, pelvic XR, FAST CT scan
		- Obtain CT in stable patient—free fluid in the absence of solid organ injury, pneumoperitoneum, bowel wall hypoperfusion, mesenteric fat stranding, inter loop fluid, and air in the mesentery should raise suspicion for bowel injury
		- If concerned for rectal injury based on mechanism, trajectory or exam and patient is stable, can consider also giving rectal contrast
		
		Penetrating abdominal trauma:
		- If unsure if penetrating wound violated the abdomen perform local wound exploration → definite violation of the anterior fascia requires operative exploration for intra-abdominal injury
		  ◦ If local wound exploration is equivocal, consider serial exam and labs in a stable patient
		  ◦ If patient develops peritonitis, leukocytosis, or hemodynamic instability → exploratory laparotomy
		
		Blunt abdominal trauma:
		- Chance fractures (transverse fractures of L4) associated with shear injuries of the small bowel and/or colon
		- Rectal injuries commonly associated with pelvic fractures, lacerated by bony fragment
			Concern for hollow viscus injury → operative exploration	**Exploratory laparotomy:**
				- Examine entire GI tract, starting at the GEJ working down to the rectum
				  ◦ Can take down left triangular ligament to mobilize the left lobe of liver and provide better exposure of the GEJ
				- Repair of gastric injuries depends on severity and location
				  ◦ Most gastric injuries are amenable to primary repair or wedge gastrectomy, injuries involving the pylorus or GEJ are more complicated
				  ◦ GEJ injury may require primary repair vs gastrectomy with creation of a Roux-en-Y esophagojejunostomy
				  ◦ Pyloric injury—if amenable to primary closure, do so in Heineke-Mikulicz fashion to prevent GOO
				    ▪ Extensive pyloric injury may require resection with Billroth I/II reconstruction
				  ◦ If there is an anterior gastric injury, posterior stomach must be examined, which requires opening the lesser sac, and if there is a posterior gastric injury, the pancreas must be examined for injury
				- Examine small bowel from LOT to terminal ileum
				  ◦ Serosal injury → can usually imbricate
				  ◦ Injury <50% bowel circumference → primarily repair, be careful not to narrow
				  ◦ Injury >50% bowel circumference → resection and anastomosis
				  ◦ Full-thickness laceration to mesentery → close to prevent internal hernias, make sure blood supply to small bowel is not compromised
				  ◦ Bucket handle injury → resect involved bowel because it is devascularized
				  ◦ Devitalized tissue must be debrided and hematomas explored to assess for underlying perforation
				- Examine the colon and rectum
				  ◦ If rectal injury suspected, patient should be placed in lithotomy
				  ◦ Blood on a DRE → concern for colorectal injury → evaluate with sigmoidoscopy
				  ◦ Important to mobilize the colon and expose the retroperitoneal portions
				  ◦ Intraperitoneal colorectal injuries:
				    ▪ Injury <50% bowel circumference → can usually primarily repair, be careful not to narrow
				    ▪ Injury >50% → resection and anastomosis vs ostomy depending on patient condition (hemodynamic status, blood loss, concomitant injuries, etc)
				  ◦ Extraperitoneal rectal injuries:
				    ▪ Fecal diversion with loop or end colostomy
				    ▪ Presacral drainage is a thing of the past and is no longer indicated!
						Esophageal injuries—see "Esophageal perforation" section in foregut chapter
						
						Major misstep: Do NOT create primary bowel anastomosis in unstable patient, just control contamination and leave abdomen open, return for second look when stabilized

Disease Process	Relevant H&P	Work-up/Staging	Treatment	Key Surgical Steps	Post-Op Care	Tips & Tidbits

Solid organ injury (core)	Initial evaluation per ATLS
	
	Most commonly injured organs with blunt abdominal trauma are liver and spleen
		Full trauma labs
		FAST Exam
		CXR, pelvic XR
		If stable, obtain trauma pan scan
			Liver or spleen laceration:
			- If stable and no extravasation on CT → nonoperative management
			  ∘ Monitor closely with serial abdominal exams, serial Hgb/Hct, bed rest, hold DVT prophylaxis
			- If extravasation seen on CT, but relatively stable → IR for embolization
			- Unstable → OR
				Techniques for controlling liver bleeding:
				- Pack around the liver to compress it together, do not pack into lacerations
				- Pringle Maneuver: transiently occlude the portal vein and hepatic artery in the hepatoduodenal ligament to differentiate liver bleeding from hepatic vein/IVC injury
				  ∘ Ongoing bleeding coming from behind the liver, despite Pringle maneuver, is likely a retro-hepatic IVC or hepatic vein injury
				- Reapproximate fractured liver capsule with 0 chromic on blunt needle, can include omental plug
				- Use hemostatic agents, cautery, argon beam, etc to help achieve hemostasis
				- Resect pulverized/devascularized liver if present
				
				Trauma Splenectomy:
				- Laparotomy
				- Pack the abdomen
				- Open the lesser sac, take down the splenic flexure of the colon
				- Mobilize spleen by taking down lateral attachments
				- Divide the short gastric arteries, taking care to avoid damaging the stomach
				- Staple across the vascular pedicle (avoid tail of the pancreas)
				- Leave drain in LUQ selectively (ie, if concerned about pancreatic injury)
					If patient had splenectomy, ensure they receive appropriate vaccines prior to discharge
					
					Complications:
					- Bile leak after liver injury—may present with abdominal pain, distention, ascites, fever
					  ∘ Treat with drainage, +/- ERCP with stent
					- Hemobilia after liver injury is due to arteriobiliary fistula
					  ∘ Treat with embolization
					- Hepatic necrosis can occur after liver injury due to devasularized tissue
					- Pancreatic fistula after splenectomy—relatively common due to proximity of pancreatic tail to splenic hilum
					  ∘ Treat with drainage, +/- ERCP with stent	

Disease Process	Relevant H&P	Work-up/Staging	Treatment	Key Surgical Steps	Post-Op Care	Tips & Tidbits

Duodenal and pancreatic injuries (core)	Initial evaluation per ATLS
	
	May present with epigastric pain, N/V
	- Initial symptoms may be minimal, if confined to retroperitoneum
	
	Blunt trauma—direct blow to the epigastrium (ie, handlebar of bike, steering wheel)
	
	Severity of duodenal injury can range from intramural hematoma to uncontained rupture
		Full trauma labs
		- Initial serum amylase is not sensitive or specific enough to confirm or rule out pancreatic injury
		- Serum amylase that remains elevated or rises during period of observation mandates further evaluation
		
		CT pan scan if stable
		
		MRCP or ERCP can be used to further evaluate pancreatic injury
			Duodenal injuries
			- Important factors to consider when choosing technique for duodenal repair:
			  ○ Patient stability
			  ○ Degree of duodenal tissue loss
			  ○ Relationship of the injury to the ampulla
			  ○ Concomitant pancreas injury?
			- Isolated blunt duodenal hematoma—can cause obstruction
			  ○ Manage nonoperatively: NGT, TPN, will usually resolve within 3 wk
			- Full thickness perforation
			  ○ Primary repair, if possible—suture repair of injuries with minimal tissue loss
			    ■ Use pedicle of omentum to buttress repair
			  ○ Roux-en-Y side-to-end duodenojejunostomy ("sucker patch")—for injuries not amenable to primary repair
			  ○ Thal/serosal patch—for duodenal injury not amenable to primary repair
			  ○ Pyloric exclusion—can be used as adjunct to suboptimal duodenal repair
			- Injury involving ampulla or distal CBD, massive disruption of duodenopancreatic complex, devascularization of the duodenum → pancreatoduodenectomy
			
			Pancreatic injuries
			- Low grade (I/II) pancreatic injuries seen on CT can be managed nonoperatively
			  ○ Operative management of low-grade injuries
			    ■ If already intra-op, can leave drain and cover with omental flap
				Exploration to evaluate for duodenal injury:
				- Medial mobilization of ascending colon and hepatic flexure
				- Extensive Kocher maneuver → exposes D2/3
				- LOT divided from lateral to medial to mobilize duodenojejunal junction → allows for visualization of D4 and anterior D3, posterior D3 can be palpated
				- Cattell-Braasch maneuver can be performed to improve visualization of posterior D3, if this is necessary to complete a duodenal repair
				  ○ Ascending colon and hepatic flexure mobilized medially
				  ○ Retroperitoneal attachments of the mesentery of small bowel are sharply divided from RLQ to duodenojejunal junction
				  ○ With evisceration of small bowel to the left, D3 and D4 can be visualized
				
				Exploration to evaluate for pancreatic injury:
				- Medial mobilization of ascending colon and hepatic flexure
				- Extensive Kocher maneuver → allows for visualization of the anterior and posterior aspects of the head and neck of the pancreas
				- Open lesser sac to visualize anterior aspect of the pancreatic body
				- If concerned for injury to posterior body, divide retroperitoneal attachments to the inferior border of the pancreas (avoid the IMV and splenic vein), gently elevate inferior border of the pancreas to visualize the posterior body
				- Divide splenorenal and splenocolic ligaments to elevate and medially mobilize spleen and tail of the pancreas
				- Hematoma of the pancreas should always be opened—could be hiding an injury
				- Intraoperative cholangiopancreatogram can be used to assess integrity of main pancreatic duct:
				  ○ Pediatric feeding tube inserted into cystic duct
				  ○ Anesthesiologist gives fentanyl to cause spasm of the sphincter of Oddi
				  ○ Inject contrast and assess duct
				  ○ Perform cholecystectomy
					Post-op pancreatic fistula—defined as drain output with amylase level > 3x upper limit of normal
					- CT scan to look for undrained collections—fluid adjacent to cut edge of the pancreas or pancreatojejunostomy → percutaneous drain
					- Antibiotic therapy if fluid culture positive
					- Nutrition—enteral nutrition via J tube, can try oral diet if fistula is low output
					- Persistent high-volume pancreatic fistula can be managed with ERCP, sphincterotomy, and placement of stent through sphincterotomy into pancreatic duct
					
					Duodenal fistula
					- Diagnose with CT with PO contrast
					- Treatment: percutaneous drain, NPO, TPN, +/- octreotide
					
					Risk of developing diabetes after pancreatectomy, especially after distal pancreatectomy
						Injuries to this area are notoriously difficult to manage for multiple reasons:
						- Shared blood supply of duodenal C-loop and head of pancreas
						- Isolated injuries to the duodenum and pancreas are rare, often have associated vascular and visceral injuries
						- Proximity of major blood vessels

Disease Process	Relevant H&P	Work-up/Staging	Treatment	Key Surgical Steps	Post-Op Care	Tips & Tidbits

Duodenal and pancreatic injuries (core) (*Cont.*)			- Can attempt ERCP with stent placement for main pancreatic duct injury in otherwise stable patient
			- Significant injury to pancreatic tail, transection of main duct to the left of the SMV → distal pancreatectomy, splenectomy
			- Pancreatic injury noted during damage control operation—control peri-pancreatic hemorrhage, leave drains, reassess on second look
			- Massive disruption of head of the pancreas, devascularization of C-loop of the duodenum, or destruction of the ampulla of Vater → pancreatoduodenectomy
			  ○ Timing depends on patient's hemodynamic status, physiologic state, and associated injuries
			  ○ Often requires use of staged procedures
			    ■ If patient unstable, control leak and return later when patient stabilized to do pancreatoduodenectomy
			    ■ It may be possible to do resection portion of pancreatoduodenectomy at the first operation, then come back for reconstruction when patient is stabilized
				Pyloric exclusion with gastrojejunostomy (Figure 7.1):
				- Duodenal perforation is closed primarily or Malecot drain is secured in duodenotomy and brought out through the skin
				- Skeletonize ~10 cm of the distal greater curve of the stomach
				- Close pylorus by firing TA stapler across pylorus or can make anterior gastrotomy and sew pylorus closed from inside with purse string, use permanent suture
				- Create antecolic gastrojejunostomy
				- Place J-tube
				- Majority of pyloric exclusions open spontaneously within 14-21 d
				
				Roux-en-Y side-to-end duodenojejunostomy:
				- Debride duodenal injury back to healthy tissue
				- Transect jejunum ~30 cm distal to LOT to create jejunal Roux limb, which is passed through avascular area of the right transverse mesocolon and brought up to the duodenal hole
				- Create 2-layer side-to-end duodenojejunostomy at site of the duodenal defect, leave drains		

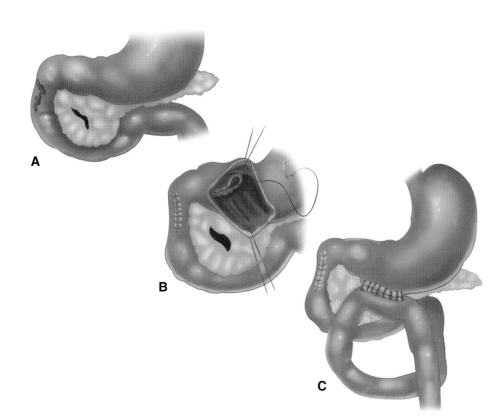

FIGURE 7.1: Primary repair of duodenal injury with pyloric exclusion and gastrojejunostomy creation. (Reproduced with permission from Brunicardi F, Andersen DK, Billiar TR, et al. *Schwartz's Principles of Surgery,* 11th ed. New York, NY: McGraw Hill; 2019, Figure 7-66.)

Disease Process	Relevant H&P	Work-up/Staging	Treatment	Key Surgical Steps	Post-Op Care	Tips & Tidbits

Diaphragmatic injuries (core)	Initial evaluation per ATLS
	
	May be noted on imaging work-up or present with symptoms due to contents herniated in chest
		CT scan—not all diaphragmatic injuries seen on CT scan, if you have high suspicion but CT is nondiagnostic, do a diagnostic laparoscopy
		
		Commonly have associated thoracoabdominal injuries—gastric, spleen, liver, lung
			Left-sided—should always be repaired
			
			Right-sided—herniation limited by liver, small defects may not require repair
				Diaphragmatic Hernia Repair:
				- Can be approached via laparotomy, laparoscopy, or thoracoscopy
				  ○ Typically approach from the abdomen in acute trauma situation so that other intra-abdominal injuries can be addressed
				- Identify location of phrenic nerve and avoid injury
				- Debride devitalized edges
				- Small defects can be repaired primarily with 0-prolene
				- Large defects may require bridging mesh
				- Place chest tube on affected side to address post-op pneumothorax or effusion
					Complications:
					- Phrenic nerve injury— elevated hemidiaphragm
					  ○ Most cases of unilateral phrenic nerve injury do not require intervention
					  ○ In severe cases, in patients with significant respiratory compromise diaphragmatic plication or pacing may be needed to improve function
						Missed diaphragm injury can lead to herniated hollow viscus incarceration, strangulation, and perforation

Disease Process	Relevant H&P	Work-up/Staging	Treatment	Key Surgical Steps	Tips & Tidbits

Pelvic fractures, Retroperitoneal hematomas (core)	Blunt etiology of pelvic fractures more common than penetrating
	
	Examine patient for:
	- Pelvic stability
	- Flank ecchymosis, umbilical ecchymosis (Cullen sign), proximal thigh ecchymosis, or scrotal ecchymosis, which can be signs of retroperitoneal hematoma
	- Signs of associated genitourinary injury (blood at urethral meatus, high-riding prostate, etc)
	- Patients with certain pelvic fractures should have vaginal and rectal exam to make sure no concomitant lacerations
		Full trauma labs
		
		Obtain portable AP pelvic XR for all blunt trauma patients—identify significant pelvic fractures, especially displaced and open-book fractures that would benefit from pelvic binder
		
		Perform FAST exam
		- Unstable, hypotensive patient with + FAST → OR
		- FAST is not a good tool to rule out RP hemorrhage
		
		Stable patient → CT is gold standard for evaluating pelvic trauma and RP hematomas
		
		Identify retroperitoneal zones:
		- Zone I (central): contains the major vessels (aorta, IVC)
		- Zone II (lateral): contains renal vessels and kidneys
		- Zone III (pelvis): contains iliac vessels
		
		CT may demonstrate hematoma or blush in any of the zones
		
		Gross hematuria associated with pelvic fracture → CT cystogram to eval for bladder injury (up to 15% of pelvic fractures have associated bladder injury)
			Initiate resuscitation in unstable patient
			
			Stabilize unstable pelvic fractures to control hemorrhage (pelvic binder, ex fix), ortho consult
			
			IR embolization or preperitoneal pelvic packing for hemorrhage control in patients with ongoing pelvic bleeding
			- IR embolization can be considered in:
			 ○ Patients who respond to initial transfusion but show evidence of active extravasation on CT
			 ○ Patients with ongoing transfusion requirement but hemodynamic stability
			 ○ Patients with persistent bleeding after preperitoneal pelvic packing
			- Unstable patient, unresponsive to initial resuscitation → OR for preperitoneal packing
			- REBOA can be placed in unstable patients as a temporizing measure until IR/OR
			
			Once in the OR:
			- Preperitoneal packing
			- Identify RP zones and know which injuries require exploration
			- Repair of associated genitourinary or rectal injuries
				Operative management of retroperitoneal hematomas:
				- Zone I—aorta and IVC
				- All zone I hematomas should be explored (blunt and penetrating)
				 ○ Extensive exposure of the entire aorta achieved with left medial visceral rotation (Mattox maneuver)
				 ○ Supraceliac aorta accessed by opening the gastrohepatic ligament
				 ○ Infrarenal aorta accessed by reflecting mesocolon cephalad, evisceration of small bowel to the right and incising through retroperitoneum overlying the aorta
				 ○ Subhepatic IVC exposure can be obtained with right medial visceral rotation (Cattell-Braasch maneuver)
				 ○ Control of bleeding at iliac vein bifurcation may require division of right common iliac artery
				 ○ Aortic repair depends on extent of injury:
				  ▪ Primary repair with 3-0 Prolene if possible without significant narrowing
				  ▪ Patch angioplasty
				  ▪ Interposition graft required in cases of significant tissue loss
				- Managment of IVC injury depends on location and patient stability
				- Primary repair if amenable
				 ○ Can ligate infra-renal IVC, if needed—will cause bilateral lower limb swelling, may require lower extremity fasciotomies
				 ○ Retro-hepatic IVC injuries— challeging injury, can attempt to manage with packing, avoid mobilizing liver to keep hematoma contained
				- Zone II—renal hilum and kidneys
				 ○ Must explore if penetrating and/or expanding
				 ○ Unstable patient with renal artery transection → nephrectomy (confirm normal contralateral kidney)
				 ○ Renal artery injury in stable patient → can attempt repair
				 ○ Renal vein injury—renal vein ligation without nephrectomy can be performed on the left (collateral venous flow), but if right renal vein is ligated patient will need nephrectomy (can do at secondary operation in setting of damage control)
				- Zone III—pelvic vessels
				 ○ Preperitoneal packing:
				  ▪ Lower midline incision, keep peritoneum intact and dissect the preperitoneal space (space is usually already dissected out by hematoma), evacuate hematoma, retract bladder out of the way, pack with laps, explore abdomen by opening peritoneum more cephalad if there is concern for intra-abdominal injury, temporary closure
				  ▪ Return to OR in 24-48 h to remove packs
				  ▪ If patient has refractory pelvic bleeding despite packs, consider taking to IR for embolization
				- Common iliac artery injury can be ligated if in extremis, will have collateral flow through internal iliac arteries
				- External iliac artery injuries must be reconstructed to prevent limb ischemia
				- Internal iliac artery injury—can ligate/embolize if unilateral, bilateral ligation/embolization can lead to pelvic ischemia
				- Consider extra-anatomical bypass for iliac artery injury if there is significant intra-abdominal contamination
					Retropertioneal hematomas that must be explored:
					- All zone I hematomas
					- All expanding hematomas
					- All penetrating retroperitoneal hematomas
					
					Some traumatic vascular injuries may be amenable to endovascular treatment in certain situations, however we would recommend sticking with the more traditional approach, unless you have extensive experience in endovascular management of traumatic injuries

Disease Process	Relevant H&P	Work-up/Staging	Treatment	Key Surgical Steps	Post-Op Care	Tips & Tidbits

Upper urinary tract injuries (kidneys and ureters) (core)	Initial evaluation per ATLS
	
	Renal injuries—blunt etiology much more common than penetrating
	
	Symptoms and signs of renal injury:
	- Hematuria, (gross or microscopic)
	- Flank ecchymosis or pain
	
	Ureteral injury—rarely due to trauma (penetrating more common than blunt), iatrogenic injury is more common (ie, ureteroscopy, hysterectomy, colectomy, etc)
	- It is best to recognize ureteral injury at the time it happens
	- Delayed recognition may present as hematuria, fever, ileus, high drain output with elevated creatinine, worsening renal function
		Trauma labs including UA
		
		CT A/P with IV contrast with delayed phase images
		
		Stable blunt trauma patients with gross hematuria, microscopic hematuria with RBCs > 100/hpf, or mechanism of exam findings concerning for renal injury should have CT to eval for GU injury
		
		There is AAST renal injury scale (grade I-V)
		
		Diagnosing a ureteral injury:
		- Retrograde pyelogram is the most accurate test to evaluate location and extent of injury
		- CT A/P with IV contrast and delayed images in patient with ureteral injury may demnonstrate
		  ∘ Perinephric stranding or hematoma
		  ∘ Low-density fluid around the kidney/ureter
		  ∘ Ureteral dilation
		  ∘ Incomplete visualization of the ureter
			Isolated renal injuries in stable patients can typically be observed
			- Even patients with urinary extravasation from renal injury can be initially observed if stable; most will stop without intervention
			
			Indications for operative intervention for renal injuries:
			- Hemodynamic instability
			- Expanding/pulsatile zone II hematoma identified intra-op
			- Grade V injury (shattered/devascularized kidney), usually need nephrectomy
			
			Options for patients with ureteral injury—choice depends on extent of injury, patient status, and timing of diagnosis
			  ∘ If detected within 72 h → immediate repair
			  ∘ >72 h → percutaneous drainage of urinoma if present, percutaneous nephrostomy and/or ureteral stent, delay definitive repair until 6 wk out
			- Surgical options
			  ∘ Cystoscopy with ureteral stent placement may be adequate for low grade injuries
			  ∘ Open repair
			    ■ Injuries to distal ureter → repair with ureteral reimplantation into bladder +/- psoas hitch and/or Boari flap
			    ■ Abdominal ureter injury—ureteroureterostomy (short segment injuries), ureteral reimplantation into the bladder with psoas hitch +/- Boari flap or transureteroureterostomy
			    ■ Ureter injury in unstable patient undergoing damage control
			      • Ligate injured ureter, place nephrostomy tube post-op
			      • Alternatively, place ureteral stent into proximal end of injured ureter and externalize to control urine drainage
			      • Definitive repair once stabilizeds
				Operative management of kidney laceration:
				- Obtain hemostasis by controlling the renal artery and vein
				- Once vascular control is established, determine severity of the laceration and if collecting system is involved
				- Determine whether primary repair, partial nephrectomy, or nephrectomy is appropriate
				- Use absorbable sutures for laceration repair
				- Confirm there is a contralateral functioning kidney prior to performing nephrectomy
				- Leave a drain if collecting system involved, to capture urine leak
				
				Trauma nephrectomy:
				- Laparotomy
				- Take down the line of Toldt to mobilize colon out of the way
				  ∘ On the left, retract descending colon medially, divide splenocolic ligament
				  ∘ On the right, retract ascending colon and duodenum medially
				- Open Gerota's fascia
				- Isolate the renal hilum, ligate and divide renal artery and vein
				- Ligate and divide the ureter
				
				Ureteroureterostomy:
				- Mobilize both ends of the ureter carefully and as minimally as possible to avoid devascularization
				- Debride devitalized tissue
				- Spatulate ends of ureter to increase size of the anastomosis
				- Use fine absorbable suture to make tension-free, watertight repair over a ureteral stent
				- Leave a Foley in place and drain near the repair
					Risk of urine leak after repair:
					- Presents with rising creatinine, increased drain output (fluid creatinine +), ileus, fever, pain
					- May require percutaneous nephrostomy, IR drain and/or cystoscopic stent placement
						If you are going to perform a ureteral injury repair on boards, it is probably best to say you would consult urology intraoperatively, although the examiner may say urology is unavailable and want you to describe the procedure.

Disease Process	Relevant H&P	Work-up/Staging	Treatment	Key Surgical Steps	Post-Op Care	Tips & Tidbits

Lower urinary tract injuries (bladder and urethra) (core)	Initial evaluation per ATLS ~80% of bladder injuries are due to blunt trauma and the majority of these are associated with a pelvic fracture
	
	Anterior urethra may be injured by penetrating trauma (GSW to penis) or blunt trauma (straddle type injury)
	
	Posterior urethra usually injured with blunt trauma, nearly always associated with pelvic fracture
	
	Patient with bladder injury will have hematuria, usually gross hematuria but sometimes just microscopic
	
	Signs of urethral injury:
	• Blood at the meatus
	• Inability to void
	• Gross hematuria
	• Perineal or scrotal swelling/ecchymosis
	• Inability to pass a Foley
	• High-riding prostate
	
	If urethral injury is suspected, do not place a Foley!
		Obtain retrograde urethrogram (RUG) in all patients with suspected urethral injury prior to attempting Foley placement
		- Inject 20-30 mL of dilute, water-soluble contrast into the urethral meatus, then obtain an XR
		
		Cystogram should be obtained in stable patients with:
		- Gross hematuria + pelvic fracture (bladder injury present in up to 50%)
		- Gross hematuria + mechanism concerning for bladder injury
		- Pelvic ring fractures with abnormal FAST
		- Important to differentiate intra- vs extra-peritoneal bladder injuries
		  ∘ With extraperitoneal rupture, contrast extravasation looks like a flame or starburst
		  ∘ With intraperitoneal rupture, contrast will outline loops of bowel and pool in the cul-de-sac
			Bladder injury management—important to understand which bladder injuries need repair and which can be managed nonoperatively:
			- Intraperitoneal bladder injuries require repair
			- Uncomplicated extraperitoneal bladder perforations do not require surgical intervention and can be treated with Foley catheter drainage
			- Patients with "complicated" extraperitoneal bladder perforations should be repaired, this includes patients with concomitant vaginal or rectal lacerations, bony fragments in the bladder, uncontrolled hematuria, undergoing surgery for another reason (open exploration, pelvic fracture repair, etc), or failure of nonoperative managementa
			
			Urethral injury management:
			- Blunt urethral injuries managed with percutaneous suprapubic tube initially, then once patient is stable, can attempt endoscopic primary realignment with Foley placement
			  ∘ If not able to realign urethra initially, leave suprapubic tube and plan for delayed urethroplasty
			- Penetrating anterior urethral injuries require exploration and primary closure at time of injury with tension-free, watertight closure with absorbable sutures, leave Foley across injury
			- Would request urology consult for assistance with urethral repair
				Intraperitoneal bladder perforation repair:
				- Lower midline laparotomy
				- Mobilize the bladder and localize the injury, will have to dissect into space of Retzius to see anterior bladder wall
				- If you are having issues localizing the injury, can always make a cystotomy and look from inside the bladder to evaluate the ureteral orifices, look for bone fragments
				- Two-layer, watertight, tension-free closure with absorbable sutures
				- Leave Foley in place post-op
					Typically obtain cystogram ~10-14 d post-op after bladder repair or non-op management of extraperitoneal injury to evaluate for ongoing leak
					- if negative, can remove Foley
					
					Most common complication after urethral injury is stricture
						The weakest portion of the bladder is at the dome. This portion is most likely to rupture with blunt trauma.
						
						How do you do a cystogram?
						- Can be done with an XR; however, a CT cystogram is now preferred in most settings
						- Patient must have a Foley (rule out urethral injury with RUG prior to placing if there is concern)
						- Instill at least 300 mL of contrast (or until patient intolerance) into the bladder via a Foley
						- Take images before filling, during filling, and after drainage

Disease Process	Relevant H&P	Work-up/Staging	Treatment	Key Surgical Steps	Post-Op Care	Tips & Tidbits

Traumatic extremity injuries (advanced)	Initial evaluation per ATLS
	
	Pulse and neurovascular exams
	
	Manual compression of active bleeding
	
	Look for hard or soft signs of vascular injury
	
	Hard signs of extremity vascular injury:
	• Pulsatile bleeding
	• Thrill or bruit
	• Pulse deficit
	• Expanding hematoma
	
	Soft signs of extremity vascular injury
	• H/o arterial bleeding at the scene or in transit
	• Neurological deficit in adjacent nerve
	• Proximity of the injury to named artery
	• Nonpulsatile hematoma over an artery
	
	Obtain ABI or BBI to evaluate extremity vascular status
		If there are hard signs of vascular injury, then patient should be taken to OR, otherwise proceed with further work-up
		
		CTA of extremity (or on-table angiogram) indicated if ABI or BBI < 0.9
		
		If there are multiple sites of injury i.e. (multiple GSW, shotgun injury, multiple fractures) need to localize the vascular defect with duplex U/S or angiogram
		
		Identify all fractures, dislocations, neurovascular injuries and soft tissue injuries
		- Obtain XR of affected limb to evaluate for bony injury
			Life over limb
			
			Hard signs of vascular injury → OR
			
			Bony fractures and dislocations
			- Call ortho for reduction of dislocations and displaced fractures ASAP
			  ∘ Compare pre- and post-reduction imaging to ensure reduction was successful
			- Repeat exam and recheck ABI after intervention
			- Antibiotics for open fractures
				Repair of extremity vascular injury:
				- Widely prep and drape, make sure GSV is accessible
				- Get proximal and distal exposure and control
				  ∘ Consider systemic heparinization prior to clamping
				- Localize the injury, debride any nonviable tissue
				- Repair of arterial injury—depends on degree of tissue loss
				  ∘ Primary repair—for partial transection, injuries with minimal tissue loss
				  ∘ End-to-end anastomosis—transection injuries with minimal tissue loss
				  ∘ Interposition graft with contralateral GSV (or PTFE if GSV not possible)—injuries with long segment tissue loss
				  ∘ In damage control situation, can place Argyll shunt and return later for definitive repair
				- Venous injury—can typically ligate (or attempt repair if patient is stable and tissue loss is minimal)
				- Close wound in layers
				  ∘ May need assistance of plastic surgery for flap creation if there is significant soft tissue loss
				- Perform completion angiogram if there is any concern and/or palpable pulses not present after repair
				- Perform fasciotomy if is patient high risk for compartment syndrome (delay in treatment, combined arterial and venous injury, significant swelling, etc)
					Frequent neurovascular checks after vascular repair	Common injury patterns
						• Posterior knee dislocation—popliteal artery injury
						• Posterior hip dislocation—sciatic nerve stretched
						• Shoulder dislocation—axillary nerve stretched
						
						- Humeral shaft fracture—radial nerve injury

Disease Process	Relevant H&P	Work-up/Staging	Treatment	Key Surgical Steps	Post-Op Care	Tips & Tidbits

Lower extremity compartment syndrome (core)	May present in association with traumatic injury, acute limb ischemia, circumferential burns
	
	Look for clinical signs of compartment syndrome
	
	Extremity is typically swollen and compartments feel tense
	
	Assess for 6Ps: pain, pallor, paresthesia, poikilothermic, paralysis, pulselessness
	
	Thigh compartment syndrome is much less common than lower leg but can occur
		Compartment syndrome is a clinical diagnosis, have a low threshold for fasciotomies
		
		Can measure compartment pressures in intubated, sedated patients
		- Compartment pressures within 30 mm Hg of diastolic pressure are diagnostic of compartment syndrome
			Emergent fasciotomy	**Four compartment fasciotomy of the lower leg (core):**
				- Lateral incision—releases the anterior and lateral compartments
				  ◦ Longitudinal incision between tibial crest and fibula—start 4-5 cm distal to fibular head (to avoid injury to peroneal nerve) and go down to 2-3 cm above the ankle
				  ◦ Dissect down to fascia and raise subcutaneous flaps
				  ◦ Make "H type" incision on the fascia to expose intermuscular septum and decompress the lateral and anterior compartments
				- Medial incision—releases the superior posterior and deep posterior compartments
				  ◦ Make longitudinal incision 1-2 cm medial to tibial margin
				  ◦ Identify and preserve saphenous vein
				  ◦ Decompress superficial posterior compartment by opening fascia
				  ◦ Decompress deep posterior compartment by dissecting soleus off of the tibia posteriorly, palpate posterior tibial pulse to confirm entry into the deep compartment
				- Place wound vac or wet to dry dressings
				
				Thigh fasciotomy:
				- The thigh has 3 compartments (anterior, posterior, adductor)
				- Perform 2 incision fasciotomy to decompress the thigh
				- Anterolateral incision to decompress anterior and posterior compartments
				- Medial incision to decompress adductor compartment
					Watch out for rhabdomyolysis
					
					Eventually close fasciotomy wounds primarily or with skin grafts
						Ischemia time > 4-6 h can cause permanent tissue damage

Disease Process	Relevant H&P	Work-up/Staging	Treatment	Key Surgical Steps	Post-Op Care	Tips & Tidbits

Traumatic brain injury (core)	Initial evaluation per ATLS
	- Typically intubate if GCS ≤ 8
	Full neuro exam—pupillary exam, calculate GCS
	Cushing's reflex (hypertension, bradycardia, irregular respiratory pattern) is a sign of elevated ICP, which should be promptly addressed
	Signs of skull base fractures: raccoon eyes, CSF rhinorrhea, Battle sign (ecchymoses over the mastoid bone), CSF otorrhea, hemotympanum
	It is very important to know if patient is on anticoagulants
		CT +/- MRI
		- Be able to recognize subdural hematomas (SDH), epidural hematomas, subarachnoid hemorrhage, and intraparenchymal hemorrhage (IPH) on imaging
		- Evaluate for midline shift
		Post-resuscitation GCS score can be used to classify TBI severity
		• Mild: 13-15
		• Moderate: 9-12
		• Severe: 3-8
			Resuscitation as needed
			Treatment of other life-threatening traumatic injuries (ie., intra-abdominal hemorrhage, peritonitis, etc)
			TXA within 3 h of moderate or severe TBI
			Prevent secondary brain injury:
			- Avoid hypoxia
			- Avoid hypotension
			- Avoid fever
			- Prevent seizures—seizure prophylaxis with levetiracetam for 7 d following TBI
			- Maintain adequate CPP (60-70 mm Hg)
			Indications for ICP monitor placement:
			- GCS ≤ 8 (after resuscitation) with abnormality on head CT
			- GCS ≤ 8 with normal head CT and ≥ 2 of following:
			  ○ Age >40 yo
			  ○ Unilateral or bilateral motor posturing
			  ○ SBP <90 mm Hg
			Therapies for elevated ICP (>20 mm Hg):
			- HOB elevation
			- Hyperventilation to PCO_2 35-40 mm Hg
			- Give hypertonic saline 30 mL over 10 min or mannitol 1 g/kg
			- Increase sedation and analgesia—fentanyl, propofol
			- Paralytics
			- CSF drainage via externalized ventricular drain, if present
			- Decompressive craniectomy
			If patient demonstrates signs of herniation (Cushing reflex, blown pupil, decline in neuro function on one side of the body), perform manuevers to decrease ICP immediately
			Emergent neurosurgical consult
			- Epidural hematomas often require immediate surgical decompression
			- SDH may require surgical decompression
			- IPH rarely require surgical evacuation
					Steroids are not recommended
					VAP prevention
					Early enteral feeding
					VTE prophylaxis within 24-72 h of stabilization of intracranial hemorrhage
						Additional reading:
						Carney N, et al. Guidelines for the management of severe traumatic brain injury, fourth edition. *Neurosurgery.* 2017 Jan 1;80(1):6-15.
						CRASH-3 trial collaborators. Effects of tranexamic acid on death, disability, vascular occlusive events and other morbidities in patients with acute traumatic brain injury (CRASH-3): a randomised, placebo-controlled trial. *Lancet.* 2019 Nov 9;394(10210):1713-1723.

Disease Process	Relevant H&P	Work-up/Staging	Treatment	Key Surgical Steps	Post-Op Care	Tips & Tidbits

Burns (core)	Initial evaluation per ATLS—don't let the burns distract you from other life-threatening issues the patient may have!
	
	Signs of inhalational injury?
	- Respiratory distress, singled nasal hairs, carbonaceous sputum, altered mental status
	- Intubate immediately if concern for airway compromise
	
	Estimate burn thickness, and total body surface area (TBSA) affected (rule of 9's)
	- Patient's palm is equal to ~1% TBSA
		Burn severity:
		- Superficial: epidermis only (ie, sunburn)
		- Superficial partial thickness, deep partial thickness: epidermis and part of dermis
		- Full thickness: through dermis
		
		Bronchoscopy if concerned for inhalational injury
		
		Watch out for CO or CN poisoning:
		- Check COHb level, treat with 100% FiO2, hyperbaric oxygen
		- No rapid test to diagnose CN poisoning, empirically treat with cyanokit (hydroxocobalamin) if concerned
			Resuscitation:
			- Parkland formula = 4 mL/%BSA/kg (½ first 8 h, ½ over next 16 h)
			- Modified Brooke formula = 2 mL/%BSA/kg (½ first 8 h, ½ over next 16 h)
			
			Good wound care, apply topical burn medications as needed
			
			Circumferential burns can cause compartment syndrome → escharotomy
			
			Early excision and grafting of burns once stabilized
			- Split thickness (STSG) vs full thickness skin graft (FTSG)
			- Usually do STSG, unless it is for coverage of a joint or cosmetically sensitive area
			- FTSG have more primary contracture but less secondary contracture
			- More donor site morbidity with FTSG
				Excision and split thickness skin grafting for burns (core):
				- Excise nonviable tissue using Goulian blade
				- Establish hemostasis, can use epi-soaked dressings
				- Select graft harvest site, lateral thigh or back are commonly used
				  ○ Donor site will regrow new skin 2-3 wk after harvesting STSG
				- Set thickness on dermatome 0.13-0.3 mm.
				- Lubricate donor site with mineral oil
				- Harvest the graft—pull tension to make the skin taut in the path of dermatome
				- Epinephrine-soaked sponge placed on donor sites following harvest to minimize blood loss
				- +/- meshing—typically mesh the graft to cover more area, unless it is being used on a cosmetically sensitive area
				  ○ 1:1-4:1 mesh depending on coverage needed
				- Place graft onto the recipient bed with the dermis side down
				- Secure graft in place
				- Leave bolster dressing or wound vac for 5-7 d, then remove and assess graft take
					Complications:
					- Seroma/hematoma build up under graft can prevent take.
					- Can develop wound contracture, which can lead to functional and aesthetic issues
						Side effects of topical antibiotics (commonly tested on ABSITE):
						- Bacitracin: hypersensitivity reaction
						- Silver sulfadiazine (Silvadene): neutropenia
						- Silver Nitrate: hyponatremia, hypokalemia
						- Mafenide Acetate (Sulfamylon): metabolic acidosis

Disease Process	Relevant H&P	Work-up/Staging	Treatment	Key Surgical Steps	Post-Op Care	Tips & Tidbits

Frostbite, Hypothermia (core)	Patient with environmental exposure
	
	May present with numbness and discoloration of fingers, toes, ears, nose, etc
	
	Signs of hypothermia—shivering, tachycardia, tachypnea, confusion in patient post environmental cold exposure
	
	Exam—skin may be hard, blistered and/or waxy looking
		Determine severity of frostbite after rewarming:
		- Frostbite classified as superficial or deep
		  ○ Superficial frostbite—clear vesicles, limited dermal involvement
		  ○ Deep injury—hemorrhagic vesicles, subdermal injury
		- Deep injury results in development of thick black eschar within 1-2 wk following injury
			Address hypothermia first
			Rewarming:
			- Critical to monitor HR, BP, and cardiac rhythm while rewarming
			- External rewarming measures—hot blankets, air-warmer, heating pads, warm water bath
			- IVF and blood products should be warmed
			- Severe hypothermia—consider peritoneal lavage, chest cavity lavage, and an intravascular warming catheter, correct acid/base and electrolyte abnormalities, may require K+ to stabilize myocardium
			- Severe hypothermia, can lead to ventricular fibrillation and cardiac arrest → CPR, can consider ECMO
			Frost bite wound management:
			- Can consider thrombolytic therapy within first 24 h of thaw time
			- Daily wound care
			- Pain control
			- Delay operative management until patient is stabilized and tissue demarcation has occurred, may require weeks to months → debridement or amputation as needed once demarcated			

Geriatric trauma (core)	Geriatric trauma = trauma patient >55 yo
	- GLF and MVC are common mechanisms
	Initial evaluation per ATLS protocol
	- ATLS recommends trauma patients > 55 yo be transported to a trauma center
	- Vital signs may not reflect severity of injury, decreased response to shock
	- Often under triaged
	Always ask about anticoagulation
		Full trauma labs
		A more extensive workup should be considered for lower energy level injuries
		Frailty score—use frailty assessment tools, frailty score more predictive of adverse outcomes and discharge disposition than actual age in geriatric trauma patients
			Most management is similar to adult trauma patients
			Warfarin reversal:
			- IV vitamin K—onset of action is 2 h, maximum effect achieved in 6-12 h
			- PO vitamin K—onset of action of oral form is 12-24 h
			- FFP—contains all coagulation factors
			  ○ Volume of 1 unit is ~250 mL
			  ○ INR of FFP is 1.4-1.6 so you will never totally correct INR with FFP
			- Prothrombin complex concentrate (PCC)—contains the vitamin K-dependent factors II, VII, IX, and X, onset of action < 10 min, recommended for emergent reversal
			DOAC reversal:
			- Dabigatran (Pradaxa)—direct thrombin inhibitor, can give idarucizumab (Praxbind) or do dialysis for reversal
			- Rivaroxaban (Xarelto), apixaban (Eliquis)—factor Xa inhibitors, can use andexanet alfa (AndexXa) or PCC for reversal
					Majority of severely injured geriatric trauma patients do not return to their pre-injury level of function; many require long-term placement in a nursing facility
					
					SNFs are the primary discharge disposition for geriatric trauma patients
						Additional tips for management of geriatric trauma patients:
						- Restart and adjust dosing of home medication when appropriate
						- Multimodal pain control, minimize narcotics, although good pain control is key in optimizing pulmonary function, mobility and avoiding delirium
						- Recognize early signs of delirium
						- Consult geriatric medicine when appropriate
						- GOC discussions should be initiated early on in hospital stay
						- Assist family in decision making that preserves patient autonomy and quality of life

Disease Process	Relevant H&P	Work-up/Staging	Treatment	Key Surgical Steps	Post-Op Care	Tips & Tidbits
Pediatric Trauma (core)	Primary trauma survey in children similar to in adults, with some adjustments Airway—When emergency surgical airway required in patient <10 yo, needle cricothyroidotomy with a 16- or 18-gauge needle and jet ventilation is preferred to open cricothyroidotomy Breathing—similar to adult patient Circulation—Pediatric patients have remarkable cardiovascular reserve and will often have relatively normal vitals until they crash, don't be tricked - If peripheral IV cannot be placed, place an IO Deficit—GCS: when <2 yo pediatric GCS is used; when >2 yo standard GCS is used	Trauma labs Selective imaging, as indicated based on exam, labs, and mechanism Recognize patterns of injury that are consistent with child physical abuse, consult social work	Typical pediatric fluid bolus: 20mL/kg Typical pediatric blood transfusion volume: 10mL/kg Most blunt liver and spleen injury managed nonoperatively, as long as patient is stable Handlebar injury—can result in duodenal hematoma, which can cause obstruction, can often be managed nonoperatively with parenteral nutrition until it resolves			

Disease Process	Relevant H&P	Work-up/Staging	Treatment	Key Surgical Steps	Post-Op Care	Tips & Tidbits
Trauma in pregnancy (core)	Initial evaluation per ATLS protocol—initial assessment remains the same as for other trauma patients Once patient has undergone initial assessment and is deemed stable, needs vaginal examination to evaluate for bleeding or leakage of amniotic fluid Measure fetal heart rate (FHR)—normal is 110 to 160 beats/min	Trauma labs, CXR, pelvic XR, FAST exam CT scan should be obtained using the same indications as in nonpregnant patients—risk of missed injury is greater than potential risk of radiation to the fetus (shield fetus when possible) Consult OB service There is no single diagnostic test for placental abruption; diagnosis based on constellation of symptoms, labs, and imaging - Presents as abdominal pain, contractions, uterine rigidity, fetal distress, and/or vaginal bleeding Kleihauer-Betke test—evaluates for fetomaternal bleeding, should be performed in all Rh(-) patients, should also be considered in Rh(+) patients who sustain blunt injury - Positive test associated with placental abruption - If test is positive, and the mother is Rh(-), a dose of Rh immune globulin should be given to prevent alloimmunization Uterine rupture can occur with severe blunt trauma or with penetrating injury - Patient would present with shock, abnormal fetal heart rate tracing, uterine tenderness, vaginal bleeding, and/or palpation of fetal parts outside the uterus	The best treatment for the fetus is treatment of the mother Continuous fetal monitoring should be performed in all trauma patients who are >24 wk gestation for a minimum of 4 h prior to discharge; may require longer monitoring if major trauma or signs of abruption Emergency C/S only considered if the fetus is >24 wk Perimortem C/S— an otherwise uninjured fetus delivered within 5 min of maternal arrest has survival rate up to 70%	**General principles for trauma surgery in pregnant patient:** - Left lateral tilt to minimize IVC compression - Make a generous vertical midline incision if exploratory laparotomy needed - Indications for emergency cesarean section are similar to in nontrauma patients **Perimortem cesarean section (resuscitative hysterotomy):** - Can be considered in situation with pregnant patient who has arrested or is peri-arrest and fetus is believed to be ≥24 wk gestation - Must be initiated within 4 min of loss of maternal pulse for maximum beneficial outcome, continue CPR during cesarean section - Make laparotomy incision - Enter the abdomen - Cut into the lower half of the uterus, use scissors to extend the incision until you reach the baby - Deliver the baby and initiate resuscitation immediately - Clamp and cut the umbilical cord - Remove the placenta and close the uterine incision to minimize ongoing hemorrhage		Amniotic fluid embolism can occur in pregnant patients - Presents with sudden onset severe respiratory difficulty, hypoxia, seizures, DIC/hemorrhage, and/or cardiovascular collapse - Tx: supportive care Trauma affects 6-8% of pregnancies Recognize red flags that may signify physical abuse—6-22% of pregnant women experience intimate partner violence!

8

Surgical Critical Care

Katherine Mandell, MD, and Gary Lucas, MD

DISEASES AND CONDITIONS

- Upper airway obstruction (c)
- Respiratory failure (c)
- Acute respiratory distress syndrome (c)
- Hypovolemic and hemorrhagic shock (c)
- Septic shock (c)

- Neurogenic shock, spinal cord injury (c)
- Cardiac failure and cardiogenic shock (c)
- Cardiac arrest (c)
- Cardiac arrhythmias (c)
- Abdominal compartment syndrome (c)

- Nutritional support (c)
- Acute kidney injury (c)
- Chronic liver disease (c)
- Upper GI bleed, stress gastritis (c)

GENERAL TIPS

- Review the ACLS algorithms.

(c) = core topic   (a) = advanced topic

Disease Process	Relevant H&P	Work-up/Staging	Treatment	Key Surgical Steps	Post-Op Care	Tips & Tidbits

Upper airway obstruction (core)	Many potential causes of emergent airway obstruction: trauma, anaphylaxis, tumor, foreign body, vocal cord paralysis, retropharyngeal abscess, angioedema, etc
	
	Hoarseness or stridor? Short neck? Prior neck surgery? C-spine precautions? Limited mobility?
	
	Palpate thyroid cartilage, cricoid cartilage, tracheal rings, and sternal notch
		Mallampati classification
		
		- Based on visualization of pharyngeal structures
		- Can be used to predict a difficult airway
			Definitive airway = cuffed tube below the vocal cords
			
			Oral tracheal intubation can be attempted initially
			
			Several attempts at intubation are typically reasonable, but if unsuccessful, surgical airway should be placed in a timely manner to avoid sustained hypoxia
			
			Procedure of choice for emergent surgical airway is cricothyroidotomy
				Intubation:
				- Make sure necessary supplies are readily available (ie, suction, lighting, bag mask, meds, ET tube, laryngoscopes, video laryngoscopy, bougies, and airway cart)
				- Preoxygenate patient, if able—can use chin tilt, oral airway, and 2-hand mask seal to help with bag masking
				- Administer medications—sedation and paralytic as appropriate, should be RSI
				  ○ Awake intubation may be required for patients with near complete airway obstruction
				- Place patient in sniffing position (if no C-spine precautions)
				- Place laryngoscope, visualize cords, insert ET tube
				  ○ Intubation over bronchoscope may help in some situations
				- Confirm appropriate tracheal position (end tidal CO_2, misting in tube, b/l breath sounds)
				- Inflate balloon, connect to ventilator, secure tube in place
				- CXR to confirm position
				
				Cricothyroidotomy:
				- Proceed with cricothyroidotomy in airway emergencies when unable to intubate from above
				- Palpate the cricothyroid membrane and other landmarks
				- Make vertical skin incision and dissect down to cricothyroid membrane
				- Incise cricothyroid membrane horizontally and dilate, can use back bend of scalpel
				- Insert tracheostomy tube or ETT
				- Confirm appropriate tracheal position (end tidal CO_2, misting on tube, b/l breath sounds)
				- Inflate balloon, connect to ventilator, secure tube in place
				- CXR to confirm position
					Typically convert cricothyroidotomy to formal tracheostomy when stabilized	Anaphylaxis (core):
						- May present with flushing, pruritis, laryngeal edema, wheezing, hypotension
						- Common causes of peri-op anaphylaxis: antibiotics, blood products, neuromuscular-blocking agents, latex
						- Treatment: remove trigger, immediately, give 0.3-0.5 mg of epinephrine (1:1000) IM, repeat q5 min as needed up to 3 times, fluids and pressors as needed for hypotension, can give albuterol, antihistamines, H2 blockers, and steroids as adjuncts
						- Intubate immediately if there is evidence of impending airway obstruction, can give racemic epinephrine via nebulizer prior to intubation to decrease edema

Disease Process	Relevant H&P	Work-up/Staging	Treatment	Key Surgical Steps	Post-Op Care	Tips & Tidbits
Respiratory failure (core)	May present with SOB, AMS, wheezing, cough Many potential etiologies can result in respiratory failure	Differential is broad and should include: pulmonary embolism, pneumonia, aspiration, ARDS, hypoventilation, pulmonary edema, diffuse alveolar hemorrhage, pleural effusion, TRALI, pneumothorax, etc Initial work-up should include CBC, BMP, ABG, ECG, and CXR Can use U/S to look for right heart strain (due to PE), pneumothorax, or effusion CT chest for further characterization of findings on CXR, if needed Obtain CTA chest if concerned for PE Consider ECHO to evaluate for CHF, pulmonary HTN, PE Bronchoscopy with BAL can be used to diagnose and guide antibiotic treatment of pneumonia - Bronchoscopy not safe in patients with very tenuous respiratory status	Treat underlying cause of respiratory failure **Criteria for intubation:** - Failure to protect airway - Unable to oxygenate and/or ventilate - Significant pulmonary hygiene requirements If patient needs respiratory support but can protect their airway, consider trial of high flow or CPAP/BIPAP prior to intubation Adjusting the ventilator: - Hypercarbic intubated patient $\longrightarrow$ increase TV or RR - Hypoxic intubated patient $\longrightarrow$ increase FiO2 or PEEP Consider tracheostomy if patient requires prolonged intubation or frequent pulmonary hygiene	**Bronchoscopy with BAL (core):** - Increase FiO2 to 100% - Sedate patient as needed, can use topical lidocaine for comfort - Insert bronchoscope but do not use suction prior to obtaining sample - Advance bronchoscope into desired lung segment - Infuse 100 mL of normal saline in 20 mL aliquots into desired bronchopulmonary segment as distally as possible and after each 20 mL aliquot aspirate fluid back - Send specimen for quantitative culture - Inspect other airways, aspirate secretions - Quantitative BAL culture with >10,000 CFU/mL is diagnostic of pneumonia **Tracheostomy (core):** - High PEEP and FiO2 are contraindications to tracheostomy - Position supine with bump under shoulders and arms tucked - Mark out landmarks—thyroid cartilage, cricoid, sternal notch - Make incision overlying second tracheal ring - Divide the platysma, strap muscles, thyroid - Avoid cautery once close to airway and have anesthesia turn down FiO2 to 30% to minimize fire risk - Make sure you have all trach supplies ready - Have anesthesia deflate the ETT balloon - Make tracheotomy at second or third tracheal ring - Can place Prolene trach sutures with long tails on either side of tracheotomy site for retraction - Have anesthesia slowly pull back ETT until they are above the tracheotomy - Dilate tracheotomy and insert the trach - Connect to ventilator, confirm correct placement (end tidal CO_2, bronchoscopy tracheostomy), secure tracheostomy	Daily SBT, extubate when appropriate Low placement of tracheostomy can result in tracheoinominate fistula, which presents as pulsatile bleeding from the tracheostomy and/or hemoptysis Tracheal stenosis can develop after prolonged intubation or tracheostomy	

Disease Process	Relevant H&P	Work-up/Staging	Treatment	Key Surgical Steps	Post-Op Care	Tips & Tidbits
Acute respiratory distress syndrome (ARDS) (core)	ARDS will present as worsening hypoxemia in a critically ill patient	CXR, ABG ARDS—Berlin Criteria: 1. Symptoms begin within 1 wk of known insult 2. CXR or CT scan with bilateral opacities 3. Respiratory status not explained by cardiac failure or fluid overload 4. PaO2/FiO2 ratio < 300 (with PEEP ≥ 5) Severity is based on PaO2/FiO2 ratio: i. Mild: 200-300 ii. Moderate: 100-200 iii. Severe: ≤100	Lung protective ventilation (LPV)—tidal volume of 6 mL/kg, plateau pressures <30 cm H20, increase PEEP and FiO2 as needed to maintain oxygenation - Shown to have mortality benefit and increased ventilator-free days Sedation—increase sedation as needed to make patient synchronous with ventilator Neuromuscular blockade—increases compliance and ensures ventilator synchrony, shown to have mortality benefit in severe ARDS and less ventilator dependent days Proning—improve V/Q mismatch, shown to have mortality benefit in severe ARDS Inhaled nitric oxide and epoprostenol—may improve oxygenation but no clear mortality or morbidity benefit, often reserved for salvage therapy Consider corticosteroids for early moderate to severe ARDS ECMO can be considered for patients with severe ARDS Consider tracheostomy if patient requires prolonged intubation (>7d) or requires frequent pulmonary hygiene - Trachestomy decreases the need for sedation, facilitates vent weaning	**Percutaneous tracheostomy:** - Patients on high PEEP and/or FiO2 are not good candidates for percutaneous tracheostomy - Patient should be sedated and paralyzed, turn FiO2 up to 100% - Palpate and mark out landmarks—thyroid cartilage, cricoid cartilage, sternal notch - Have another provider performing bronchoscopy and transluminate while you palpate to identify the ideal spot (usually around second tracheal ring), pull ETT back over bronchoscope as needed to visualize the spot - Make skin incision - Insert needle through incision into trachea under direct bronchoscopic visualization - Insert wire into trachea and remove needle - Pass short dilator and then tapered dilator (blue rhino horn) over wire to dilate trachea to appropriate size - Insert tracheostomy tube over the wire with dilator - Remove wire and dilator from tracheostomy and insert inner cannula, connect to ventilator and confirm ETCO2, can also insert bronchoscopy through tracheostomy to confirm location - Secure tracheostomy in place	Daily SBT Early tracheostomy dislodgement is an airway emergency and should be managed with reintubation from above, attempts to reinsert trach before track has formed may result in false passage	Additional reading: Acute Respiratory Distress Syndrome Network, Brower RG, et al. Ventilation with lower tidal volumes as compared with traditional tidal volumes for acute lung injury and the acute respiratory distress syndrome. *N Engl J Med.* 2000; 342(18): 1301-1308. Guérin C, et al; PROSEVA Study Group. Prone positioning in severe acute respiratory distress syndrome. *N Engl J Med.* 2013; 368(23): 2159-2168. National Heart, Lung, and Blood Institute PETAL Clinical Trials Network, Moss M, et al. Early neuromuscular blockade in the acute respiratory distress syndrome. *N Engl J Med.* 2019 May 23;380(21):1997-2008.

Disease Process	Relevant H&P	Work-up/Staging	Treatment	Key Surgical Steps	Post-Op Care	Tips & Tidbits
Hypovolemic and hemorrhagic shock (core)	Patient presents with hypotension, tachycardia, AMS, cold extremities, diaphoresis Potential causes include trauma, nontraumatic hemorrhage (GIB bleed, obstetric bleeding, etc), or increased insensible losses (emesis, diarrhea, etc)	Ensure patient has good IV access Full labs—CBC, CMP, ABG with lactate, coagulants, TEG Use history and exam +/- imaging/adjuncts (ECG, CXR, bedside U/S, CT) to determine source of hypovolemic shock - Hypotension in a trauma patient is hemorrhagic shock until proven otherwise - Postoperative hypotension must be assumed to be due to surgical bleeding ◦ Consider other etiologies as well: hypovolemia, MI, other cardiac issues, pneumothorax, adrenal insufficiency, over sedation Pulse pressure variation (PPV) and stroke volume variation (SVV) can be used to assess fluid responsiveness	For management of specific causes, see sections on GIB, trauma, etc Resuscitation (choice of fluid depends on patient scenario): - Blood products—use balanced resuscitation (1:1:1) or whole blood for patients in hemorrhagic shock - Crystalloid—hypovolemia from other fluid losses - Colloid (ie, albumin)—may be preferred for volume replacement in patients with hypoalbuminemia (ie, liver failure) but not ideal for acute resuscitation A patient with ongoing postsurgical bleeding should be taken back to the OR ASAP During the resuscitation for hypovolemic/hemorrhagic shock monitor vitals, lactate, pH, base excess, SVV, PPV, and urine output, and use these metrics to determine whether ongoing resuscitation is needed and when systemic perfusion is adequate Correction of acidosis, coagulopathy, and hypothermia are key adjuncts for the treatment of hemorrhagic shock			You may get a scenario with patient with post-op tachycardia - Differential: bleeding, PE, MI, anastomotic leak, sepsis/infection, withdrawal, atrial fibrillation, etc - Ensure patient is attached to monitors and get full set of vitals, perform focused exam - Obtain CBC, BMP, ABG, lactate, ECG, cultures if concerned for sepsis - Consider imaging with CXR, KUB, U/S, and/or CT depending on clinical picture - Treat etiology, as indicated Additional reading: Holcomb JB, et al; PROPPR Study Group. Transfusion of plasma, platelets, and red blood cells in a 1:1:1 vs a 1:1:2 ratio and mortality in patients with severe trauma: the PROPPR randomized clinical trial. *JAMA*. Feb 2015; 313(5): 471-482.

Disease Process	Relevant H&P	Work-up/Staging	Treatment	Key Surgical Steps	Post-Op Care	Tips & Tidbits

Septic shock (core)	May present with tachycardia, hypotension, tachypnea, fever, and/or altered mental status
	
	Variety of potential sources including pneumonia, UTI, intra-abdominal source, soft tissue infection, meningitis, bacteremia, osteomyelitis, etc
	
	Perform exam, assess wounds, lines, Foley, medical devices, or other potential sources
		Initial tests—CBC, CMP, ABG, lactate, U/A, CXR, CRP, procalcitonin
		
		Blood cultures x 2 from separate peripheral blood draws
		
		Consider further imaging to work-up suspected source once patient is stabilized
			Early goal directed resuscitation—continuous monitoring of physiological targets (CVP, MAP, ScvO2, PPV, SVV) used to guide initial resuscitation and pressor use
			- Initial crystalloid bolus of 30 mL/kg
			- Assess fluid responsiveness/volume status—passive leg raise, SVV, PPV, bedside U/S of IVC
			- Additional fluid and pressors as needed to maintain MAP >65 mm Hg
			  ○ Norepinephrine is pressor of choice in septic shock
			    ■ Can add vasopressin at set rate
			    ■ Epinephrine is second line
			Broad spectrum antibiotics should be started within 1hr of sepsis recognition
			Place Foley, central line, intubate if needed
			Treat underlying cause, obtain source control
			Consider steroid supplementation in patients with refractory hypotension despite fluids and pressors and suspicion for adrenal insufficiency
			- 50 mg hydrocortisone IV q6h for at least 3 d
				Central line placement:
				- Position patient in slight Trendelenburg with head turned away from chosen site
				- Access internal jugular vein with needle under U/S guidance, thread wire into vein
				- Confirm intravenous location of wire with U/S in two dimensions prior to dilating
				- Pass the dilator over the wire
				- Once dilated, thread the preflushed catheter over the wire into the vein
				- Remove the wire, secure the catheter, obtain CXR to confirm location and rule out PTX
					Follow-up culture results and narrow antibiotics as appropriate
					
					Can trend inflammatory markers (CRP, procalcitonin) to assess response to treatment
						Additional reading:
						Rivers E, et al; Early Goal-Directed Therapy Collaborative Group. Early goal-directed therapy in the treatment of severe sepsis and septic shock. *N Engl J Med*. 2001 Nov 8;345(19):1368-1377.
						ARISE Investigators; ANZICS Clinical Trials Group, et al. Goal-directed resuscitation for patients with early septic shock. *N Engl J Med*. 2014 Oct 16;371(16):1496-1506.
						Singer M, et al. The Third International Consensus Definitions for Sepsis and Septic Shock (Sepsis-3). *JAMA*. 2016 Feb; 315(8): 801-810.
						Annane D, et al. Guidelines for the Diagnosis and Management of Critical Illness-Related
						Corticosteroid Insufficiency (CIRCI) in Critically Ill Patients (Part I): Society of Critical Care Medicine (SCCM) and European Society of Intensive Care Medicine (ESICM) 2017. *Crit Care Med*. 2017 Dec; 45(12): 2078-2088.

Disease Process	Relevant H&P	Work-up/Staging	Treatment	Key Surgical Steps	Post-Op Care	Tips & Tidbits

Neurogenic shock, Spinal cord injuries (SCI) (core)	Initial evaluation per ATLS
	
	Patients with neurogenic shock are usually trauma patients with cervical or high thoracic spinal cord injuries (must be T6 or above), occurs due to loss of sympathetic tone
	
	May have hypotension, bradycardia, warm extremities, loss of motor function and/or sensation
	
	Perform full neurologic exam with motor function, sensory function, and reflexes (Babinski/plantar, bulbocavernosus, cremasteric, anal wink)
		Trauma labs
		
		CT spine is initial imaging of choice in a stable patient
		
		- ~25% of patients with 1 spine fracture have another noncontiguous spinal fracture → image entire spine in patient with known spine fracture
		
		MRI should be considered in patients with possible SCI and concern for cord compression due to disk herniation, bone fragments, or hematoma
		
		Injuries above T1 typically result in some degree of quadriplegia
			Respiratory failure common with high C-spine injury, intubate if needed
			
			Neurogenic shock → initiate resuscitation immediately
			
			- Even if neurogenic shock is suspected, must rule out concomittant hemorrhagic shock
			- If patient remains hypotensive, even once they are felt to be volume replete, start pressors
			- Norepinephrine is the first line vasopressor for neurogenic shock
			- Keep MAP > 65 mm Hg—important to maintain adequate spinal perfusion and prevent secondary injury
			
			Avoid aggravating SCI:
			
			- Immobilization with backboard and cervical collar in blunt trauma patients
			- Maintain in-line cervical stabilization when intubating or examining neck of patient with suspected C-spine injury
			- Correct hypotension to maintain spinal perfusion
			- Maintain normothermia
			- Trend neuro exam (with ASIA score)
			- Avoid succinylcholine
			
			Consult neurosurgery/ortho spine ASAP
			
			- In patients with SCI, recognize injury patterns that require surgical intervention:
			  - Significant spinal cord compression and neurologic deficits
			  - Unstable spine fractures
			  - Acute thoracolumbar compression fractures causing kyphosis >35%
			- Patients with stable vertebral fractures without neurologic deficits typically managed nonoperatively with immobilization (c collar or brace)
			
			Bradycardia → atropine, cardiac pacing if ongoing
			
			- Bradycardia associated with SCI usually resolves within 2-5 wk
					Patients with spinal cord injury can develop neurogenic bladder, severe constipation common after SCI—bowel regimen important
					
					High risk of VTE after SCI—ensure patient is on DVT ppx
						Hemorrhagic shock should be assumed before neurogenic shock in a hypotensive trauma patient.
						
						Trauma patient with hypotension and relative bradycardia should always raise concern for neurogenic shock.
						
						Neurogenic shock ≠ "spinal shock"—spinal shock refers to transient flaccid paralysis and areflexia that can occur after SCI, not necessarily associated with hemodynamic collapse

Disease Process	Relevant H&P	Work-up/Staging	Treatment	Key Surgical Steps	Post-Op Care	Tips & Tidbits
Cardiac failure and cardiogenic shock (core)	Patients with heart failure may have leg edema, dyspnea on exertion, angina, orthopnea, pulmonary congestion, etc Patients in cardiogenic shock will be hypotensive and may present with diaphoresis, cold/clammy extremities, JVD, pulmonary congestion, and/or decreased capillary refill	CBC, CMP, troponin, ABG with lactate, ScvO2 BNP elevated in CHF, but nonspecific Patients in cardiogenic shock may have elevated lactic acid, base deficit, and decreased pH Central venous O2 (ScvO2) or mixed venous O2 (SvO2) will be decreased in cardiogenic shock CXR—may show pulmonary vascular congestion ECG ECHO	Cardiac support with medications: - Inotropes can be beneficial in cardiogenic shock (dobutamine, milrinone, and epinephrine) - Beta-blockers may improve chronicity and contraction of ventricle - Treat hypervolemia with diuretics or dialysis, if needed Cardiac ischemia due to CAD should be identified and treated with PCI Consider cardioversion in hypotensive patients with cardiogenic shock 2/2 arrhythmia (afib with RVR, SVT, VT) Cardiac surgery consult for consideration of intra-aortic balloon pump, LVAD, ECMO, etc		Heart failure treatment for surgical patients: - Judicious fluid and volume status management - Continue home meds (beta-blockers, ACEI, diuretics) as appropriate	Takotsubo cardiomyopathy (stress cardiomyopathy)—mimics acute coronary syndrome, reversible left ventricular apical ballooning in the absence of significant coronary artery stenosis - Transient, typically precipitated by acute physiologic or emotional stress
Cardiac arrest (core)	May happen in surgical patients for a variety of reasons Start CPR and call for back-up ASAP Establish an airway, ensure patient has IV access and is hooked to monitors and pads Obtain focused history and details regarding time of arrest MI symptoms: chest discomfort/pressure, shoulder pain, SOB, women and diabetics may have atypical symptoms	Initiate ACLS algorithm immediately—check pulse/rhythm q2min, epinephrine 1 mg q3-5min - May also give amiodarone (first dose 300 mg, second dose 150 mg) and lidocaine (first dose 1-1.5 mg/kg, second dose 0.5-0.75 mg/kg) Obtain initial work-up: CBC, BMP, calcium, ABG, lactate, troponin, ECG, bedside ECHO Work-up the 4 "H's" and 4 "T's" and treat accordingly: - Hypoxia, Hypovolemia, Hypothermia, H+ (acidosis), Hyper/hypokalemia - Thrombosis (MI, PE), Tension pneumothorax, Tamponade, Toxins	Shockable rhythms—ventricular fibrillation and pulseless ventricular tachycardia - Defibrillate at 360 J Nonshockable rhythms—PEA, asystole Rapidly identify and treat causes of nonshockable arrest (H's & T's) STEMI Tx—aspirin 325 mg, 80 mg atorvastatin, heparin drip (if appropriate), cardiology consult ASAP for consideration of PCI		If ROSC obtained, next step is to identify and treat cause of arrest	

Disease Process	Relevant H&P	Work-up/Staging	Treatment	Key Surgical Steps	Post-Op Care	Tips & Tidbits

Cardiac arrhythmias (core)	Arrhythmia symptoms: palpations, hypotension, SOB, chest pain, dizziness
	
	Get full set of vitals, ensure patient has good IV access and is hooked up to monitors and pads
	
	Obtain focused history including recent surgery, pertinent medical history, home meds
	
	Post-op afib often occurs due to fluid overload, pain, sepsis, or missed home beta-blocker doses
	
	Does patient have history of atrial fibrillation/arrhythmia or is it new?
		ECG, attach patient to cardiac monitors
		
		CBC, BMP, Ca, Mg, Phos, Troponin, ABG
		
		CXR
			Atrial fibrillation:
			
			- Stable → IV beta-blocker (5 mg metoprolol IV q5min), amiodarone (bolus dose and then drip), or calcium channel blocker (diltiazem 15-25 mg q15min), monitor closely
			  ○ Prefer amiodarone for new afib and beta-blockers or CCBs for chronic afib not well rate controlled
			- Unstable → sedate and perform synchronized cardioversion with 120-200 J for biphasic or 200 J for monophasic
			
			Address underlying causes of arrhythmia:
			
			- Correct electrolytes—K > 4 mEq/L, Mg > 2 mEq/L
			- Judicious use of fluid, diuresis if fluid overloaded
			- Resume home antiarrhythmic meds if held
			- Treat infection/sepsis if present
			
			Cardiac pacing:
			
			- Indications: symptomatic bradycardia, acute MI, cardiogenic shock, prevention of tachyarrhythmias post cardiac surgery
			- Noninvasive cardiac pacing = transcutaneous pads placed on chest
			- Invasive cardiac pacing
			  ○ Epicardial—pacing leads placed in myocardium and brought out through chest wall at conclusion of cardiac surgery
			  ○ Transvenous—access obtained via IJ or subclavian vein, sheath placed, and lead advanced through right atrium using fluoro or U/S until it makes contact with right ventricle
			
			If at any point patient loses a pulse, initiate CPR
					In patient with atrial fibrillation >48 h, consider starting therapeutic anticoagulation based on CHADS-VASc score for stroke prevention	Treatment of other arrhythmias:
						- SVT—can try vagal maneuvers (ie, Valsalva), adenosine (6 mg IV rapid)
						  ○ If unstable—immediately treat with synchronized cardioversion, 50-100 J
						- Symptomatic bradycardia—IV atropine (0.5 mg q3-5min), transcutaneous pacing if refractory
						- Stable ventricular tachycardia—give amiodarone, procainamide, or sotalol
						- Unstable arrhythmias requiring defibrillation:
						  ○ Pulseless ventricular tachycardia
						  ○ Ventricular fibrillation
						- Unstable arrhythmias potentially requiring synchronized cardioversion:
						  ○ Narrow complex tachyarrhythmia (SVT, atrial fibrillation, atrial flutter)
						- Unstable arrhythmias potentially requiring transcutaneous pacing:
						  ○ Bradycardia
						  ○ Heart block

Disease Process	Relevant H&P	Work-up/Staging	Treatment	Key Surgical Steps	Post-Op Care	Tips & Tidbits
Abdominal compartment syndrome (ACS) (core)	Patient presents with hypotension, tachycardia, tensely distended abdomen, increasing airway pressures, and/or progressive oliguria Can occur after trauma, intra-abdominal catastrophe, retroperitoneal hemorrhage, and/or massive resuscitation (ie, pancreatitis, ruptured AAA, burns)	Measure intra-abdominal pressure (IAP) by instilling 25 mL saline into bladder and measuring pressure through Foley with pressure transducer - Patient must be intubated and paralyzed for bladder pressure to be accurate Intra-abdominal HTN = IAP > 12 mm Hg ACS = IAP > 20 mm Hg with organ dysfunction (elevated airway pressures, worsening renal failure, etc)	NG tube, Foley catheter, rectal tube to decompress Sedation and paralysis Consider paracentesis if patient has large volume of ascites Decompressive laparotomy	**Decompressive laparotomy:** - Midline laparotomy extending the length of the abdomen - Explore for perforation, bleeding, or ischemia - Address specific intra-abdominal findings as appropriate - Apply temporary abdominal closure - Once patient stabilizes, can return to OR to attempt abdominal closure 　○ Watch out for high airway pressures when attempting to re-close 　○ Earlier time to first takeback (≤ 48h) associated with greater likelihood of primary fascial closure 　○ Rarely able to close abdomen primarily after having open abdomen for > 2 wk		Additional reading: Pommerening MJ, et al. Time to first take-back operation predicts successful primary fascial closure in patients undergoing damage control laparotomy. *Surgery*. 2014 Aug;156(2):431-438.

Disease Process	Relevant H&P	Work-up/Staging	Treatment	Key Surgical Steps	Post-Op Care	Tips & Tidbits
Nutritional support (core)	Many different reasons that patient may require nutrition support (intubated, intestinal failure, critically ill, PO intolerance, etc) Signs of malnutrition: muscle wasting, ≥ 10% body weight loss over 6 mo, BMI < 18.5	Nutrition labs: albumin, prealbumin, transferrin, retinol-binding protein, CRP Indirect calorimetry is preferred method for determining patient's nutritional needs, however it is expensive and not widely available Determine if patient can have enteral nutrition and if they will be able to take in adequate calories	Enteral nutrition is preferred over parenteral when possible, start as soon as possible Enteral access: - Intubated patients need OGT/NGT/Dobhoff feeding tube 　○ Always verify NGT placement with XR prior to use 　○ Place postpyloric tube if concern for reflux or poor gastric emptying - Gastrostomy tube can be placed for long-term feeding access needs (ie, stroke with dysphagia, esophageal stricture, etc) 　○ Can be PEG vs IR placed gastrostomy vs surgical gastrostomy - GJ or surgical jejunostomy tube for patients with a contraindication to gastric feeding or postpyloric feeding needed Parenteral Nutrition (TPN) - For patients who cannot have enteral nutrition - In a well-nourished patient, NPO status can be tolerated for 7d prior to starting TPN 　○ Start sooner for malnourished patients - Central venous access required (PICC vs central line) - Complications: 　○ Hyperglycemia 　○ Access complications 　○ Cholestasis Monitor for refeeding syndrome in patients with severe malnutrition - Start feeds slowly, replace electrolytes - Refeeding presents with low K, Mg, Phos - Can lead to cardiac, pulmonary, and neurologic complications or even death	See gastrostomy and jejunostomy tube placement in general surgery section		Nutrition sources: • Glucose—3.7 kcal/g • Protein—4 kcal/g • Lipids—9 kcal/g Nonprotein caloric needs: 25-30 kcal/kg/d Protein needs: 1-2 g/kg/d Vitamin A supplementation can be used to aid with wound healing in patients on chronic steroids Additional reading: Compher C, et al. Guidelines for the provision of nutrition support therapy in the adult critically ill patient: The American Society for Parenteral and Enteral Nutrition. *JPEN J Parenter Enteral Nutr.* Jan 2022; 46(1): 12-41.

Disease Process	Relevant H&P	Work-up/Staging	Treatment	Key Surgical Steps	Post-Op Care	Tips & Tidbits

Acute kidney injury (core)	Will present as patient with decreased UOP, rising creatinine
	
	Ask about underlying kidney disease and risk factors (DM, HTN, etc)
		Oliguric vs non-oliguric renal failure
		- Oliguria = UOP < 0.5 mL/kg/h
		- Anuria = UOP < 50 mL/d
		Flush Foley, make sure not clogged/kinked, bladder scan
		CBC, BMP, U/A, urine sodium, urea and creatinine
		- Calculate FENa—determine prerenal vs renal vs postrenal
		  ○ Prerenal FENa < 1%— can be due to hypovolemia, heart failure, abdominal compartment syndrome
		  ○ Renal FENa > 1% — due to intrinsic glomerular disease, ATN, AIN, nephrotoxic drugs
		  ○ Postrenal FENa > 4%— due to clogged Foley, ureter injury, BPH causing retention
		- Muddy brown casts = ATN
		Renal U/S
		Nephrology consult
			Initial fluid challenge with 1-2L NS → fluid responsive?
			Can try trial of diuresis for patients with AKI and fluid overload
			Avoid nephrotoxins
			Initiate renal replacement therapy if not improving
			- Indications for emergent dialysis—hyperkalemia, metabolic acidosis, volume overload, uremia, toxins (methanol, ethanol)
			Hyperkalemia—can cause mild ECG changes (peaked T waves) to severe arrhythmias and arrest
			- Treatment—give IV calcium gluconate immediately to stabilize the myocardium
			- Shift potassium intra cellularly with insulin + glucose, β-agonists, sodium bicarb
			- Decrease total body potassium—lasix, kayexalate, dialysis			

Disease Process	Relevant H&P	Work-up/Staging	Treatment	Key Surgical Steps	Post-Op Care	Tips & Tidbits

Chronic liver disease (core)	Patient may present acutely with complications of liver disease including SBP, encephalopathy, jaundice, variceal bleeding, renal failure
	
	Many etiologies for chronic liver failure (alcohol, HCV, HBV, NASH, Wilson's disease, hemochromatosis, alpha-1 antitrypsin deficiency, autoimmune, etc)
		Obtain CBC, CMP, LFT's, INR, coagulants, blood cultures, ammonia level, type and screen, CXR
		
		Calculate MELD-Na score
		
		Bloody emesis in a cirrhotic is variceal bleeding until proven otherwise
		
		Creatinine elevated ⟶ consider hepatorenal syndrome
		
		Spontaneous bacterial peritonitis (SBP)—will present with abdominal pain and large volume ascites ⟶ paracentesis with fluid assessment (PMN, culture)
		
		- PMN > 250 in ascites fluid is diagnostic of SBP
		
		Hepatology consult, evaluation for transplant
			Variceal bleeding
			
			- Resuscitation, blood products as needed, PPI, vasopression, octreotide, ceftriaxone for SBP ppx, intubate if needed
			- GI consult for EGD—banding, sclerotherapy, epinephrine injection
			  ○ Use Blakemore tube for tamponade until GI available to perform EGD, if needed
			- Refractory bleeding ⟶ repeat EGD vs TIPS
			- Portosystemic shunt is a last resort option, rarely done
			
			Encephalopathy—lactulose, rifaximin
			
			Hepatorenal syndrome—treat underlying liver disease, can try trial of octreotide for splanchnic vasoconstriction
			
			Spontaneous bacterial peritonitis—perform paracentesis and send fluid studies, start empiric antibiotics
						Acute liver failure
						
						- May present with malaise, abdominal pain, jaundice, encephalopathy
						- Potential etiologies include acetaminophen overdose, drug-induced liver injury, viral hepatitis, Wilson's disease, autoimmune hepatitis
						- Work-up should include: serum acetaminophen, viral serologies, toxicology screen, serum ceruloplasmin, autoimmune markers (ANA, anti-smooth muscle Ab, anti-liver microsomal Ab), liver U/S +/- liver biopsy
						- Management of ALF:
						  ○ Treat underlying cause:
						    ■ N-acetylcysteine for acetaminophen toxicity
						    ■ Hepatitis B ⟶ antiviral therapy with entecavir
						    ■ Autoimmune hepatitis ⟶ high dose steroids
						    ■ Budd-Chiari ⟶ anticoagulation, TIPS
						  ○ Serial neuro exams to monitor for development of cerebral edema, treat elevated ICP as needed, may need for intubation due to severe encephalopathy
						  ○ Serial LFTs, INR, ABG, lactate and NH_3 levels
						  ○ Coagulopathy treated only if the patient is bleeding
						  ○ Referral for transplant if indicated

Disease Process	Relevant H&P	Work-up/Staging	Treatment	Key Surgical Steps	Post-Op Care	Tips & Tidbits
Upper gastrointestinal bleeding (UGIB), Stress gastritis (core)	Patient may present with unexplained drop in hemoglobin, hematemesis, hematochezia, melena, blood in NGT, or overt hemorrhage History of peptic ulcer disease, NSAIDS, H. pylori, or cirrhosis? Start with the ABCs—make sure patient has good access Perform an abdominal exam, look for signs of cirrhosis and portal hypertension Many potential etiologies of UGIB including PUD, bleeding mass, varices, stress gastritis, etc	Peptic ulcer disease is MCC of UGIB Other causes: esophageal varices, Mallory-Weiss tear, cancer, stress gastritis, etc CBC, BMP, LFTs, coagulants, type and cross NGT to aspirate for blood if source unclear (determine upper vs lower GI source) EGD—can be diagnostic and therapeutic CTA—bleeding rate $\geq$ 0.35 mL/min detectable IR mesenteric angiography—requires bleeding rate at $\geq$0.5 mL/min to be detectable, can embolize at the same time Tagged RBC scan—can detect slower bleeds, requires bleeding rate $\geq$0.2 mL/min to be detectable	Stress gastritis prevention—enteral nutrition, PPI, or H2 blocker prophylaxis Resuscitation/blood transfusion, PPI Correct coagulopathy EGD ASAP Consider IR intervention, if EGD unsuccessful Proceed with surgery if unstable or continued bleeding and endoscopic and IR options have been exhausted	See EGD in "Barrett's esophagus" section in Chapter 2. **Surgery for bleeding due to stress gastritis:** - Anterior gastrostomy with oversewing of lesions, +/- vagotomy and pyloroplasty or GJ - Partial gastrectomy—doesn't work well because stress gastritis is usually multifocal - Total gastrectomy—a last resort for life-threatening, refractory hemorrhage, nearly 100% mortality	Continue PPI Monitor for signs of rebleeding Enteral nutrition as soon as able H. pylori testing with treatment as indicated	Stress gastritis occurs in critically ill, ICU patients - Two biggest risk factors for significant bleeding are coagulopathy and prolonged mechanical ventilation (>48 h) - Other risk factors: history of GI ulceration and bleeding, TBI, burns, sepsis, steroids

9

Pediatric Surgery

Richy Lee, MD

DISEASES AND CONDITIONS

- Hypertrophic pyloric stenosis (c), pyloromyotomy (c)
- Malrotation with volvulus and Ladd's procedure (c)
- Intussusception (c)
- Duodenal atresia
- Jejunoileal atresia
- Gastrointestinal bleeding (c), Meckel's diverticulum (c)

- Inguinal hernia (c)
- Umbilical hernia (c)
- Tracheoesophageal malformations (a)
- Necrotizing enterocolitis (a)
- Gastroschisis and omphalocele (a)
- Meconium disease of the newborn (a)
- Hirschsprung disease (a)

- Anorectal malformations (a)
- Biliary atresia (a)
- Congenital diaphragmatic hernia (a)
- Cryptorchidism (a), orchiopexy (a)
- Thyroglossal duct cyst, brachial cleft anomalies (a)
- Aerodigestive tract foreign bodies (a)
- Chest wall deformity repair (a)

(c) = core topic   (a) = advanced topic

GENERAL PEDIATRIC SURGERY TIPS

- There are many potential pediatric surgery topics—focus on the core topics first and then expand your studying from there.
- In a neonatal patient with emesis, it is important to determine if it is bilious or nonbilious as this can help guide you toward the correct diagnosis.
- Abdominal x-rays are frequently used to evaluate intra-abdominal processes in neonates. It may be helpful to have supine AP and lateral decubitus views.
- Bilious vomiting in neonate is a surgical emergency!
  ○ Bilious emesis indicates an obstruction distal to the ampulla of Vater with a differential including:
    ■ Malrotation with midgut volvulus
    ■ Hernias with bowel incarceration
    ■ Duodenal atresia
    ■ Jejunoileal atresia

  ■ Meconium disease of the newborn
  ■ Hirschsprung's disease
  ■ Anorectal malformations
  ■ Small left colon syndrome
  ○ You must rule out malrotation with volvulus
  ○ Up to 50% of neonates with bilious emesis end up requiring surgical intervention.

- Abdominal mass is listed as a core topic on the curriculum. The most common pediatric malignant intra-abdominal masses are neuroblastoma, nephroblastoma, and hepatoblastoma. The management of these masses is very nuanced and most likely too detailed for the boards, so we will just provide the basic information on these topics:
  ○ Neuroblastoma
    ■ Most common intra-abdominal solid tumor in children

  ■ May present with HTN, abdominal pain, diarrhea, weight loss, failure to thrive, racoon eyes, unsteady gait, usually <2 yo
  ■ Will have elevated urine catecholamines (VMA, HVA)
  ■ Treat with surgery if resectable
  ○ Nephroblastoma (Wilm's Tumor)
    ■ May present as abdominal mass, hematuria, HTN
    ■ "Claw sign" on CT with replacement of renal parenchyma
    ■ Treat with nephrectomy if resectable
  ○ Hepatoblastoma
    ■ May present as rapidly enlarging abdominal mass
    ■ AFP (elevated)
    ■ Treat with surgery if resectable

Disease Process	Relevant H&P	Work-up/Staging	Treatment	Key Surgical Steps	Post-Op Care	Tips & Tidbits
Hypertrophic pyloric stenosis (core)	Feeding intolerance, nonbilious emesis in an infant Usually presents at 4-10 wk old May feel olive-shaped mass in RUQ Look for signs of volume depletion on exam	CBC, BMP Will have hypokalemic, hypochloremic metabolic alkalosis and aciduria U/S—pylorus ≥ 3-mm thick, ≥ 14 mm in length, no passage of fluid through pyloric channel for 15-20 min Can get UGI if U/S unclear—will show string sign	First step—resuscitation, do not rush these patients to the OR - Bolus 20 mL/kg (bolus with NS) - D5 1/2NS with K at 1.5x maintenance (4:2:1 rule) - Make sure metabolic alkalosis and electrolytes are corrected - Make sure patient is making adequate urine (UOP 1.5-2 mL/kg/h) Keep NPO, but NGT not necessary NOT a surgical emergency—wait to take patient for pyloromyotomy until they are stabilized and adequately resuscitated	**Laparoscopic pyloromyotomy (core):** - Place NGT prior to induction - Make pyloromyotomy beginning on antrum extending on to duodenum 　○ Pyloromyotomy should not extend past vein of Mayo to avoid duodenal perforation 　○ Pyloric vein of Mayo travels transversely across distal pyloric channel (junction of pylorus and duodenum) - Spread between muscle fibers until you see mucosa bulge - If you make full thickness defect, close and cover with omental patch and make pyloromyotomy on other side - Leak test by insufflating NG tube. - Convert to open if issues with completing procedure	- Start routine feeding post-op - Common to have emesis post-op, keep hydrated with IVF - If vomiting persists beyond 2-wk post-op, may have incomplete myotomy → get UGI contrast study to evaluate for passage of contrast through pyloric channel, redo pyloromyotomy, if needed	Major misstep: Rushing a patient with hypertrophic pyloric stenosis to the OR prior to adequately resuscitating the patient.

Disease Process	Relevant H&P	Work-up/Staging	Treatment	Key Surgical Steps	Post-Op Care	Tips & Tidbits
Malrotation, Midgut volvulus (core)	Bilious emesis, abdominal pain/distention Look for signs of hypovolemia: sunken fontanelle, dry mucus membranes. Neonatal bowel obstruction differential diagnosis: malrotation with midgut volvulus, duodenal atresia, jejunal atresia, incarcerated hernia, imperforate anus, meconium disease of the newborn, NEC, Hirschsprung's	Labs Abdominal XR UGI—duodenal sweep does not cross midline, corkscrew appearance U/S: SMV to the left of SMA	IV access, resuscitation, NGT placement Surgical emergency! Take to OR ASAP	**Ladd's Procedure (core):** - Transverse laparotomy - Detorse bowel by rotating it counterclockwise (turn back time) - Resect any bowel if it is frankly necrotic - Lyse Ladd's bands - Widen mesentery by scoring anterior leaflet - Perform appendectomy - Put small bowel in the right abdomen and colon on the left - Second look laparotomy, if needed	Start enteral feeds when NGT output appropriate and having bowel function May result in short bowel syndrome - Treat with long-term TPN, anti-diarrheals, intestinal rehab, referral for small bowel transplant	Bilious vomiting in neonate is a surgical emergency! Normal embryologic development: - Fifth week—bowel herniates out of abdomen and turns 90° counterclockwise - 10-11th week—bowel goes back in abdomen and rotates 180° counterclockwise
Intussusception (core)	May present with episodic abdominal pain during which child is inconsolable, N/V, currant jelly (bloody mucoid) stools Usually happens between 3mo and 3 y Frequently had a recent viral illness 85% idiopathic On exam, may have abdominal distention, sausage-like mass Rule out incarcerated inguinal hernia	Labs KUB U/S—target sign Usually ileocolic	Resuscitation—20 mL/kg crystalloid Fluoroscopic reduction—if patient is stable and well-appearing, can attempt reduction with air enema: - Air enema under fluoroscopy - Successful 80% of the time - <1% perf rate - Intussusception may recur (15%), can repeat fluoroscopic reduction up to 3x. If recurs again, then take to OR. If patient has peritonitis, hemodynamic instability, free air, unable to reduce fluoroscopically → do not attempt fluoroscopic reduction, take to OR	**Open or laparoscopic reduction of intussusception:** - If open, milk intussusceptum out of intussuscepted portion by manually compressing intussuscipiens. If laparoscopic, gently pull on the afferent and efferent limbs. - If laparoscopic and having issues reducing the intussusception, convert to open - Only resect bowel if unable to reduce, doesn't appear viable, or if you find a pathologic lead point ○ Perform end-to-end handsewn anastomosis if resection is needed	Observe for at least 4-6 h after air enema reduction and trial diet prior to discharge	Intussusception in adults is managed differently so do not get the management confused. Transient entero-enteral intussusception is a normal physiologic finding and no intervention is needed.

Disease Process	Relevant H&P	Work-up/Staging	Treatment	Key Surgical Steps	Post-Op Care	Tips & Tidbits

Duodenal atresia	Newborn with bilious emesis (sometimes nonbilious if atresia is proximal to ampulla of Vater) and feeding intolerance, usually presents within first few hours after birth
	
	Examine abdomen, evaluate for hernias, verify patient has patent anus, look for any features suggesting Down syndrome
		Frequently diagnosed on prenatal ultrasound
		Place NGT for decompression
		Abdominal XR: double-bubble sign with lack of distal gas
		Must get pre-op ECHO to look for any cardiac issues (present in up to 50%)
			Resuscitation—20 mL/kg crystalloid
			Surgical repair
				Open Duodenoduodenostomy:
				- Transverse supraumbilical, RUQ, or periumbilical incision
				- Thoroughly explore the abdomen to rule out malrotation or additional sites of atresia/stenosis/obstruction
				- Perform Kocher maneuver
				- Make transverse duodenotomy on antimesenteric border just proximal to the atresia
				- Investigate for multiple sites of obstruction due to webs or stenoses. Place catheter into distal duodenum and flush with saline to rule out concomitant distal intestinal atresia
				  ○ Sometimes, obstruction is due to elongated web (type 1 atresia), which can be treated with resection of web alone
				- Make longitudinal duodenostomy on antimesenteric border distal to atresia in area that will reach for anastomosis without significant tension
				- Perform diamond duodenoduodenostomy
				  ○ Anastomosis is made by approximating the apices of each incision to the midportion of the other incision to create a large diamond-shaped anastomosis
				- Close the abdomen
					Initiate feeds when NGT output appropriate	Duodenal atresia is the most common gastrointestinal defect in children with Down syndrome.

Jejunoileal atresia	May initially present as polyhydramnios and bowel dilation on prenatal ultrasound and then, after birth, newborn may present with bilious emesis, abdominal distension, failure to pass meconium
	
	Examine abdomen, look for hernias, and confirm presence of anal opening
		May be suspected/diagnosed on prenatal imaging (U/S, MRI)
		Full labs
		Abdominal XR—supine and left lateral decubitus, will demonstrate dilated bowel loops
			IV fluid resuscitation, NGT decompression, electrolyte replacement
			Surgical repair:
			- If unable to rule out malrotation with volvulus, patient should be brought to the OR emergently
			- Once diagnosis of ileal or jejunal atresia is made take patient to OR urgently
			  ○ Not able to achieve effective decompression with NGT when atresia is distal to LOT
			  ○ Progressive abdominal distention can result in respiratory compromise
				Surgical management of small bowel atresia:
				- Transverse laparotomy
				- Evaluate all bowel for viability, perforation, malrotation, and identify all sites of atresia/stenosis
				- Come up with a plan to preserve as much bowel as safely possible
				- Resect nonviable, severely atretic, and severely dilated bowel
				- Rule out additional atretic segments (~5% have second atresia) → irrigate distal segment with warm saline solution
				- Create anastomoses
				  ○ Handsewn technique may make it easier to deal with size discrepancy
				  ○ Can do tapering enteroplasty or Cheatle slit (extension of distal enterostomy along antimesenteric border) to help compensate for size discrepancy
				- Confirm colonic patency by irrigating intraoperatively
						Likely due to vascular ischemia, whereas duodenal atresia is likely due to failure of recanalization.

Disease Process	Relevant H&P	Work-up/Staging	Treatment	Key Surgical Steps	Post-Op Care	Tips & Tidbits
GI bleeding in child (core)	Presentation variable depending on location and source—ask about details of bleeding episodes (frequency, severity, duration), stool color, and associated symptoms Assess vital signs and ABCs Assess mental status Abdominal and rectal exam	Ensure adequate IV access and resuscitation CBC, coagulation panel, CMP, stool studies Initial imaging should be XR, then get U/S, Meckel's scan, CTA, and/or tagged RBC scan, as indicated Endoscopy if unable to localize with imaging Differential diagnosis: - Neonates: anal fissure, milk protein allergy, NEC, malrotation, Hirschsprung's associated enterocolitis, coagulopathy - Infants: anal fissure, milk protein allergy, Meckel's diverticulum, intussusception, infectious colitis, medical causes (ie, thrombocytopenia) - Children: polyps, Meckel's diverticulum, intussusception, infectious colitis, GI duplication, vascular malformations, trauma/foreign body - Adolescents: IBD, infectious colitis, Meckel's, trauma/foreign body, vascular malformations, GI duplication, hemorrhoids - Meckel's diverticulum—MCC of clinically significant LGIB in children - Intestinal polyps (usually solitary juvenile hamartomatous polyps)—frequent cause of small-volume, LGIB bleeding that is self-limited in children	Resuscitation Some causes may be managed medically For bleeding due to Meckel's diverticulum take to OR for diverticulectomy vs bowel resection	**Surgical treatment of GI bleed due to Meckel's diverticulum (core):** - Can be done open or laparoscopic - Explore entire abdomen and run bowel - Locate Meckel's - Remove with small bowel resection vs diverticulectomy ○ Can perform diverticulectomy if narrow base, no mass is palpated, and not inflamed		Blood transfusion is weight based in pediatrics (10 mL/kg), rather than units of blood product

Disease Process	Relevant H&P	Work-up/Staging	Treatment	Key Surgical Steps	Post-Op Care	Tips & Tidbits
Pediatric inguinal hernia (core)	Groin bulge, worse with straining and crying Reducible? Try to reduce if incarcerated (sedate, if needed) More common in males and premature infants	Often diagnosed on exam—examine both sides and abdomen Can get U/S if diagnosis unclear	Emergent operation if unable to reduce If reducible but difficult, repair within 48 h If easily reducible, elective repair within 6-8 wk - Can be done open or laparoscopic Laparoscopic repair allows for assessment of both sides, but laparoscopy may be contraindicated in patients that are unstable, very small, and/or cannot tolerate general anesthesia or insufflation (ie, cardiopulmonary issues)	**Pediatric open inguinal hernia repair (core):** - Oblique incision over internal ring - Dissect down to external oblique fascia - Identify and open the external ring obliquely up towards the internal ring - Identify and preserve cord structures while mobilizing hernia sac from cord - Inspect sac for contents and reduce if present - Perform high ligation of the hernia sac, do not have to resect distal sac - Do not use mesh - Close in layers - Consider exploring contralateral side if low-birth weight, premature, poor access to medical care, VP shunt **Pediatric laparoscopic inguinal hernia repair:** - General anesthesia required - Laparoscopic entry at umbilicus - Inspect peritoneum and both sides for inguinal hernia - Place purse string around the hernia defect from intra-abdominal approach for high ligation of the sac ○ Many different techniques used to do this laparoscopically - Repeat on contralateral side as needed	If done electively, it is typically an outpatient procedure	
Pediatric umbilical hernia (core)	Umbilical bulge Reducible? More common in premature infants and African Americans	Diagnosed on exam	Can observe asymptomatic umbilical hernias in patients <5yo Surgery if incarcerated, patient has VP shunt, or failure to close by ~5 yo	**Pediatric umbilical hernia repair (core):** - Transverse infraumbilical incision - Identify hernia sac and dissect from umbilical stalk and subcutaneous tissue - Invert and reduce sac or ligate and excise - Free up fascial edges and close defect with interrupted suture ○ Primary suture repair, do not use mesh - Reapproximate underside of umbilicus to fascia - Close	Typically done as an outpatient procedure	

Disease Process	Relevant H&P	Work-up/Staging	Treatment	Key Surgical Steps	Post-Op Care	Tips & Tidbits

Tracheoesophageal malformations (advanced)	Polyhydramnios
	Symptoms depend on type of malformation
	- Newborn may present with feeding intolerance, excessive drooling, recurrent pneumonia (H-type)
	Inability to pass NGT
		Full labs
		NGT placement
		XR: evaluate bowel gas pattern, look for presence of gas in stomach
		Esophageal atresia with distal fistula (Type C) is most common type (can't pass NGT but has distal bowel gas)
		Echo— look for associated cardiac abnormalities, assess which side of the chest the aortic arch is located, important to do prior to taking the patient for surgery
		Investigate for other VACTERL abnormalities
			NGT decompression, elevate head of bed, resuscitation
			Operative repair options:
			- Primary repair possible if esophageal gap is short
			- If gap length >3 vertebral bodies → delay repair (usually 6-8 wk), place G-tube and NGT for decompression while waiting
			  ○ May have to use gastric, jejunal or colonic conduit if gap remains too long
			- If premature or unstable → NGT, place G-tube, and delay definitive repair, may need urgent OR to clip TEF if that is the cause of instability
				Tracheoesophageal malformation repair:
				- Begin with rigid bronchoscopy to confirm diagnosis
				- Variety of approaches
				  ○ Right posterolateral thoracotomy vs thoracoscopy
				- May need to approach via left posterolateral thoracotomy if patient has right-sided aortic arch
				  ○ Extrapleural vs transpleural approach
				- Identify proximal and distal portions of esophagus
				- Identify fistula, then mobilize and ligate
				- Close the tracheal defect
				- Mobilize esophagus and bring the ends together to create single-layer (full-thickness) end-to-end anastomosis
				- Leave NGT across anastomosis
				- Consider placing tissue flap between anastomosis and tracheal closure
				- Leave drain next to anastomosis
					Can start feeds via NGT in 48-72 hrs
					Consider contrast study of anastomosis prior to oral feeds
					Complications:
					- GERD is common
					- Anastomotic leak—diagnosed on contrast study, most controlled by surgical drain and will heal without intervention
					- Stricture— common long-term complication, can be treated with endoscopic balloon dilation
					- Tracheomalacia
						VACTERL syndrome - complex syndrome that involves abnormalities of multiple organ systems
						- **V**ertebral defects
						- **A**nal atresia
						- **C**ardiac abnormalities
						- **T**racheoEsophageal abnormalities
						- **R**enal abnormalities
						- **L**imb defects

Necrotizing enterocolitis (advanced)	Risk factors: prematurity, low birth weight, formula feeds, maternal exposure to NSAID, congenital cardiac anomaly Typically 2-3 weeks old May present with feeding intolerance, abdominal distention, vomiting, bloody stools, lethargy, discoloration of abdominal wall, increased oxygen requirement, increase in apnea/bradycardia episodes, temperature instability	Full labs—may see leukopenia, thrombocytopenia, metabolic acidosis, elevated inflammatory markers Abdominal XR—look for dilated bowel loops, fixed bowel loops on serial AXR, pneumatosis, portal venous gas, pneumoperitoneum Do **NOT** do contrast enema	Medical/supportive treatment initially, unless there is perforation or uncontrolled sepsis - Stop feeds, place NGT, IV antibiotics (ampicillin, gentamicin, metronidazole), parenteral nutrition, serial abdominal exams and XRs Surgery for perforation or failure to improve with medical management - Options: laparotomy vs peritoneal drain (for very small neonates)	**Laparotomy for necrotizing enterocolitis:** - Transverse laparotomy - Assess all bowel for viability and sites of perforation - Remove grossly necrotic bowel, save viable or questionable bowel - Make ostomies (rather than anastomoses) - Leave bowel in discontinuity and place silo for temporary abdominal closure if unstable	Continue antibiotics, resuscitation, and parenteral nutrition Delay reconstruction until NEC has resolved and neonate growing Long-term complications: - Post-NEC stricture - Short bowel syndrome	Early diagnosis and treatment are key.

Disease Process	Relevant H&P	Work-up/Staging	Treatment	Key Surgical Steps	Post-Op Care	Tips & Tidbits
Gastroschisis and omphalocele (advanced)	Omphalocele—has a sac covering it (unless it has ruptured) - Associated with chromosomal abnormalities, Beckwith-Weidemann syndrome, Prune-Belly syndrome Gastroschisis—no sac, occurs to the right of the umbilicus - Can be associated with intestinal atresia	Typically seen on obstetric U/S Preterm delivery not recommended Planned C-section not required unless other issues are present (placenta previa, abnormal lie and presentation, fetal hypoxia, etc.) Rule out other abnormalities - Omphalocele: get echo to rule out cardiac abnormalities, renal ultrasound, karyotyping 　○ Omphalocele is more commonly associated with other abnormalities (50%)	IV access, resuscitation, keep patient warm, cover exposed bowel or sac with petroleum gauze to decrease heat/fluid losses Place NGT, Foley Surgical management - Gastroschisis 　○ First, determine if primary closure is feasible or if silo placement and delayed closure will be required 　　■ Primary closure—suture fascial defect closed vs cover with umbilical cord remnant and petroleum gauze for sutureless repair 　　■ For patients with large gastroschisis place silo and gradually reduce bowel until abdomen can eventually be closed - Omphalocele 　○ Reduce bowel and primary repair, if able, but typically there is significant loss of abdominal domain so most cases are managed with "paint and wait" and then manage ventral hernia down the road		Watch out for abdominal compartment syndrome after closure TPN for nutrition Enteral feeds when NGT output appropriate and bowel function present If patient has ongoing feeding tolerance issues consider delayed motility and/or missed atresia	

Disease Process	Relevant H&P	Work-up/Staging	Treatment	Key Surgical Steps	Post-Op Care	Tips & Tidbits

Meconium disease of the newborn (advanced)	Newborn presenting with abdominal distention, bilious emesis, failure to pass meconium
	
	May be suspected based on prenatal U/S—may show hyperechoic abdominal mass (inspissated meconium in the terminal ileum), bowel dilation, polyhydramnios
		Meconium plug vs meconium ileus
		- Meconium plug—distal colonic or rectal obstruction caused by plug of inspissated meconium
		  ○ More common in low birth weight neonates
		  ○ Abdominal XR—nonspecific, air fluid levels
		  ○ Contrast enema—can be diagnostic and therapeutic
		  ○ Usually occurs in otherwise healthy neonates, loose association with cystic fibrosis and Hirschsprungs
		- Meconium ileus—inspissated meconium causes obstruction at terminal ileum and patient often has microcolon due to disuse, strong association with cystic fibrosis
		  ○ May have associated perforation, volvulus, intestinal atresia
		  ○ Abdominal XR—distended small intestine loops, "soap-bubble" appearance, may see calcifications if perforation has occurred
		  ○ Contrast enema—will show microcolon (due to disuse)
		    ■ Obstruction is usually at terminal ileum
		    ■ If contrast does not reach the dilated intestine → concern for atresia or volvulus
		  ○ Test for cystic fibrosis—most patients who present with meconium ileus have CF
			Resuscitation, antibiotics, NGT
			
			Meconium plug—almost all cases resolve with gastrograffin enemas, rarely require surgery for complications
			
			Meconium ileus—initial management for uncomplicated cases is nonoperative with gastrograffin enema (successful in 2/3 of patients), N-acetylcysteine via NGT, serial abdominal XRs
			
			- OR if patient has complete obstruction, perforation, volvulus, or fails nonoperative management
				Operation for meconium ileus:
				- Make a transverse RLQ incision (overlying terminal ileum where obstruction most common occurs)
				- Run the bowel and identify transition point
				- Resect bowel if compromised
				- Make a small enterotomy and milk out the meconium as much as possible
				- Irrigate with N-acetylcysteine
				- Do not need to be overly aggressive in debriding meconium material if perforation occurred (it is sterile)
				- Create end ostomy and separate mucous fistula
					Meconium ileus—NAC irrigation via ostomy, enemas, or NG tube
					
					Stoma reversal in 6-12 wk when obstruction resolved	

Disease Process	Relevant H&P	Work-up/Staging	Treatment	Key Surgical Steps	Post-Op Care	Tips & Tidbits

Hirschsprung's disease (advanced)	Newborn fails to pass meconium
	
	Can also present in older children as chronic constipation
	
	Can develop Hirschsprung's-associated enterocolitis: rapidly progressive abdominal distention, foul smelling diarrhea, lethargy, sepsis
	
	Explosive release of watery stool with anorectal exam
		Abdominal XR
		
		Contrast enema: rectosigmoid index ≤ 1
		
		Suction rectal biopsy—to confirm diagnosis
		
		- Biopsy with absence of parasympathetic ganglia, presence of hypertrophied nerve trunks
			Treat with flagyl and rectal irrigation while awaiting confirmative biopsy results prior to surgery, as long as patient is stable
			
			Must do full thickness biopsies to determine length of aganglionic section prior to pull through procedure surgery
			
			Surgery—pull through procedure (Soave, Swenson or Duhamel)
			
			- Can be transanal and/or transabdominal
			
			May need diverting ostomy prior to definitive repair if patient presents with severe colitis or severe dilation
				Pull-Through Procedure:
				- Can be done open or laparoscopic-assisted
				- Place NGT and Foley
				- Obtain full thickness biopsies of colon wall with intraoperative pathology performed to determine proximal extent of aganglionosis
				- Aganglionic colon resected and normal bowel anastomosed to just above the anal sphincter
				- Three commonly used procedures:
				  ○ Swenson: excision of aganglionic bowel with end-to-end anastomosis
				  ○ Soave: excision of aganglionic bowel with mucosectomy of the distal rectum and pull through of the normal bowel with a cuff of aganglionic muscle
				  ○ Duhamel: retains a short segment of aganglionic rectum with posterior pull-through of normal bowel and side-to-side stapled anastomosis
				- If additional length is needed, perform splenic flexure mobilization +/- division of middle colic vessels
					Anastomotic leak presents with abdominal pain, distention, fever, vomiting
					
					- Usually requires revision of anastomosis and stoma
					
					Can develop postop enterocolitis
					
					- Treat with rectal irrigations and metronidazole
					
					Perineal excoriations are common—barrier creams can help
					
					Start dilations with Hegar dilators 3 wk after surgery to prevent strictures	

Disease Process	Relevant H&P	Work-up/Staging	Treatment	Key Surgical Steps	Post-Op Care	Tips & Tidbits

Anorectal malformations (advanced)	Often discovered immediately after birth due to lack of anal opening or failure to pass meconium
	
	Exam—may have abdominal distention, lack of patent anus, look for fistula in perineum and other urogenital malformations, spinal/sacral defects
		Determine the anatomy of the anorectal malformation (ARM):
		- In females, rectum can end blindly (no fistula) or fistulize to vestibule or perineal skin, or be part of complex malformation (cloaca—confluence of urethra, vagina, and rectum)
		- In males, distal rectum can end blindly (no fistula) or fistulize to urethra
		- Obtain A/P and lateral sacral XR
		  ○ Calculate sacral ratio—helps predict potential for bowel control
		  ○ Measure distance from end of bowel to skin
		Screen for other abnormalities associated with VACTERL
			NPO, IV fluids, NG tube
			Surgery (colostomy vs primary anoplasty):
			- Perineal fistula present → primary anoplasty
			  ○ Allow 24 h for fistula to form
			- No fistula, other types of fistula, cloaca, or end of bowel >1.5 cm from skin → end colostomy with mucous fistula, then anorectoplasty in 1-2 mo
			  ○ Mucus fistula is used for distal colostogram prior to reconstruction
				Colostomy in a pediatric patient:
				- Procedure can be performed via laparoscopy or through LLQ incision
				- End colostomy created using proximal sigmoid
				- Create mucous fistula so that distal colostogram can be obtained and can irrigate distal pouch to clear the meconium
				
				Posterior sagittal anorectoplasty (PSARP):
				- Place Foley
				- Prone position
				- Incision in midline of buttocks
				- Identify sphincter complex with muscle stimulator
				- Circumferentially mobilize rectum so that it can reach perineum and be pulled into center of the sphincter complex without tension
				  ○ Separate rectum from posterior vagina in females or urethra in males
				- Ligate fistula
				- Fix rectum to muscle complex, close in layers, and perform anoplasty, with circumferential interrupted sutures
				- If patient has a high malformation (ie, fistula proximal to membranous urethra on distal colostogram), then start operation with laparotomy or laparoscopy to mobilize the rectum and decrease the risk of ureter injury
				- Temporary colostomy creation, as indicated (most patients already have one)
					Start anal dilations at 2 wk to prevent anal stenosis.
					Reverse colostomy when neo-anus is appropriately healed and dilated (usually in 3-4 mo)
					Constipation is very common—need bowel regimen to ensure daily evacuation
						Patients with high malformations, poor sphincter muscles, and/or associated spinal/sacral anomalies are more likely to have issues with incontinence.

Biliary atresia (advanced)	Jaundice in newborn that starts ~3-6 wk of age Light-colored stools, dark urine More common in Asian patients Liver edge may be palpable on exam	Full labs—CMP will show direct hyperbilirubinemia Serology to rule out hepatitis A, hepatitis B, hepatitis C, TORCH infections (toxoplasmosis, rubella, CMV, HSV) Alpha 1-antitrypsin level Abdominal U/S HIDA scan with phenobarbital pretreatment, if U/S unclear Liver biopsy—ductular proliferation, inflammatory infiltrate, cholestasis Work-up is time sensitive, ideal to perform Kasai ASAP	Kasai procedure (portoenterostomy) Liver transplant if Kasai procedure fails	**Kasai Procedure (Portoenterostomy):** - Right subcostal incision - Cholangiogram via gallbladder to define anatomy and confirm diagnosis - Dissect out distal CBD (fibrous/scar) and divide above junction with duodenum - Dissect out proximal CBD at the level of portal vein bifurcation and open flush with liver parenchyma - Remove gallbladder - Transect jejunum ~10-15 cm distal to LOT and bring up a Roux limb - Construct the portoenterostomy anastomosis and then jejunojejunostomy ~40 cm distal on Roux limb - Leave drain adjacent to anastomosis	Common complications: - Cholangitis—treat with antibiotics - Fat malabsorption—vitamins A, D, E, K supplementation, formula with medium chain triglycerides - Portal HTN	Outcomes after the Kasai Procedure: - >50% 5-y survival - Two-thirds go on to require transplant (usually in first 20 y)

Disease Process	Relevant H&P	Work-up/Staging	Treatment	Key Surgical Steps	Post-Op Care	Tips & Tidbits
Congenital diaphragmatic hernia (advanced)	Polyhydramnios Newborn will present with respiratory distress hypoxia/hypercarbia, often requiring ventilatory support Varying degree of pulmonary hypoplasia and pulmonary HTN based on degree of herniation and size of hernia	Often initially diagnosed on fetal U/S and can be characterized further on fetal MRI - CDH diagnosed prenatally in 50-80% of cases ABG, full labs Karyotyping CXR—Intestinal, gastric, and/or liver herniation into hemithorax, mediastinal shift away from the defect ECHO—Identify cardiac defects, assess for pulmonary hypertension Types of CDH: - Bochdalek—right or left posterolateral diaphragmatic hernia - Morgagni—anterior diaphragmatic hernia	First priority when patient is born is to stabilize them from a cardiopulmonary standpoint - Needs range from nasal cannula to CPAP to intubation to ECMO in severe cases OGT decompression, IV fluid resuscitation Repair delayed until patient is stabilized Repair can be done via MIS (usually thoracoscopy) or open surgery	**Open congenital diaphragmatic hernia repair:** - Supine positioning - Subcostal incision - Reduce herniated contents - Expose the posterior rim of the diaphragm - Assess the defect—resect any residual hernia sac or associated pulmonary sequestration - Create primary, tension-free repair with interrupted sutures, if possible - Larger defects may require patch repair with Gore-Tex mesh - Place chest tube - Closure - If unable to close abdomen, then use bridging Vicryl mesh	Complications: respiratory failure, PTX, recurrence	
Cryptorchidism (advanced)	More common in preterm infants (affects up to 30%) Perform exam, including palpation of areas where an undescended testis may be located (scrotum, inguinal canal, base of the penis, thigh, perineum) - Most common location is at external ring	Check for associated anomalies: inguinal hernia, hypospadias, epididymal abnormalities, Prune-Belly syndrome, posterior urethral valves, anomalies of upper urinary tract Testis not palpable bilaterally → hCG administration test → Elevated FSH is indicative of anorchia; normal FSH suggests undescended testicles Nonpalpable testis → laparoscopy to localize	Orchiopexy recommended if remains undescended after 6 mo of age - Open inguinal orchiopexy if testicle is palpable - Laparoscopic orhiopexy for intra-abdominal testicle	**Open inguinal orchiopexy (advanced):** - Examine under anesthesia to see if you can palpate testicle - Make transverse incision at inguinal skin crease - Incise external oblique over inguinal canal and extend to the external ring - Mobilize spermatic cord and testis, divide the gubernaculum - Mobilize hernia sac off the cord and perform high ligation - Divide transversalis fascia to get length for spermatic cord - Make scrotal incision and create sub-dartos pouch that tunnels to inguinal incision - Bring testis down into scrotal pouch and pexy in place - Close	Complications: hematoma, wound infection, testicular atrophy	Main goals of orchiopexy are to prevent infertility and allow for future testicular examination

Disease Process	Relevant H&P	Work-up/Staging	Treatment	Key Surgical Steps	Post-Op Care	Tips & Tidbits
Brachial cleft anomalies, thyroglossal duct cyst (advanced)	Brachial cleft anomaly (cyst, sinus, fistula): - Off midline mass and/or external sinus - Often asymptomatic but can become tender, enlarged, or inflamed with superinfection or abscess, especially during upper respiratory tract infections - Avoid probing or injecting with dye if opening found Thyroglossal duct cyst: - Midline, anterior neck mass - Mass moves with protrusion of tongue and swallowing. Can present with fever, erythema, and drainage if infected - Most present within the first 5 y of life	Neck U/S should be the initial test—look for presence of normal thyroid in case of thyroglossal duct cyst CT/MRI of second branchial cysts may show characteristic beak sign between external and internal carotid arteries Barium esophagogram, CT, and/or endoscopy may be helpful in identifying third or fourth branchial fistula/sinus	Branchial cyst, sinus, or fistula: - Elective excision is indicated to minimize risks of recurrence, infection, or malignancy - Infected → antibiotics, aspiration or incision and drainage. Avoid doing definitive resection operation when acutely infected to minimize the risk of damage to nearby structures, wound infection, or incomplete resection Thyroglossal duct cyst: - Infected → Antibiotics +/- I&D - Elective resection when not infected	**Excision of branchial cyst/sinus/fistula:** - Position supine, with shoulder roll and head turned to contralateral side - Mark or cannulate tract if possible - Make horizontal elliptical skin incision along Langer's lines around the cutaneous opening or over palpable cyst - Dissect along the tract - Manual palpation with a finger in the pharynx may facilitate identification of the upper extent of the fistula - Ligate fistula tract with an absorbable suture - If the tract is very long, may need to make a second, more cephalad, "step ladder" incision for exposure - Excise cyst and entire fistula tract - Irrigate and close in layers - Excision of first branchial lesion is more complex because it requires mobilization of parotid gland and identification and preservation of facial nerve **Excision of thyroglossal duct cyst (Sistrunk procedure):** - Position supine, with shoulder roll - Make an infrahyoid transverse skin incision directly over the cyst - Dissect through platysma and down to the cyst - Dissect out the cyst and trace tract cephalad and posterior up to hyoid bone - Cut hyoid bone to resect central portion - Trace tract up to base of tongue then ligate and divide, resect en bloc with hyoid bone and cyst - Irrigate and close in layers	May recur if excision incomplete - Recurrence <7% after branchial anomaly excision and <10% after Sistrunk procedure Monitor for hypothyroidism, if thyroid tissue is identified within the specimen	Branchial cleft lesions: - First—fistulas occur between mandible and hyoid bone - Second—fistulas occur at anterior border of SCM - Third—fistulas occur at junction of SCM and clavicle

Disease Process	Relevant H&P	Work-up/Staging	Treatment	Key Surgical Steps	Post-Op Care	Tips & Tidbits
Aerodigestive tract foreign body (advanced)	Symptoms of aspiration: cough, stridor, hemoptysis, respiratory compromise, asphyxia Symptoms of ingestion: dysphagia, odynophagia, emesis, drooling, chest pain, refusal to eat Children 6 mo to 3 y most likely to ingest foreign bodies Coins are the most commonly ingested objects Parents may report history of choking episode Immediately assess airway and breathing	PA and lateral XRs of the neck and chest—lateral view may help distinguish coin vs disc battery Airway foreign bodies usually lodge in the right mainstem bronchus 60% of ingested foreign objects pass into the stomach Objects that get stuck in the esophagus usually get stuck at the cricopharyngeus, aortic crossover, or LES If nothing seen on XR, but patient has persistent symptoms of foreign body ingestion contrast esophagogram or CT should be obtained	**Ingestion:** - Most ingested foreign objects pass spontaneously (~80%), 15-20% retrieved endoscopically, <1% require operative intervention. - Coins lodged in the esophagus should be removed endoscopically. Rigid or flexible esophagoscopy may be required. - Coins in the stomach or small bowel can be allowed to pass per rectum. get repeat XR in 1-2 wk to confirm passage. - Button battery stuck in the esophagus is a surgical emergency. Asymptomatic button batteries in the stomach can be allowed to pass. - Ingestion of multiple magnets requires removal by endoscopy or surgery. **Aspiration:** - In a child with symptoms consistent with airway obstruction, perform immediate direct laryngoscopy to evaluate for object in oropharynx. Retrieve with Magill forceps - Emergent surgical airway if necessary—trach or needle cricothyroidotomy preferred in children (avoid cricothyroidotomy in children <8 yo) - Bronchoscopy under general anesthesia for objects lodged in more distal airway		Monitor for complications, PO challenge prior to discharge	

Disease Process	Relevant H&P	Work-up/Staging	Treatment	Key Surgical Steps	Post-Op Care	Tips & Tidbits
Chest wall deformities (advanced)	Pectus excavatum (concave sternal plate): - Most common chest wall defect - Usually presents during puberty, worsens during growth spurts - More common in males (75%) - Can affect cardiopulmonary function and cause chest pain and SOB during exercise - Ask about history of metal allergy Pectus carinatum (convex chest): - Often presents at time of pubertal growth spurt - Commonly asymptomatic, but patient may have pain in affected costal cartilages Obtain psychosocial history from patient and parents Examine for cardiac conditions and scoliosis	Chest CT for patient with pectus excavatum → calculate Haller index, calculate correction index - Haller index = (transverse distance of chest) / (distance from sternum to vertebra) ○ ≥3.25 is severe PFTs, ECG ECHO, if cardiac symptoms	Consider Nuss repair for patients with severe pectus excavatum and physiologic impairment (ie, symptomatic, abnormal PFTs, associated cardiac abnormality). - Optimal age for the Nuss procedure is ~15 yo, leave bar in place for 2-3 y		CXR in PACU to document bar position, expected to have trace PTX Bar rotation or migration should be recognized by new onset of pain or visibly recurrent excavatum - Reoperation is usually required for repositioning/ stabilization - Rotation up to 45° can be observed Pectus bar removed within 3 y after insertion	Patients post repair of pectus excavatum been shown to have improvement in psychosocial testing, body image, and report improved exercise tolerance.

10

Head and Neck Surgery

Joseph Sniezek, MD, MBA, FACS, and Gary Lucas, MD

DISEASES AND CONDITIONS

- Hyperparathyroidism (c), parathyroidectomy (c)
- Thyroid nodule (c)
- Well-differentiated thyroid cancer (c), partial thyroidectomy (c), selective neck dissection
- Medullary thyroid cancer (c), total thyroidectomy (c)
- Thyroiditis (c)
- Hyperthyroidism (c)
- Neck mass evaluation (c), head and neck cancer (a), lymph node biopsy (c)
- Parotidectomy (a)
- Neck abscess

GENERAL HEAD AND NECK SURGERY TIPS

There is a risk of recurrent laryngeal nerve (RLN) injury when operating in the neck

- Unilateral injury results in weak/breathy voice
- Bilateral injury can result in upper airway obstruction

If you are given a patient with history of prior neck surgery who needs to undergo another neck surgery (ie, thyroidectomy, parathyroidectomy, etc), obtain preoperative flexible laryngoscopy to ensure the RLNs are intact bilaterally.

(c) = **core topic**   (a) = **advanced topic**

Disease Process	Relevant H&P	Work-up/Staging	Treatment	Key Surgical Steps	Post-Op Care	Tips & Tidbits

Hyperparathyroidism (core)	May present with fatigue, headaches, anxiety/depression, bone/muscle pain, kidney stones
	
	Oftentimes, hypercalcemia is incidentally found on routine labs
	
	History of MEN syndrome (I, IIa)?
	
	Perform neck exam
		Serum calcium, PTH level, BMP
		- Elevated PTH and calcium suggests diagnosis of primary hyperparathyroidism
		- Elevated PTH and creatinine with low calcium suggests secondary hyperparathyroidism
		Vitamin D level—in patients with low vitamin D, start patient in vitamin D supplementation and then recheck PTH and calcium in several months (low vitamin D can artificially elevate PTH)
		24-h urine calcium to rule out familial hypocalciuric hypercalcemia
		Renal U/S to look for nephrolithiasis
		DEXA bone scan
		Consider genetic counseling if genetic syndrome suspected
		In cases of primary hyperparathyroidism 80% is due to single gland disease (adenoma), 15-20% due to multigland disease, <1% due to parathyroid malignancy
		Localization studies—if planning to operate, obtain one or more of these studies to localize the abnormal gland:
		- U/S—usually the initial localization test, obtain others if not diagnostic
		- Sestamibi scan
		- 4D CT
		- PET-CT
		- MRI
		- Selective venous sampling
			Indications for parathyroidectomy:
			- Symptomatic
			- Age <50 yo
			- Serum Ca >1 mg/dL above upper limit of normal
			- Renal involvement—nephrolithiasis, nephrocalcinosis, GFR <60 mL/min
			- Hypercalciuria—urine calcium >400 mg/24 h
			- Osteoporosis (T-score ≤ -2.5 or vertebral compression fracture)
			- Poor follow-up
			Single adenoma → parathyroidectomy
			Parathyroid hyperplasia → 3.5 gland excision
			Treatment of hypercalcemic crisis:
			- Normal saline bolus until rehydrated
			- Lasix, calcitonin, and/or bisphosphonates, as needed
				Parathyroidectomy (core):
				- Ideally, abnormal gland has been localized with preoperative imaging so that focused parathyroidectomy can be performed; however, if unable to localize then need to do 4 gland exploration
				- Check preoperative PTH
				- +/- Recurrent laryngeal nerve (RLN) monitoring during case
				- Make collar incision, create sub-platysma skin flaps, split strap muscles and dissect them off the thyroid
				- Retract thyroid gland medially, identify and ligate middle thyroid vein
				- Identify and preserve recurrent laryngeal nerves
				  ○ Use location of RLN to assist in parathyroid exploration:
				    ■ Superior parathyroid gland is located superficial (ventral) to the RLN
				    ■ Inferior parathyroid gland is located deep (dorsal) to the RLN
				- Identify target parathyroid gland and remove
				- Check PTH 10-15 min after removal of gland
				  ○ PTH should drop by 50%
				  ○ If not, proceed with 4 gland exploration
				- If performing 4 gland exploration, identify all 4 parathyroids
				  ○ Can confirm parathyroid tissue with frozen section
				  ○ Excise clearly abnormal appearing gland and recheck PTH
				  ○ If all glands appear normal, may need to excise 3.5 glands
				- Confirm recurrent laryngeal nerve function prior to closure
				
				Reimplantation of parathyroid:
				- May be required for normal parathyroid with disrupted vascular pedicle
				- Confirm it is parathyroid tissue with frozen section, if needed
				- Parathyroid divided into 1-3-mm sections
				- Create several pockets in SCM with blunt dissection
				- Place pieces of parathyroid into each pocket
				- Mark pockets with a clip or Prolene suture
					Check PTH and calcium levels
					
					Postoperative hypocalcemia
					- Classic calcium nadir occurs within 24-48 h after parathyroidectomy
					- May present as perioral numbness, tetany, muscle spasms
					- Treat with calcium supplementation and calcitriol as needed
						<1% of cases of hyperparathyroidism are due to parathyroid carcinoma → resect en bloc with hemithyroidectomy
						
						MC location of missed gland is the normal anatomic location
						
						Most common nonanatomic locations:
						- Thymus
						- Carotid sheath
						- Intrathyroidal
						- Paraesophageal space
						
						Additional reading:
						Wilhelm SM, Wang TS, Ruan DT, et al. The American Association of Endocrine Surgeons Guidelines for Definitive Management of Primary Hyperparathyroidism. *JAMA Surg.* 2016;151(10):959-968.

Disease Process	Relevant H&P	Work-up/Staging	Treatment	Key Surgical Steps	Post-Op Care	Tips & Tidbits
Thyroid nodule (core)	Ask about compressive symptoms, hypo- or hyperthyroidism symptoms Family history of thyroid cancer? History of XRT? Previous neck surgery? Examine thyroid and cervical lymph nodes	Thyroid nodules are common, only ~5% end up being malignant Check TSH Thyroid ultrasound—concerning features: - Hypoechoic - Microcalcifications - Irregular borders - Extra-thyroidal extension - Taller than wide Indications for FNA of thryoid nodule: - ≥2 cm - ≥1.5 cm with low suspicion on U/S - ≥1 cm with intermediate to high suspicion on U/S - History of XRT - Family history of thyroid cancer - Hoarseness No need to biopsy simple cysts Bethesda classification of thyroid cytopathology used to categorize thyroid FNA results	Next steps depend on Bethesda classificaton: 1. Nondiagnostic (5-10% malignancy risk) ⟶ repeat FNA 2. Benign (0-3% malignancy risk) ⟶ follow-up imaging in 12 mo 3. FLUS/AUS (10-30% malignancy risk) ⟶ repeat FNA or obtain molecular testing 4. Follicular neoplasm (25-40% malignancy risk) ⟶ diagnostic lobectomy, can consider molecular testing ▪ Cannot diagnose follicular thyroid cancer based on FNA alone 5. Suspicious for malignancy (50-75% malignancy risk) ⟶ lobectomy or total thyroidectomy 6. Malignant (97-99% malignancy risk) ⟶ total thyroidectomy	**FNA of thyroid nodule:** - Localize the nodule using ultrasound - Anesthetize the skin with local anesthetic - Pass a 25-gauge needle through the mass multiple times while aspirating		

Disease Process	Relevant H&P	Work-up/Staging	Treatment	Key Surgical Steps	Post-Op Care	Tips & Tidbits

Well-differentiated thyroid cancer (core)	Patient may present with nonpainful anterior neck mass
	
	History of XRT? Symptoms of hypo- or hyperthyroidism?
	
	Compressive symptoms, rapid growth, hoarseness raise concern for anaplastic thyroid cancer
	
	Examine thyroid and cervical nodes
		TSH, T4
		
		Thyroid U/S with FNA
		- Psammoma bodies on pathology = papillary thyroid cancer
		- FNA cannot distinguish follicular adenoma from follicular carcinoma
		
		Papillary, follicular and Hürthle cell thyroid cancer are considered "differentiated thyroid carcinomas"
		
		Staging for follicular or papillary thyroid cancer:
		- Cervical U/S to assess LNs, FNA any suspicious LNs
		- CT/MRI used in select patients with clinical suspicion for advanced locoregional disease
		
		Patients <55 yo with differentiated thyroid carcinomas have a good prognosis, even widely metastatic tumors get a maximum stage II
			Papillary and follicular thyroid cancer:
			
			- Tumor <1cm, LN (-), no extrathryoidal extension (ETE) → lobectomy preferred
			- Tumor 1-4 cm, LN(-), no ETE → lobectomy vs total thyroidectomy
			- >4 cm, LN(+), distant metastases, history of head and neck radiation, **or** ETE present → total thyroidectomy
			- If you do lobectomy and patient is found to have tumor >4 cm, LN(+), ETE, vascular invasion, *or* positive margin → completion thyroidectomy
			- Total thyroidectomy preferred if planning to treat with radioactive iodine
			
			No routine neck dissection required for papillary or follicular cancer with clinically negative LN, however:
			- If a positive central neck lymph node (level VI) is identified → central neck dissection
			- If a positive lateral neck lymph node (levels II-VI) is identified → lateral and central neck dissection should be performed
			
			Hürthle cell cancer—more aggressive variant of follicular thyroid cancer, managed similarly
				Thyroid lobectomy (core):
				- Patient positioned in semi-Fowler position with shoulder-bump
				- +/- Recurrent laryngeal nerve monitoring during case
				- Collar incision ~2 fingerbreadths above sternal notch
				- Raise subplatysmal flaps
				- Split the strap muscles
				- Ligate and divide the middle thyroid vein
				- Free superior pole of thyroid by dividing the anterior suspensory ligament and superior pole vessels, staying close to the gland and preserving the external branch of the superior laryngeal nerve
				- Mobilize the inferior pole
				- Identify and preserve the RLN, ligate the inferior thyroid artery close to the gland
				- Identify and preserve the parathyroid glands
				- Free thyroid lobe from the trachea
				- Divide thyroid at the isthmus, ensure excellent hemostasis
				- Central and/or lateral neck dissection if indicated by positive LN
				
				Total thyroidectomy: see Medullary thyroid cancer section
				
				Selective neck dissection:
				- Remove all fatty and lymphoid tissue in affected LN compartment(s) (Figure 10.1)
				  ◦ Lateral compartment = anterior triangle (II, III, IV) and posterior triangle (V)
				  ◦ Central compartment (VI) = between sternohyoid muscle, hyoid bone, and suprasternal notch
					Complications:
					- Post-op neck hematoma—if causing airway obstruction, it should be opened immediately at bedside
					- Recurrent laryngeal nerve injury
					
					Check TSH level ~6-wk post-op → levothyroxine dose adjusted accordingly
					- All patients after total thyroidectomy will require thyroid hormone supplementation
					  ◦ Initial dose: 1.6 mcg/kg/d
					  ◦ Repeat TSH in 4-6 wk, adjust dose as needed
					- ~20% of patients post thyroid lobectomy develop subclinical hypothyroidism (elevated TSH, normal T4) and should have TSH checked
					- Symptoms of post-op hypothyroidism: fatigue, weakness, cold intolerance, weight gain, constipation, dry skin
					
					Radioactive iodine ablation therapy used to treat microscopic disease if:
					• Tumor >4 cm
					• Gross extrathyroidal extension
					• Thyroglobulin >10 ng/mL
					• >5 positive LNs
					
					Surveillance: check thyroglobulin level in 6-12 wk and neck U/S in 6-12 mo
						Papillary thyroid cancer is the most common type of thyroid cancer and has an excellent survival rate.
						
						Papillary thyroid cancer tends to spread via lymph nodes, whereas follicular thyroid cancer tends to spread hematogenously.
						
						Anaplastic thyroid cancer— all are stage IV, can do thyroidectomy with LN dissection if R0/R1 resection possible, otherwise just give palliative XRT
						
						Thyroid lymphoma— nonsurgical treatment, CHOP + XRT
						
						Additional reading:
						
						Patel KN, et al. The American association of endocrine surgeons guidelines for the definitive surgical management of thyroid disease in adults. *Ann Surg.* 2020 Mar;271(3):e21-e93.
						
						Haugen BR, et al. 2015 American thyroid association management guidelines for adult patients with thyroid nodules and differentiated thyroid cancer: the American thyroid association guidelines task force on thyroid nodules and differentiated thyroid cancer. *Thyroid.* 2016 Jan;26(1):1-133.

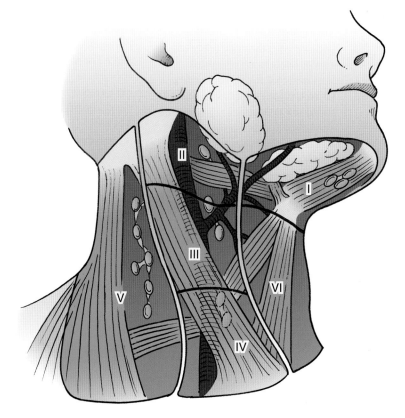

FIGURE 10.1: Cervical lymph node levels I-VI

Level Ia: Submental triangle

Level Ib: Submandibular triangle

Level II: Upper jugular nodes

Level III: Middle jugular nodes

Level IV: Lower jugular nodes

Level V: Posterior triangle

Level VI: Nodes of the central compartment

Modified with permission from Minter RM, Doherty GM. *Current Procedures: Surgery.* New York, NY: McGraw Hill; 2010, Figure 1-5.

Disease Process	Relevant H&P	Work-up/Staging	Treatment	Key Surgical Steps	Post-Op Care	Tips & Tidbits
Medullary thyroid cancer (MTC) (core)	Family history? MEN IIa/b? - 25% of MTC is hereditary Symptoms? History of XRT? Neck and LN exam	TSH Thyroid U/S with biopsy Neck U/S with FNA of suspicious nodes Calcitonin, CEA RET proto-oncogene testing Hyperparathyroidism and pheochromocytoma screening - Serum Ca, PTH, plasma metanephrines If elevated CEA or very high calcitonin (>400) obtain staging CT neck, chest, and liver	Patients with known RET mutation should undergo prophylactic thyroidectomy: • MEN 2A → by 5 yo • MEN 2B → by 1 yo MTC treated with total thyroidectomy with central neck dissection - Also do modified lateral neck dissection if lateral LN involved If MTC diagnosed after lobectomy, have to go back for completion thyroidectomy if there is residual disease or +RET mutation	**Total thyroidectomy with central neck dissection (core):** - Patient positioned in semi-Fowler position with shoulder-bump - +/- RLN monitoring during case - Collar incision ~2 fingerbreadths above sternal notch - Raise subplatysmal flaps - Split the strap muscles - Ligate and divide the middle thyroid vein, allowing lobe to be medially rotated - Free superior pole by dividing the anterior suspensory ligament and superior pole vessels, staying close to the gland and preserving the external branch of the superior laryngeal nerve - Mobilize the inferior pole - Identify and preserve the RLN - Ligate the inferior thyroid artery close to the gland - Identify and preserve the parathyroid glands - Repeat on the other lobe of the thyroid - Free the thyroid from the trachea, ensure excellent hemostasis - Confirm nerve function prior to closure - Perform central neck dissection for MTC ○ Remove all fatty and lymphoid tissue between sternohyoid muscle, hyoid bone, and suprasternal notch	Levothyroxine supplementation, monitor TSH levels Can develop hypocalcemia after total thyroidectomy—monitor PTH and Ca levels Surveillance: - Check calcitonin and CEA 2-3 mo post-op, then annually - Obtain neck U/S if tumor markers are elevated - CT neck, chest, and liver if calcitonin ≥ 150 pg/mL	MTC arises from parafollicular c cells Parafollicular c cells are not iodine-avid, therefore radioactive iodine is not used for MTC. If a patient is found to have MTC and a pheochromocytoma, operate on the pheo first

Disease Process	Relevant H&P	Work-up/Staging	Treatment	Key Surgical Steps	Post-Op Care	Tips & Tidbits

Thyroiditis (core)	May present with pain and/or swelling of thyroid
	
	Ask about symptoms of hyper or hypothyroidism
	
	Ask about recent URI, pregnancy, medications
	
	On examination, palpate thyroid and cervical nodes, look for signs of hyper- or hypothyroidism
		Check TSH, T3/T4—thyroiditis may be associated with hyper- or hypothyroidism
		
		Can check anti-TPO and anti-thyroglobulin antibodies
		
		ESR, CRP—significantly elevated in infectious thyroiditis
		
		Thyroid U/S—FNA should be done when there is a discrete thyroid nodule
		
		+/- Thyroid uptake scan
		
		Inflammation of the thyroid may be due to a number of causes:
		
		- Hashimoto's thyroiditis—autoimmune disease due to antibodies against the thyroid gland
		  ○ Most common cause of hypothyroidism in the United States
		  ○ Painless goiter that appears hypoechogenic on U/S
		  ○ + Anti-TPO and anti-thyroglobulin antibodies
		
		- Reidel's (fibrosing) thyroiditis—thyroid may feel firm and "woody," due to progressive fibrosis of the thyroid
		  ○ Diagnosed by open biopsy
		- Suppurative thyroiditis—acute infection, pain and swelling of thyroid, may have fever, usually due to GPC (staph, strep)
		- Subacute thyroiditis—thyroid is painful, usually preceded by viral upper respiratory infection
		- Postpartum thyroiditis—autoimmune, antibodies formed against fetal thyroid cells accumulate in mother's thyroid gland
		- Drug-induced thyroiditis—common drugs implicated include lithium, amiodarone, and tyrosine kinase inhibitors
			Hashimoto's—treat with thyroid hormone replacement (levothyroxine)
			
			- Surgery only indicated if rapidly enlarging mass with suspicion of malignancy, cosmetic issue, or compressive symptoms
			
			Reidel's thyroiditis—thyroidectomy for symptomatic disease
			
			Suppurative thyroiditis—antibiotics (ampicillin), NSAIDS, incision and drainage for abscess
			
			Subacute thyroiditis—NSAIDs and symptomatic treatment
			
			Postpartum thyroiditis—usually transient, supplement with levothyroxine as needed for hypothyroidism
						Myxedema coma—severe hypothyroidism
						
						- Medical emergency, mostly seen in older patients
						- May present with hypothermia, hyponatremia, bradycardia
						- Initiate treatment immediately with steroids and levothyroxine

Disease Process	Relevant H&P	Work-up/Staging	Treatment	Key Surgical Steps	Post-Op Care	Tips & Tidbits
Hyperthyroidism (core)	Patient may present with weight loss, palpitations, tremor, heat intolerance, visual changes Examine for thyromegaly, tracheal deviation, tremor, tachycardia/atrial fibrillation, Graves ophthalmopathy	Three most common etiologies of hyperthyroidism: • Graves disease (70%) • Toxic multinodular goiter (25%) • Solitary toxic nodule (5%) TSH—will be low in hyperthyroidism T3/4—increased Thyroid U/S Thyroid scintigraphy—determine solitary toxic nodule ("hot nodule") vs toxic multinodular goiter (heterogeneous uptake) vs Graves hyperthyroidism (diffuse, increased uptake) vs thyroiditis (decreased or no uptake) - Hot nodules are almost always benign, do not warrant FNA - Cold nodules need further workup with thyroid U/S and FNA TSH receptor antibodies—elevated in Graves disease	Many patients can be managed medically Medical management of thyrotoxicosis: - Anti-thyroid medications—propylthiouracil (PTU), methimazole ○ PTU or methimazole can be used for short term prior to definitive treatment (surgery or RAI ablation) or as long-term treatment for Graves thyroiditis - Adjuncts: beta-blockers, Lugol's (KI) solution, steroids - Critical to treat hyperthyroidism preoperatively to prevent thyroid storm Some patients will be refractory or develop adverse reactions to the medications Can do thyroidectomy or radioactive iodine ablation for definitive treatment Surgery is preferred for the following: - Pregnant patients - Moderate or severe Graves ophthalmopathy (RAI can cause worsening of ophthalmopathy) - Issues with access to medical care - Massive goiter or compressive symptoms - Concern for malignancy - Surgery preferred for toxic MNG and toxic adenoma because radioactive iodine (RAI) ablation is less effective and antithyroid meds not effective for long-term management Recheck T3/4 prior to surgery to ensure patient is euthyroid with medical treatment	**Total thyroidectomy:** see medullary thyroid cancer section	Stop anti-thyroid medications and start levothyroxine when euthyroid (POD#0-7)	Thyroid storm: - Medical emergency - Occurs in patients with long-standing hyperthyroidism (commonly Graves) and is usually triggered by physiologic stress (surgery, illness, etc) - May present with fever, tachycardia, agitation, psychosis - Will have low TSH, high T3/T4 - Requires prompt treatment with beta-blockers, PTU, steroids, sedatives

Disease Process	Relevant H&P	Work-up/Staging	Treatment	Key Surgical Steps	Post-Op Care	Tips & Tidbits

Neck mass (core), head and neck cancer (advanced)	May present as cervical mass, adenopathy, or oropharyngeal mass
	
	Associated symptoms include odynophagia, dysphagia, hoarseness, airway obstruction, otalgia, hearing loss, etc
	
	Ask about social and sexual history (HPV, HIV, tobacco, EtOH), prior XRT exposure, recent URI, travel history, TB exposure, "B" symptoms (malaise, night sweats, fatigue)
	
	Examine head and neck, lymph node basins, oral cavity, skin exam
	
	Perform fiberoptic nasopharyngoscopy
		Neck mass—observation may be appropriate for up to 4 wk if high index of suspicion that neck mass is related to infection (recent URI, tender, mobile, etc)
		- If the mass fails to resolve after 4 wk, grows rapidly, or changes during the observation period, further workup indicated
		CBC, BMP, ESR, CRP
		Viral serologies as indicated (EBV, CMV, HIV), if concerned for infection
		U/S with FNA of mass/LN:
		- Obtain CNB or excisional biopsy if FNA inconclusive
		- P16 testing for oropharyngeal cancer
		- LN imaging characteristics suspicious for malignancy:
		  ○ Central necrosis
		  ○ >1.5 cm in diameter
		  ○ Irregular borders
		  ○ Round shape (vs oval)
		  ○ Peripheral vascularity
		- FNA of LN shows SCC and primary unknown ⟶ further work-up:
		  ○ HPV, EBV testing of tumor
		  ○ CT (or MRI) head/neck with IV contrast
		  ○ CT chest
		  ○ PET, if CT or MRI fails to localize
		  ○ Pan-Endoscopy (EUA, flexible nasolaryngoscopy, esophagoscopy, +/-bronchoscopy)
		  ○ If still unable to find primary, consider tonsillectomy
		  ○ If still unable to find primary, consider selective neck dissection
		- FNA of LN shows adenocarcinoma, primary unknown ⟶ CT neck, CT C/A/P, mammogram, EGD, colonoscopy to look for source
		- FNA of abnormal LN shows thyroid tissue ⟶ this is thyroid cancer, proceed with thyroid cancer work-up and treatment
			Treat according to primary source
			Head and Neck SCC (simplified):
			- Smoking cessation
			- Treatment algorithm is complex and based on primary location
			- Review in multidisciplinary tumor board, referral to medical and radiation oncology
			- Options for treatment with surgery, XRT, and/or chemotherapy
			  ○ Surgery is generally preferred treatment when amenable: resection of primary +/- selective neck dissection
			  ○ Many will receive XRT as well
			  ○ Chemo/XRT for unresectable disease
			- Management of oral cavity SCC differs based on p16 status of tumor
			- Nasopharyngeal primary ⟶ chemo/XRT
				FNA Biopsy of abnormal lymph node (core):
				- Locate abnormal lymph node on U/S
				- Anesthetize with local anesthetic
				- Pass 25-gauge needle through mass multiple times while aspirating
				- Put sample onto slide with 95% ethyl alcohol
				
				Excisional Cervical Lymph Node Biopsy (core):
				- Identify and mark the targeted LN by palpation or U/S
				- Make incision directly over lesion and dissect out the node, avoid nearby neurovascular structures
				- Clip the lymphatic pedicle and remove the LN
				- Ensure hemostasis, close wound
					Airway (ie, trach) and nutrition (ie, feeding tube) management, as needed
					
					Monitor for nerve injury (ie, facial, recurrent laryngeal, hypoglossal, spinal accessory) and lymphatic leak
					
					Oncology surveillance (exam in 1-2 mo, CT in 3-4 mo)
						SCC is the most common primary malignancy of the head and neck
						
						Types of neck dissections: Radical neck dissection—removal of level I-V nodes along with the SCM, internal jugular vein (IJV), and CN XI
						- Rarely performed these days, typically reserved for neck metastases that involve the SCM, IJV and CN XI
						
						Modified radical neck dissection—removal of level I-V nodes but spares at least 1 nonlymphatic structure (SCM, IJV, or CN XI)
						- Gold standard for head and neck SCC with clinically positive resectable neck disease
						
						Functional neck dissection—removal of level I-V nodes but spares SCM, IJV, and CN XI
						
						Selective neck dissection—any procedure with removal of one or more levels of the cervical nodes based on pattern of cervical metastasis, which is typically predictable based on location of primary malignancy

Disease Process	Relevant H&P	Work-up/Staging	Treatment	Key Surgical Steps	Post-Op Care	Tips & Tidbits

Parotid Mass	May present as asymptomatic enlarging mass
	
	Ask about history of HIV, smoking, prior XRT, skin cancer of scalp or face
	
	Examine for cervical lymphadenopathy
	
	Assess facial nerve function—the facial nerve runs through the parotid gland and tumor invasion can cause deficit
		Parotid U/S with FNA biopsy
		
		If malignant, obtain:
		- CT (or MRI) neck
		- CT chest
		
		Types of salivary gland neoplasms include:
		- Benign: ~80% of parotid masses are benign
		  ○ Pleomorphic adenoma—most common salivary gland tumor
		  ○ Warthin's tumor—can be bilateral
		- Malignant: ~20% of parotid masses are malignant
		  ○ Mucoepidermoid carcinoma (MEC)—most common malignant salivary gland tumor
		  ○ Adenoid cystic carcinoma
		  ○ Acinic cell carcinoma
			Parotidectomy, also do selective neck dissection if LN+
			
			Unresectable (T4b) → definitive XRT
				Parotidectomy (advanced):
				- Can perform superficial lobe or total parotidectomy depending on type of tumor
				- Position patient supine with shoulder roll and head turned away from operative side
				- Use facial nerve monitoring during case
				- Make a Blair incision—sickle-shaped preauricular incision curved under the earlobe, and along the hairline of the neck
				- Develop sub-platysma flap
				- Identify and preserve greater auricular nerve
				- Parotid gland mobilized and dissected away from anterior aspect of SCM, external jugular vein, and tragal cartilage
				- Identify main trunk of the facial nerve and trace it anteriorly to find the branches, preserve if possible
				- If facial nerve is directly invaded by malignant tumor, then it should be sacrificed
				- If doing total parotidectomy, branches of facial nerve are gently retracted and deep lobe delivered
				- Test facial nerve prior to closure
					Complications of parotidectomy:
					- Facial nerve injury
					- Auriculotemporal syndrome (Frey syndrome)—gustatory sweating
					  ○ Treatment: antiperspirants or Botox injection
					- Salivary fistula	

Neck abscess	Patient may present with fever, dysphagia, and/or dyspnea Can lead to airway compromise, secure airway if needed Ask about recent dental or pharyngeal (tonsil) infection	CBC, BMP CT neck with IV contrast	Initial trial of IV antibiotics may be reasonable if patient is stable, mildly symptomatic (no airway compromise), and abscess is small Treat with incision and drainage if symptomatic Refer to dentist if dental etiology suspected			Swelling of the submental area may represent Ludwig's angina and warrants immediate evaluation of the floor of mouth, ensure airway is patent - Treat with antibiotics and timely drainage of abscess

11

Thoracic Surgery

Andrew Feczko, MD

DISEASES AND CONDITIONS

- Pneumothorax (c), chest tube placement (c), blebectomy and pleurodesis (c)
- Pleural effusion/empyema (c), thoracentesis (c), VATS decortication

- Chylothorax (c), thoracic duct ligation
- Solitary pulmonary nodule, VATS wedge resection (a)
- Malignant tumors of the lung (a), mediastinoscopy, thoracotomy (c)

- Mediastinal mass (a)
- Mediastinitis (a)
- Superior vena cava syndrome (a)

GENERAL TIPS

- Some of the advanced topics (ie, lung cancer, mediastinal mass) can get quite complex and you are not expected to know all of the intricacies. Focus on the core topics.

(c) = core topic   (a) = advanced topic

Disease Process	Relevant H&P	Work-up/Staging	Treatment	Key Surgical Steps	Post-Op Care	Tips & Tidbits

Pneumothorax (PTX) (core)	SOB, chest pain
	
	Traumatic—penetrating or blunt injury, often associated with rib fractures
	
	Primary spontaneous pneumothorax (PSP)—tall, thin, young, males, smokers
	
	Secondary spontaneous pneumothorax—COPD, interstitial lung disease, catamenial pneumothorax, lymphangioleiomyomatosis (LAM), cystic fibrosis, etc
		CXR
		
		CT chest—better anatomic definition, evaluate for blebs, occult pneumothorax (PTX seen on CT but no CXR)
			Traumatic PTX—place chest tube
			- If it is a small/occult pneumothorax and patient is stable, can consider observation with repeat upright CXR in 6 h
			PSP management:
			- Place chest tube
			  ○ For small PTX (<3 cm to apex) can consider observing and getting repeat CXR in 6 h
			- Surgery can be performed to decrease risk of recurrence, discuss with patient
			  ○ PSP recurrence rate without surgery:
			    ■ First time → 20-30%
			    ■ Second time → 60-75%
			  ○ Surgery includes VATS blebectomy with pleurodesis and/or pleurectomy
			    ■ 5-10% risk of recurrence after surgery
			  ○ Indications for surgery after first episode:
			    ■ Bilateral PTX
			    ■ Complete PTX
			    ■ High-risk occupation or hobbies (diver, pilot)
			    ■ Live in remote area
			Secondary spontaneous pneumothorax management:
			- Place chest tube for acute management
			- Surgical blebectomy and pleurodesis may be considered in appropriate candidates
			  ○ Avoid large wedge resections because the residual space may lead to prolonged air leak
			- Consider chemical or talc pleurodesis for high risk surgical patients (ie, COPD with significant bleb disease)
			Smoking cessation
				Chest tube placement (core):
				- Select 16-24 Fr chest tube or 14 Fr pigtail
				- Position patient supine with arm raised above head, drape anatomic landmarks into the field, prep the field
				- Inject local anesthetic, make skin incision in fifth or sixth ICS between mid to anterior axillary line
				- Divide subcutaneous tissue and muscle down to the level of the rib
				- Enter the pleural space bluntly just above the rib and palpate lung/pleural space to confirm chest entry
				- Insert chest tube far enough that sentinel hole is several centimeters in the chest
				- Suture tube to the skin and place occlusive dressing
				- Connect tube to atrium, initially at -20 cm H2O, evaluate for tidaling and air leak
				- Obtain CXR to confirm tube position and assess lung expansion
				
				VATS blebectomy and pleurodesis (core):
				- Double lumen ETT → single lung ventilation
				- Lateral decubitus, typically place 3 ports with the camera low in the chest and working ports triangulated to access the apex and major fissure
				- Perform blebectomy using linear stapler, usually at the apex
				  ○ Limit the extent of resection to avoid an apical space and increased risk of prolonged post-op air leak
				- Perform pleurodesis (talc, D50, doxycycline, mechanical) or pleurectomy
				- Reinflate lung and look for air leak
				- Leave chest tube in place
					CXR in PACU
					
					Keep chest tube to suction x 48 h if pleurodesis performed
						Large, persistent air leak and/or unresolved PTX after chest tube is placed for traumatic PTX should raise concern for tracheobronchial tree injury

Disease Process	Relevant H&P	Work-up/Staging	Treatment	Key Surgical Steps	Post-Op Care	Tips & Tidbits

Parapneumonic effusion, empyema (core)	May present with cough, fever, pleuritic chest pain, SOB	CXR, CT scan
		
		Chest tube/thoracentesis with pleural fluid analysis—check LDH, pH, protein, glucose, cytology, gram stain, and culture
		- Light's criteria—determine whether pleural effusion is exudative or transudative
		  ○ Protein (effusion)/Protein (serum) >0.5
		  ○ LDH (effusion)/LDH (serum) >0.6
		  ○ LDH (effusion) >2/3 upper limit of normal
		  ○ If any of the above criteria are met, it is exudative
		Stages of parapneumonic effusion and empyema:
		- Acute phase: 1-3 d, no loculations yet
		- Fibrinopurulent: 4-14 d
		- Organized: >14 d, fibrinous rind, nonexpansile lung
			Antibiotics
			
			Drainage via chest tube(s), then reimage to assess for remaining collections
			
			If drainage is inadequate after chest tube, will need surgical decortication vs lytics
			- Early surgical washout and decortication typically preferred for good operative candidates
			  ○ Allows for removal of fluid and semisolid material with good drainage and lung reexpansion
			- Intrapleural fibrinolytics may be a good option for poor surgical candidates
			  ○ t-PA-DNase q12 x 3 d, followed by repeat CT scan to assess response (MIST2 protocol)
			  ○ Not effective for organized effusion/ trapped lung
				Thoracentesis (core):
				- Position patient sitting upright
				- Use U/S to identify the posterior rib space above the diaphragm and look for a good pocket to target
				  ○ For nonloculated, free-flowing effusion, can puncture posteriorly somewhere above the ninth rib, 1-2 rib spaces below where breath sounds are decreased
				- Sterilize chosen site, inject local
				- Insert a 20-gauge needle over the top of chosen rib, aspirate until you get fluid return
				- Withdraw desired amount of fluid, send for analysis
				- Withdraw needle and place dressing
				- Get CXR
				
				VATS Decortication:
				- Primary goals:
				  ○ Remove fibrinous rind
				  ○ Reexpand lung
				  ○ Establish good drainage of the thoracic cavity
				- Use single lung ventilation, place patient in lateral decubitus
				- Place ports
				- Remove fluid and semisolid material
				- Fully mobilize the lung from the chest wall and mediastinum, open the fissures
				- Decorticate the lung by peeling away the thickened rind to promote reexpansion
				- If unable to perform thoracoscopically convert to thoracotomy
				- Place 2-3 chest tubes for drainage
					Daily CXR
					
					Common to have postoperative air leak
					- Remove tube when air leak has resolved and infection is controlled
						In patients with large effusions, rapid drainage can result in reexpansion pulmonary edema
						- Avoid this by placing chest tube to water seal initially (rather than suction)
						- Clamp tube intermittently if patient develops chest discomfort, cough, or amount of fluid initially removed exceeds 1000-1500 mL
						Patients with recurrent malignant pleural effusions may benefit from talc pleurodesis vs palliative indwelling catheter placement (pleurX)
						
						- If the lung reexpands with drainage, talc pleurodesis via VATS can be attempted, can also obtain pleural biopsy at same time if needed
						- If there is a persistent space despite drainage (trapped lung), an indwelling (pleurX) catheter may be a good palliative option for symptomatic relief
						Additional reading:
						Rahman NM, et al. Intrapleural use of tissue plasminogen activator and DNase in pleural infection. *N Engl J Med*. 2011 Aug 11;365(6):518-526.

Disease Process	Relevant H&P	Work-up/Staging	Treatment	Key Surgical Steps	Post-Op Care	Tips & Tidbits
Chylothorax (core)	Patient presents with pleural effusion, which appears milky when sampled - Fluid may not look milky if patient is NPO Etiologies include malignancy (causing lymphatic obstruction), penetrating trauma, and iatrogenic injury from thoracic or cervical operations	Place pleural drain if patient does not already have one Send pleural fluid for analysis, including triglyceride and chylomicron levels - Triglyceride level >110 mg/dL and lymphocyte predominance highly suggestive of chylothorax - Chylomicron detection is confirmatory	Chylothorax can lead to electrolyte abnormalities, nutritional depletion, and compromised immune function Nonoperative management should be attempted initially: - Fluid resuscitation, bowel rest, TPN - If output low/leak resolving, can try low fat or medium-chain fatty acid diet - +/- Octreotide - Malignant chylothorax management involves treatment of underlying malignancy Consider intervention if nonoperative management unsuccessful or for high output chyle leaks in the postoperative setting: - IR lymphangiogram can be diagnostic (identify site of leak) and potentially therapeutic (thoracic duct embolization with gelfoam, coils, or glue) - Can treat surgically with thoracic duct ligation (thoracotomy vs VATS) + pleurodesis procedure	**Thoracic duct ligation:** - Can be done via MIS or lower posterolateral thoracotomy - Cream can be administered to stimulate chyle production and aid in leak identification and confirmation of successful ligation - Perform mass ligation of tissue between azygous vein (lateral), spine (posterior), aorta (medial), and esophagus (anterior) as far down on diaphragm as possible - Can also do chemical or mechanical pleurodesis - Decortication may be needed if lung is entrapped - Leave chest tube(s) in place	Continue NPO/TPN or low-fat diet initially post-op, monitor chest tube output	It is important to understand the typical course of the thoracic duct to minimize risk of injury: - Thoracic duct begins in the abdominal cavity at the cisterna chylii, transits through the aortic hiatus and crosses from the right to left hemithorax near T5-6, before emptying into the junction of the left IJ and subclavian vein - Anatomy of the thoracic duct is highly variable, with potential for duplicated and secondary ducts

Disease Process	Relevant H&P	Work-up/Staging	Treatment	Key Surgical Steps	Post-Op Care	Tips & Tidbits

Solitary pulmonary nodule (SPN) (advanced)	Smoking history?
	
	Occupational exposure?
	
	Family history?
	
	Underlying lung disease?
	
	USPSTF Recommendation: Screening low-dose chest CT for patients 50-80 yo with 20+ pack-year smoking history who currently smoke or have quit in the past 15 years
	
	Differential: lung cancer, metastatic cancer, infectious (granuloma), hamartoma, AVM, carcinoid
		Solitary pulmonary nodule defined as a discrete, well-marginated, spherical lesion or opacity ≤ 3 cm in diameter surrounded by normal lung parenchyma
		- If >3 cm, then it is a mass
		CT scan—size? location? density (solid vs sub-solid)?
		Compare to prior imaging
		Sample pleural effusion if present
		Fleischner guidelines—for management of indeterminate pulmonary nodules, we recommend reading them; however, this is a general simplification for practical purposes that should give you safe answers for the boards:
		- Solitary solid nodule <6 mm
		  ○ Low-risk patients: no routine follow-up required
		  ○ High-risk patients: optional CT at 12 mo
		- Solitary solid nodule 6-8 mm
		  ○ Low-risk patients: CT at 6-12 mo, then consider CT at 18-24 mo
		  ○ High-risk patients: CT at 6-12 mo, then CT at 18-24 mo
		- Solitary solid nodule >8 mm
		  ○ Consider CT at 3 mo, PET-CT, or tissue sampling
		  ○ If PET avid, obtain biopsy (transthoracic IR biopsy vs EBUS vs VATS wedge resection)
		- Single ground glass nodule < 6mm—no routine follow-up
		- Singe ground glass nodule ≥ 6mm—CT at 6-12 mo, repeat in two years if persistent
			Treatment based on diagnosis
			If performing VATS wedge resection for suspicious nodule, can get frozen section and plan to proceed with oncologic resection if positive for carcinoma
				VATS wedge resection (advanced):
				- Pre-op wire localization, if needed
				- Have anesthesia use double-lumen ETT for single lung ventilation, position patient in lateral decubitus
				- Place ports—typically 3 ports triangulated to the area of interest
				- Localize the lesion
				- Perform wedge resection using linear stapler
				- Leave chest tube
					Post-op air leak:
					- Can try decreasing suction to see if lung drops
					- If prolonged, consider reexploration with pleurodesis and/or pleurectomy
						Additional reading: MacMahon H, et al. Guidelines for management of incidental pulmonary nodules detected on CT images: from the Fleischner Society 2017. *Radiology.* 2017 Jul;284(1):228-243.

Disease Process	Relevant H&P	Work-up/Staging	Treatment	Key Surgical Steps	Post-Op Care	Tips & Tidbits

Malignant tumors of the lung (advanced)	Leading cause of cancer death in the United States
	
	May present with cough, DOE, hemoptysis, recurrent pneumonia, chest wall pain
	
	Most are asymptomatic at presentation, incidentally noted on imaging obtained for other reason or screening CT
	
	Risk factors: smoking, air pollution, asbestos, occupational exposures
	
	Exam: listen to lungs, palpate nodal stations (supraclavicular, cervical)
		Major histologic subclasses of lung cancer:
		- Non-small cell lung cancer (NSCLC)
		  ○ Adenocarcinoma—most common type of NSCLC (45%), often peripherally located
		  ○ Squamous cell carcinoma (SCC)
		  ○ Large cell
		- Small cell lung cancer (SCLC)—early metastatic spread frequently precludes surgical resection
		- Pulmonary carcinoid tumors
		
		Lung cancer staging (Table 11.1):
		- CT C/A
		- PET
		- MRI brain—obtain in patients with neuro complaints, SCLC, and/or ≥ stage II disease
		- Bronchoscopy—can be done at same time as resection
		- Pre-resection nodal staging (Figure 11.1)
		  ○ Mediastinoscopy—access to nodal stations 2R/L, 4R/L, 7, 10, 11
		  ○ EBUS +/- transbronchial biopsy—access to nodal stations 2R/L, 4R/L, 7, 10R/L, 11
		  ○ Chamberlain—left second ICS anterior thoracotomy to access nodal stations 5 and 6
		  ○ Mediastinoscopy or EBUS can be done with frozen section analysis prior to formal resection under same anesthetic
		- +/- tissue biopsy—patients with strong clinical suspicion of stage I/II lung cancer do not require biopsy before surgery; however, intra-op frozen section should be used to confirm diagnosis
		- Pulmonary function testing—determine if patient can tolerate planned resection
		  ○ Can get lung perfusion scan, if borderline
			Discuss all patients at multidisciplinary tumor board
			Simplified treatment of lung cancer:
			- Node negative → surgical resection vs stereotactic body radiation therapy (SBRT) (for poor operative candidate)
			- +N1 nodes → upfront surgery followed by adjuvant therapy
			- +N2 nodes → neoadjuvant therapy possibly followed by surgery
			- +N3 nodes, unresectable tumor, or metastatic disease → definitive chemoXRT
			Surgical resection:
			- May entail wedge resection, lobectomy, or pneumonectomy based on tumor
			- Mediastinal lymphadenectomy should be performed during all lung cancer resections
			Most chemo regimens include paclitaxel and platinum-based (carboplatin, cisplatin) therapy
			- May also be treated with targeted therapy and/or immunotherapy (ie, PDL1 inhibitors)
			Smoking cessation
				Mediastinoscopy:
				- Position patient supine with neck extended
				- Make 2-3 cm incision ~2 cm above sternal notch
				- Dissect through platysma, deep cervical fascia, and pre-tracheal fascia
				- Enter into mediastinum with blunt dissection down along the anterior trachea, which will lead to tract into the superior mediastinum, posterior to great vessels and anterior to trachea
				- Insert mediastinoscope into tract and biopsy nodal stations, send for frozen if planning to potentially perform resection in the same setting
				
				Thoracotomy (posterolateral) (core):
				- Position in lateral decubitus with single lung ventilation
				- Perform posterolateral thoracotomy in the fifth ICS
				- Divide the latissimus dorsi
				- Divide vs mobilize and spare the serratus anterior
				- Divide fibers of trapezius and rhomboid encountered posteriorly
				- Retract scapula and count ICS to ensure you are in the fifth ICS
				- Make incision along the top edge of the sixth rib
				- Ensure patient is on single lung ventilation prior to entering pleura
				- Insert rib spreader, may resect posterior segment of sixth rib prior to spreading ribs to prevent uncontrolled fracture
					Surveillance:
					- Stage I/II → H&P + chest CT q6mo for 2-3 y, then annually thereafter
					- Stage III/IV → H&P + chest CT q3-6mo for 3 y, then q6-12mo thereafter
						Tip for remembering the nodal stations:
						- Mediastinal (N2) nodes are single digits (stations 2-9)
						- Hilar/intrapulmonary (N1) nodes are double digits (stations 10-14)
						
						Metastatic lesions to the lung:
						- Metastatic sarcomas and melanoma often present as single pulmonary nodule
						- Metastatic head & neck, breast, colon, and renal cell cancer typically metastasize to the lungs as multifocal lesions
						- Patient with lung metastases and an unknown primary:
						  ○ Check tumor markers (CEA, CA 19-9, AFP, β-HCG)
						  ○ CT C/A/P +/- PET
						  ○ Colonoscopy and mammogram should be up to date
						  ○ CT-guided biopsy of accessible lesions
						  ○ Positive napsin A or TTF-1 can help differentiate primary lung cancer from metastatic lesion

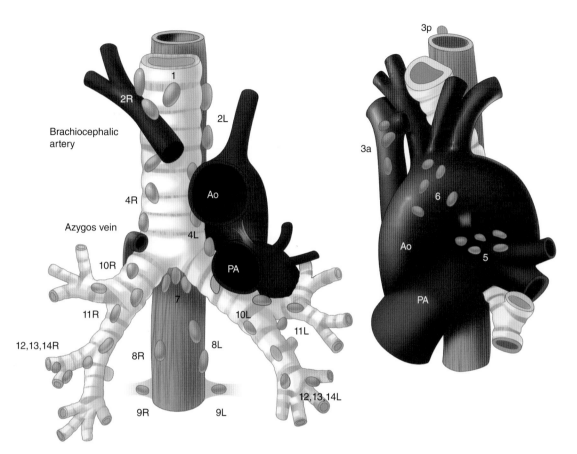

FIGURE 11.1: Mediastinal lymph node stations (stations 12, 13, and 14 not shown in their entirety). Taken from but not original to: Dangleben DA, Madbak FG. ABSITE Slayer, 2e. McGraw Hill, 2021. Figure 27-5. (Modified with permission from Ferguson MK. *Thoracic Surgery Atlas*. Philadelphia, PA: WB Saunders; 2007.)

Table 11.1: TNM staging of lung cancer	
T staging	T1: ≤ 3 cm
	T2: 3-5 cm
	T3: 5-7 cm or invading parietal pleural, phrenic nerve, or pericardium, or two tumors in same lobe
	T4: > 7 cm or invading mediastinum, diaphragm, heart, great vessels, trachea/carina, esophagus, RLN, or spine, or separate nodules within same lung but separate lobes
N staging	N1: Ipsilateral hilar/intrapulmonary LN+ (stations 10-14)
	N2: Ipsilateral mediastinal LN+ (stations 2-9)
	N3: Contralateral mediastinal or supraclavicular LN+
M staging	M0—no metastasis
	M1—metastasis
Stage	I—T1-2N0M0
	IIA—T1N1M0
	IIB—T2N1M0, T3N0M0
	III—T1-4N2-3M0, T3N1M0, T4N0-2M0
	IV—M+, malignant pleural effusion

Disease Process	Relevant H&P	Work-up/Staging	Treatment	Key Surgical Steps	Post-Op Care	Tips & Tidbits

Mediastinal mass (advanced)	Most patients are asymptomatic, masses incidentally found on imaging
	
	Patients with larger lesions may present with cough, chest pain, SOB, Horner syndrome, SVC syndrome
	
	Thymomas: most common anterior mediastinal tumor, can be associated with myasthenia gravis (MG)
	
	- Patients with MG may present with weakness, ocular symptoms (ptosis, diplopia), fatigue
		The mediastinum is separated in to anterior, middle, and posterior compartments and differential depends on which compartment the mass is in (Figure 11.2)
		
		Cross-sectional imaging—CT or MRI
		
		- Determine which compartment mass is in and that will help guide the differential
		For anterior mediastinal mass check AFP, hCG to evaluate for germ cell tumor
		
		Biopsy—multiple options for biopsy if tissue diagnosis needed
		
		- Transthoracic biopsy
		- VATS biopsy
		- Can do mediastinoscopy or EBUS for biopsy of middle mediastinal mass
		- Chamberlain procedure—open biopsy of anterior mediastinal masses or masses in aortopulmonary window, if needed
		
		Thymoma
		
		- 30-50% of patients with thymoma have MG
		- Masaoka staging system used to classify tumors, has prognostic value and helps determine need for adjuvant treatment
		  ○ Benign vs malignant nature determined by presence of metastasis, gross invasion into adjacent structures, and microscopic evidence of capsular invasion
		
		Work-up for thymoma/thymic carcinoma
		- CT scan—to evaluate primary tumor and pleural spaces
		- PFTs
		- +/- Sniff test—assessment of diaphragmatic function if there is concern for phrenic nerve involvement
		- Pre-op biopsy not needed for small thymic tumors with no evidence of invasion beyond the thymus, but biopsy is required prior to starting chemo
			MG management
			
			- Medical management with anticholinesterases (pyridostigmine, neostigmine), glucocorticoids, plasmapheresis
			- Thymectomy—studies have demonstrated improved outcomes with surgical thymectomy versus medical management alone
			
			When taking a patient with MG to OR:
			- Coordinate with patient's neurologist
			- Consider pre-op plasmapheresis for patients with poorly controlled MG
			- Consider stress dose steroids for steroid-dependent patients
			- Judicious use of neuromuscular blocking agents due to potential for delayed emergence
				Operative approaches for anterior mediastinal tumors:
				- Median sternotomy
				- Transcervical
				- Hemi-clamshell thoracotomy with or without neck extension or a clamshell thoracotomy
				  ○ May be necessary for large, advanced stage tumors
				- Minimally invasive—VATS vs robotic
				
				Operative approaches for middle and posterior mediastinal tumors:
				- Posterolateral thoracotomy
				- Minimally invasive—VATS vs robotic
				
				Thymectomy:
				- Can be done open or minimally invasive
				- Boundaries of dissection: phrenic nerves laterally, innominate vein superiorly, diaphragm inferiorly
				- Thymic gland is indistinguishable from mediastinal adipose tissue → take all tissue anterior to the pericardium within the dissection boundaries
				- Preserve phrenic nerves
					Patients with MG are at risk of post-op myasthenic crisis, respiratory failure
					
					Tx: urgent plasmapheresis or IVIG
						Borders of the mediastinum:
						- Sternum—anteriorly
						- Vertebral column—posteriorly
						- Parietal pleura—laterally
						- Thoracic inlet—superiorly
						- Diaphragm—inferiorly
						
						Additional reading:
						Kuo HC, et al; MGTX Study Group. Randomized trial of thymectomy in myasthenia gravis. N Engl J Med. 2016 Aug 11;375(6):511-522.

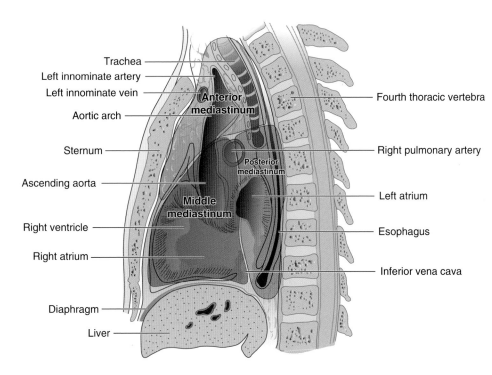

Trachea
Left innominate artery
Left innominate vein
Anterior mediastinum
Aortic arch
Sternum
Ascending aorta
Right ventricle
Right atrium
Diaphragm
Liver
Middle mediastinum
Posterior mediastinum
Fourth thoracic vertebra
Right pulmonary artery
Left atrium
Esophagus
Inferior vena cava

FIGURE 11.2: The anterior, middle, and posterior divisions of the mediastinum.
Mediastinal mass differential:
- Anterior mediastinal mass: thymoma, thymic carcinoma, thymic hyperplasia, ectopic thyroid/ substernal goiter, lymphoma, teratoma/germ cell tumor (the terrible Ts)
- Middle mediastinum: bronchogenic cyst, pericardial cyst, foregut duplication cyst, lymphoma, esophageal, lung, and tracheal malignancies
- Posterior mediastinum: neurogenic tumors (neuroblastoma, Schwannoma, ganglionoma, etc)

(Reproduced with permission from Doherty GM. *Current Diagnosis & Treatment Surgery*, 15th ed. New York, NY: McGraw Hill; 2020, Figure 19-6.)

Disease Process	Relevant H&P	Work-up/Staging	Treatment	Key Surgical Steps	Post-Op Care	Tips & Tidbits
Mediastinitis (advanced)	May present with fever, tachycardia, chest pain, dysphagia, crepitus, edema of the chest wall, septic shock May be related to recent cardiothoracic surgery, esophageal or tracheal perforation, descending infection from oropharyngeal source (retropharyngeal or peritonsillar abscess, dental abscess)	Full labs Determine etiology CT neck and chest with PO and IV contrast +/- esophagogram if worried about esophageal perforation as source	Antibiotics Source control—typically done via percutaneous drains or surgical washout - Esophageal perforation—see section in foregut chapter - Odontogenic/peritonsillar abscesses with mediastinal extension—can typically be controlled via cervical incision and placement of drains into the mediastinum			

Disease Process	Relevant H&P	Work-up/Staging	Treatment	Key Surgical Steps	Post-Op Care	Tips & Tidbits
Superior vena cava syndrome (advanced)	Due to extrinsic compression or intrinsic abnormality causing obstruction of venous return from the head, neck, and upper extremities May present with swelling of the face, neck, arms, and upper chest, dilated neck and chest veins, headache, cough and dyspnea from laryngeal edema, Horner's syndrome Symptoms vary depending on speed of progression of SVC obstruction	CXR CT—may identify causative mass, non-opacification of the SVC inferior to the site of obstruction with chest wall collaterals Venography can be used if further characterization required Biopsy mass to determine etiology Differential: - Malignant mass—MCC (~ 60% of cases) ○ Lung cancer (especially small cell), lymphoma, malignant thymoma, esophageal cancer, germ cell tumors, teratomas - Fibrosing mediastinitis from infectious process (histoplasmosis, TB, fungal disease) - Thyroid goiter - Indolent lymphoproliferative diseases (Castleman disease) - Sarcoidosis - Intravascular devices causing vessel scarring/thrombosis	Initial maneuvers: treatment of underlying cause, supplemental oxygen, elevate the head, diuretics, consider steroids Consider anticoagulation, XRT, and chemo depending on etiology Substernal goiter → surgical resection Fibrosing mediastinitis → mediastinal XRT and antifungal, possible intravascular intervention Disease caused by intravascular device → remove device, treat stenosis with venoplasty +/- stent		In cases of SVC syndrome caused by malignancy, overall survival poor due to advanced stage of underlying disease	

12

Skin and Soft Tissue

Shelby Reiter, MD, and Danielle Hayes, MD

DISEASES AND CONDITIONS

- Melanoma (c), wide excision (c), sentinel lymph node biopsy (c), inguinal lymphadenectomy (a)
- Nonmelanoma skin cancers (c)
- Pilonidal disease (c)

- Soft tissue sarcomas (c), resection of soft tissue sarcoma (a)
- Necrotizing soft tissue infections (c)
- Paronychia and felon (c)

- Hidradenitis (c)
- Pressure ulcers (c)
- Merkel cell carcinoma
- Dermatofibrosarcoma protuberans

(c) = core topic   (a) = advanced topic

Disease Process	Relevant H&P	Work-up//Staging	Treatment	Key Surgical Steps	Post-Op Care	Tips & Tidbits

Melanoma (core)	History of sun exposure
	
	Family history?
	
	Perform thorough ROS to elicit symptoms of metastatic disease
	
	Full skin and nodal basin exam
	
	- ABCDE of melanoma—asymmetry, irregular borders, color variation, diameter >6 mm, evolving
	- Lesion ulcerated?
		Punch or excisional biopsy
		
		If concerning LN on exam, get U/S w/ biopsy of suspicious LNs
		
		TNM staging
		- T stage
		  ○ Tis—melanoma in situ
		  ○ T1 ≤ 1 mm
		    ■ T1a ≤ 0.8 mm without ulceration
		    ■ T1b ≤ 0.8 mm with ulceration or 0.8-1.0 mm without ulceration
		  ○ T2 > 1-2 mm
		  ○ T3 > 2-4 mm
		  ○ T4 > 4 mm
		- N stage
		  ○ N1 1 LN(+)
		  ○ N2 2-3 LN(+)
		  ○ N3 ≥ 4 LN(+)
		Do full staging if LN+ or to assess specific signs or symptoms:
		• CT C/A/P and/or PET
		• Brain MRI
		• BRAF testing
		• LDH (for stage IV)
			Wide local excision of lesion:
			- Recommended margins based on tumor thickness
			  ○ Melanoma in situ → 0.5 cm margins
			  ○ ≤1 mm thick → 1 cm margins
			  ○ >1-2 mm thick → 1-2 cm margins
			  ○ >2 mm thick → 2 cm margins
			- Consider preoperative plastic surgery consult if excision will be in cosmetically sensitive area (ie, face, foot, etc) or will result in large defect requiring flap coverage
			
			Nodal staging:
			- SLNB for clinically node negative patients with tumor ≥1 mm thick or ≥0.8 mm thick with ulceration
			  ○ +SLNB → U/S surveillance vs lymphadenectomy (MSLT-II)
			- Clinically positive lymph nodes → lymphadenectomy
			
			All patients with LN+ disease should be considered for systemic therapy—immunotherapy or targeted therapy:
			- Anti-PD1—pembrolizumab, nivolumab
			- BRAF mutation—dabrafenib
			- Anti-CTLA-4—ipilimumab
			M1 disease → systemic therapy
				Wide local excision (core):
				- Mark out needed margins (based on thickness)
				- Excise as 3:1-4:1 (length:width) ellipse to allow for closure
				- Excision shoud be down to, but not including, the fascia
				- Close in layers
				
				Inguinal sentinel lymph node biopsy (core):
				- Send to nuclear medicine for tech-99 injection the night before or morning of surgery (requires at least 8 h), confirm activity in nodal basin with gamma probe
				- +/- Intradermal injection of isosulfan blue or methylene blue
				- Borders of inguinal basin are inguinal ligament, adductor longus, sartorius
				- Make vertical or oblique incision in groin below inguinal ligament
				- Dissect down through subcutaneous issue, use gamma probe to localize hot nodes
				- Remove hot, blue, and grossly abnormal nodes, clip/ligate associated lymphatics
				- Do background count (should be <10% of hottest sentinel node)
				- Close in layers
				
				Inguinal lymph node dissection (advanced):
				- Vertical or curvilinear incision below inguinal crease, overlying femoral vessels
				- Remove all nodal tissue in the femoral triangle down to the fascia
				- Take care to identify and skeletonize femoral vein and artery
				- Beware of saphenous vein medially
				- May also need to perform deep/pelvic lymphadenectomy, if involved
				  ○ Extend skin incision cephalad
				  ○ Incise external and internal oblique above inguinal ligament, parallel to the fibers
				  ○ Skeletonize lymphatic tissue off iliac vessels
				- Close in layers +/- sartorius flap if concerned about exposure of vessels
				  ○ Divide proximal attachment of sartorius off ASIS and transpose to cover vessels by securing to external oblique or inguinal ligament
				- Leave drain
					Refer to medical oncology and radiation oncology for consideration of systemic therapy and XRT, depending on pathological stage
					
					Surveillance of nodal basin with + SLN per MSLT-II:
					- U/S and exam q4mon x 2 y, q6mo x 3-5 y, annual PET/CT
					- Abnormal LN → FNA of LN
					  ○ If positive, re-stage → lymphadenectomy if no M1 disease +/- systemic therapy, XRT
					
					Surveillance: H&P q3-12mo, obtain imaging PRN to further evaluate any concerning findings
						Axillary lymph node dissection for melanoma includes levels I-III, unlike for breast cancer which typically includes only levels I-II
						
						Major misstep: Doing a shave biopsy of suspected melanoma. You must have a full-thickness biopsy of the lesion.
						
						Additional reading:
						Morton DL, et al. Final trial report of sentinel-node biopsy versus nodal observation in melanoma. *N Engl J Med*. 2014 Feb 13;370(7):599-609.
						
						Faries MB, et al. Completion dissection or observation for sentinel-node metastasis in melanoma. *N Engl J Med*. 2017 Jun 8;376(23):2211-2222.

Disease Process	Relevant H&P	Work-up//Staging	Treatment	Key Surgical Steps	Post-Op Care	Tips & Tidbits
Nonmelanoma skin cancer (core)	Risk factors: UV light, old age, fair skin, immunosuppression Basal cell carcinoma (BCC)—most common type of skin cancer, will look nodular, raised with rolled edges and pearly appearance Actinic keratosis (AK)—precursor to SCC erythematous, scaly lesions Squamous cell carcinoma (SCC)—second most common skin cancer, raised edges, ulcerated Do full skin exam, examine lymph node basins	Biopsy—punch vs incisional vs excisional	Topical imiquimod, 5-FU, or cryotherapy can be used for actinic keratoses Treat with local excision with 4mm margins for low-risk lesions, 4-6 mm margins recommended for high-risk lesions - High risk lesion: >2 cm, immunosuppressed patient, prior XRT, perineural involvement Can consider Mohs surgery (serial frozen section analysis of margins) for BCC or SCC in cosmetically sensitive area	**Wide local excision:** - Mark out needed margins - Excise as 3:1-4:1 (length:width) ellipse to allow for closure - Close in layers	SCC and BCC have >90% cure rate with adequate surgical resection Skin examinations q6-12mo x 5 y Minimize UV exposure	

Pilonidal disease (core)	Most common on young, hirsute patients
	
	On exam will see midline pits and sinuses within natal cleft
	
	Can present as abscess/acute infection with intergluteal pain, fluctuant mass, cellulitis, drainage
		Clinical diagnosis	Hair removal for prevention
			
			If patient presents with abscess, treat with incision and drainage
			
			Treat chronic or recurrent disease with surgical resection, many options:
			
			- Excision with wound left open and healing by secondary intention
			- Excision with primary closure
			  ○ Excision with off midline closure
			    ■ Off midline closure associated with lower recurrence rates
			  ○ Advanced techniques:
			    ■ Bascom cleft lift, Rhomboid flap, Karydakis flap, VY flap, Z-plasty
				Bascom cleft lift:
				- Position patient in prone jack-knife
				- Mark "safety lines" of natal cleft by pushing buttocks together and marking where they touch
				- Mark out incision for off-center excision of disease then make incision on medial side first to excise mid-line disease
				- Raise skin flap on contralateral side
				- Cut contractures/scars and scrub out granulation tissue
				- Irrigate and assure hemostasis
				- Leave drain, close in layers
					Avoid excessive sitting
					
					Post-op seroma and dehiscence are fairly common
						Additional reading: Johnson EK, Vogel JD, Cowan ML, Feingold DL, Steele SR. The American Society of Colon and Rectal Surgeons' clinical practice guidelines of the management of pilonidal disease. *Dis Colon Rectum.* 2019; 62(2): 146-157.

Disease Process	Relevant H&P	Work-up//Staging	Treatment	Key Surgical Steps	Post-Op Care	Tips & Tidbits
Soft tissue sarcoma (core)	Painless, enlarging mass that can arise in a variety of locations (extremity, abdomen, retroperitoneum, etc)	CT or MRI of primary site Core needle biopsy: - Determine histology and grade - CNB tract should be in an area that can be excised during resection - Not required for retroperitoneal sarcomas CT chest to rule out pulmonary metastases once sarcoma diagnosis confirmed	Resectable → resection with goal of microscopically negative margins Neoadjuvant XRT and/or systemic therapy: consider for borderline resectable tumors, high grade tumors, and/or tumors with high risk for recurrence Adjuvant XRT for extremity sarcoma if margins positive, >5 cm, and/or high grade Adjuvant XRT for abdominal/ RP sarcomas discouraged due to proximity of bowel Unresectable or not a surgical candidate → definitive XRT and/or systemic therapy	**Wide local excision of soft tissue sarcoma (advanced):** - Aim for 2 cm gross margins - Include CNB tract in specimen - Orient specimen - If large wound requiring flap closure and/or concerning for positive margins, can place wound vac and wait for final pathology report prior to reconstruction, in case additional margins are needed	Surveillance: H&P and imaging q3-6mo x 3 y, then q6mon x 2 y, cross-sectional imaging q3-6mo x 2-3 y for abdominal/RP sarcomas	Sarcomas typically spread hematogenously, rather than via the lymphatics, therefore lymph node biopsy/ dissection is typically not required
Necrotizing soft tissue infection (NSTI) (core)	Risk factors: diabetes, immunocompromised, history of MRSA, IVDU Exam findings: rapidly spreading erythema, hemorrhagic bullae, exquisite tenderness to palpation, necrotic tissue, crepitus, numbness, or motor weakness	Clinical diagnosis Send full labs—labs are nonspecific but may demonstrate: • Leukocytosis or leukopenia • Anemia • Hyponatremia • Elevated CRP • Hyperglycemia • Elevated creatinine Plain films or CT may show air tracking in soft tissues, abscess, or fascial separation/tracking fluid Intra-op may see murky "dishwater fluid," thrombosed vessels, and/or devitalized tissue that easily dissects from adjacent fascia with blunt dissection	Early initiation of resuscitation, broad-spectrum antibiotics (vancomycin + zosyn + clindamycin), and surgical consultation Surgical debridement ASAP— debride all nonviable, necrotic tissue - Delayed surgery leads to increased mortality Infections involving the perineum may ultimately necessitate diverting colostomy Infections involving the extremities may require amputation	**Wide surgical debridement:** - Prep and drape widely - Aggressively debride back to healthy tissue, excise all necrotic and nonviable tissue - Test muscle for stimulation and resect if nonfunctional - Irrigate and establish hemostasis - Pack and dress wounds	ICU care with continued antibiotics, resuscitation, and monitoring Evaluate wound frequently post-op Plan for early return (24-48 h) to OR for further debridement, as needed Consider skin grafting/ wound reconstruction once sepsis and infection resolved	

Disease Process	Relevant H&P	Work-up//Staging	Treatment	Key Surgical Steps	Post-Op Care	Tips & Tidbits
Paronychia, Felon (core)	Pain, erythema, swelling of finger Paronychia—infection of the soft tissue fold on either side of the fingernail Felon—infection in the soft tissue of the fingertip pad Risk factors for development: • Hangnail, nail biting, splinter, cut, or other nail injury • Diabetes • Psoriasis • Occupation with frequent immersion in water (bartenders, swimmers, dishwashers, etc)	Diagnosis based on exam Staph aureus is most common cause	Antibiotics (cephalexin, trimethoprim-sulfamethoxazole, or clindamycin) Drainage of abscess, if present, is essential for effective treatment Treatment with antibiotics and warm compresses alone may be appropriate in the absence of an abscess	**Paronychia drainage:** - Digital block - Can often be drained without an incision - Elevate lateral edge of the nail from nail bed using a freer elevator, excise that part of the nail plate if necessary - Irrigate wound **Felon drainage:** - Digital block - Longitudinal incision made on the center or ulnar side of volar pad - Blunt dissection to release all involved septa in the pulp to adequately decompress abscess - Irrigate and pack wound	Continue antibiotics for 7-10 d	
Hidradenitis suppurativa (core)	Chronic painful nodules, sinus tracts, abscesses, and scarring found in axilla, inguinal region, inframammary fold, buttocks, or gluteal cleft Risk Factors: obesity, mechanical stress, smoking, hormones	Clinical diagnosis Hurley Staging: - Stage 1: recurrent abscesses and nodules without scarring or sinus tracts - Stage 2: recurrent abscesses and nodules with limited sinus tracts and scarring - Stage 3: diffuse or multiple interconnected sinus tracts, abscesses, and scarring across the entire area	Prevention: treatment of comorbidities (ie, diabetes), maintain a healthy weight, smoking cessation, avoid excessive heat/perspiration, avoid deodorants/antiperspirants If abscess present → incision and drainage Medical treatment—can try topical clindamycin (initial therapy), PO doxycycline, retinoids, infliximab or adalimumab Wide local excision for refractory disease	**Wide local excision of hidradenitis suppurative:** - Excise any abnormal tissue down to normal appearing subcutaneous tissue - Allow to heal by secondary intention, high recurrence rates with primary closure - Consider wound vac placement - Skin grafting vs local or flap reconstruction for large wounds once it is healing and free of infection or recurrence		

Disease Process	Relevant H&P	Work-up//Staging	Treatment	Key Surgical Steps	Post-Op Care	Tips & Tidbits
Pressure ulcers (core)	Most commonly seen in bed-bound or wheelchair-bound patients Most common over bony prominences, especially sacrum and greater trochanter May be missed source of infection/sepsis in chronically hospitalized or ICU patient	Clinical diagnosis CBC, ESR, CRP Consider CT or MRI to evaluate for underlying fluid collection or osteomyelitis if concerned - Stage 1: skin redness/darkening - Stage 2: partial-thickness skin loss including epidermis and/or dermis - Stage 3: full-thickness skin loss down into the subcutaneous tissue - Stage 4: full-thickness skin loss, damage to muscle, bone, or tendon	Off-load pressure (air-fluidized bed, frequent repositioning), aggressive local wound care, treat with antibiotics if cellulitis present, frequent reevaluation Early-stage ulcers may heal with time and good wound care Necrotic and infected tissue should be debrided Biopsy if question of osteomyelitis For large wounds (stage III/IV), can consider flap coverage when infection cleared and healthy wound bed is present - Do not try to close wound primarily or with split-thickness skin graft		Aggressive wound care, continue to off-load pressure Optimize nutrition for prevention and wound healing Avoid lying on wound for 2-8 wk after grafting or flap coverage	
Merkel cell carcinoma	Rare, aggressive tumor Rapidly growing, flesh or purple-colored nodule Associated with UV exposure, more common in immunocompromised patients Do full skin and nodal basin exam	Obtain excisional or punch biopsy—biopsy will demonstrate small, round blue cells Immunohistochemistry: CK20(+), TTF-1(-), CAM 5.2(+), Cytokeratin(+) If LN(+), high risk features, or symptoms concerning for metastases → whole-body PET/CT or CT C/A/P +/- brain MRI (if suspicious symptoms)	Wide local excision with 1-2 cm margins and SLNB (if clinically LN-) Clinically LN + or SLNB + → lymphadenectomy, consider XRT M1 → XRT and/or chemotherapy Immunotherapy may be helpful for patients with metastatic and recurrent disease Patients should be reviewed by multidisciplinary tumor board and considered for clinical trial	Wide local excision with sentinel lymph node biopsy (see melanoma section)	Surveillance: H&P with skin and nodal exam q3-6mo x 3 y	If patient requires major reconstruction after excision, delay until after negative margins confirmed

Disease Process	Relevant H&P	Work-up//Staging	Treatment	Key Surgical Steps	Post-Op Care	Tips & Tidbits
Dermatofibrosarcoma protuberans (DFSP)	Slow-growing, painless, violet or pink, cutaneous lesion	Biopsy shows spindle cell in storiform pattern - CD34(+), vimentin(+), factor XIIIa(-) Can get an MRI for surgical planning, if needed If patient has DFSP with fibrosarcomatous changes, should get CT of chest to rule out mets	Wide local excision with 2-4 cm margins Clear surgical margins are most important aspect of treatment If patient requires major reconstruction after excision, delay until after negative margins confirmed Positive margin or recurrence → repeat resection XRT considered for persistently positive margins or if not a candidate for resection Consider imatinib if unresectable	Wide local excision (see melanoma section)	High risk for local recurrence Surveillance: H&P q6-12mo	Arise from neuroendocrine cells of the skin

13

Transplant Surgery

Shelby Reiter, MD, and Danielle Hayes, MD

DISEASES AND CONDITIONS

- Brain death (c), organ donation (a)
- Renal transplant (a)
- Liver transplant (a)

GENERAL TIPS

- There are no core diseases or operations for this specialty, other than brain death, listed on the curriculum; therefore, it would be best to devote relatively less time studying transplant topics.

(c) = core topic   (a) = advanced topic

Disease Process	Relevant H&P	Work-up/Staging	Treatment	Key Surgical Steps	Post-Op Care	Tips & Tidbits

Brain death (core), Organ donation (advanced)	May present after stroke, TBI, anoxic brain injury, etc
	
	All patients with severe brain injuries who are brain dead or likely to progress to brain death should be considered potential organ donors → referral to local organ procurement organization
		Brain death = irreversible, catastrophic brain injury causing total cessation of brain function
		Criteria for brain death declaration:
		- Irreversible, unresponsive coma with known cause
		- Exclude potentially reversible medical conditions (ie, acid-base or electrolyte derangements, endocrine function, paralytic or CNS depressant meds, hypothermia, etc)
		- Brain death exam
		  ○ Fixed and dilated pupils
		  ○ Absence of brainstem reflexes—corneal, oculocephalic, oculovestibular, gag, cough
		    ■ Spinal reflexes are NOT a sign of brain activity
		  ○ No motor response to noxious stimuli
		  ○ No spontaneous respirations
		  ○ Some states require two brain death exams by different physicians with defined time interval between the two
		- Confirmatory apnea test—the most definitive finding supporting the diagnosis of brain death
		  ○ $PaCO_2$ normalized to 40 mm Hg, patient preoxygenated with 100% FiO_2 and then disconnected from ventilator and placed on 100% FiO_2 delivered passively to ETT via T-piece
		  ○ ABG drawn after ~10 min
		  ○ If there is no evidence of spontaneous respiratory activity, $PaCO_2$ ≥ 60 mm Hg, and pH is acidotic, this is considered evidence of brain death
		  ○ If there is any evidence of respiratory activity, patient is not brain dead, return to vent immediately
		  ○ Apnea test not valid for patients with cervical fracture above C4 or on substances that depress respiratory drive
		- Adjuncts: Cerebral angiography (gold standard), cranial doppler, CTA, MRA, and nuclear cerebral blood flow scan
		  ○ Can be obtained to evaluate for brain death if brain death exam and/or apnea test cannot be performed
		Donation after cardiac death—a way for patients with severe brain injury who do not technically meet the criteria for brain death to be donors
		Must have family consent before patient can be an organ donor
			Patients with severe brain injury develop physiologic derangements that must be treated to prevent cardiovascular collapse and loss of useable organs
			- Autonomic dysregulation → profound vasodilation and hypotension
			  ○ Increased ICP initially causes catecholamine storm, but patient eventually loses sympathetic tone causing peripheral vasodilation and hypotension
			- Depletion of ADH → diabetes insipidus → inappropriate diuresis, hypovolemia, hyperosmolality, and hypernatremia
			Without intervention, brain death is usually followed by severe injury to all organs and circulatory collapse within 48 h			

Disease Process	Relevant H&P	Work-up/Staging	Treatment	Key Surgical Steps	Post-Op Care	Tips & Tidbits
Renal transplant (advanced)	Patient may have ESRD due to a variety of different causes (DM, HTN, nephrotic syndrome, polycystic kidney disease, glomerulonephritis, etc) Ask about any potential contraindications to transplant—lack of necessary social support, active substance use, poor cardiopulmonary status, active malignancy, active infection, etc	Patient evaluated by multidisciplinary transplant committee to determine candidacy ABO determination, HLA typing, PRA testing, type and screen CXR, ECG, stress test CBC, CMP, liver function, coagulation panel Serology for hep B and C, HIV, CMV, EBV, TB test, RPR or VDRL	Renal transplant—may be from living or deceased donor	**Renal transplant:** - Back bench preparation—clear perinephric fat, mobilize renal vein and artery, and ligate gonadal, adrenal, and lumbar vessels - Curvilinear incision made extending from 1 cm above pubic symphysis to 2-4 cm lateral to the ASIS - Dissect down through fascia without entering the peritoneum, contents of the peritoneum are retracted medially to expose the retroperitoneum - Divide round ligament/retract spermatic cord - External iliac artery and vein identified and exposed - Clamp external iliac vein, make a venotomy, suture renal vein to external iliac vein in end to side fashion, unclamp - Clamp external iliac artery, make arteriotomy, suture renal artery to external iliac artery, unclamp - Fill bladder with saline via Foley, make incision on the bladder, and sew the ureter to the bladder using absorbable suture +/- stent - Ensure good renal perfusion and hemostasis, close abdominal wall in layers	Post-op immunosuppression—usually on steroids, tacrolimus, cyclosporine, mycophenolate +/- thymoglobulin Ensure good diuresis with close attention to fluid management Monitor electrolytes Complications: - Vessel thrombosis → diagnosis on renal U/S → can attempt revascularization, often results in graft loss - Urine leak → test fluid collection for creatinine → for small leak just decompress bladder, drain collection and observe, large leak may require percutaneous nephrostomy or operative intervention - Lymphocele → can cause compression of kidney, ureter, vessels, or bladder → small, asymptomatic collections often resolve without intervention, symptomatic collections may require treatment with sclerosing agent or peritoneal fenestration - Renal artery stenosis → delayed complication, diagnose on U/S → treat with angioplasty and stent Monitor for signs of organ rejection—can be acute or chronic Lifelong immunosuppression required, at risk of opportunistic infections	

Disease Process	Relevant H&P	Work-up/Staging	Treatment	Key Surgical Steps	Post-Op Care	Tips & Tidbits
Liver transplant (advanced)	Patient will present with acute or chronic liver failure or malignancy (HCC, cholangiocarcinoma) Ask about any potential contraindications to transplant—lack of necessary social support, active substance use, poor cardiopulmonary status, uncontrolled extrahepatic malignancy, active infection, etc	Multidisciplinary team evaluates patient for transplant eligibility MELD-NA—stratifies severity of ESLD, used to prioritize patients listed for transplant: - Score based on: creatinine, total bilirubin, INR, sodium, dialysis - MELD exception points given for certain conditions (HCC, cholangiocarcinoma, hepatopulmonary syndrome, cystic fibrosis, hepatic artery thrombosis within 2 wk of transplant) Milan criteria—transplant eligibility criteria for patients with HCC: - One lesion <5 cm or up to 3 lesions each <3 cm - No major hepatic vascular invasion by tumor - No metastatic disease	Liver-directed therapy to control HCC while patient awaits transplant Transplant with deceased donor liver or living donor graft	**Deceased donor liver transplant:** - Donor procurement and back table preparation - Bilateral subcostal incision - Recipient hepatectomy and portal dissection - Implantation of donor liver - Caval (piggyback, bicaval, or cavocavostomy), portal, arterial, and biliary anastomoses ○ Maintain close communication with anesthesia during reperfusion - Ensure hemostasis, leave drains	Initially taken to ICU post-op Post-op immunosuppression, serial labs Complications: - Post-op hemorrhage - Early hepatic artery thrombosis → can attempt revascularization, often require re-transplantation - Bile leaks → drain, ERCP with stent, or surgical revision - Primary graft nonfunction—poor graft function without identifiable cause → re-transplantation or death within 7 d - Acute cellular rejection—most common in first 90 d, diagnosed by liver biopsy, treat with additional immunosuppression - Infectious complications—abscesses, cholangitis, nosocomial infections, CMV, EBV, fungal infections Lifelong immunosuppression required	

14

Gynecology and Obstetrics

Michelle Marieni, MD

DISEASES AND CONDITIONS

- Ectopic pregnancy (c), laparoscopic salpingostomy and salpingectomy
- Pelvic inflammatory disease (c)

- Ovarian cancer (a), hysterectomy and salpingo-oophorectomy (a)

- Surgical considerations of the pregnant patient (c), cesarean section (a)

GENERAL TIPS

- Request OB/GYN consult if you encounter any of these topics on the boards; however, examiners will likely tell you that they are not available.

- Differential for acute pelvic pain in a female patient should include appendicitis, ectopic pregnancy, ovarian torsion, PID, and hemorrhagic ovarian cyst.

- Always check hCG in female patients of reproductive age who present with abdominal pain.

(c) = core topic   (a) = advanced topic

Disease Process	Relevant H&P	Work-up/Staging	Treatment	Key Surgical Steps	Post-Op Care	Tips & Tidbits

Ectopic Pregnancy (core)	~ 1 in 50 pregnancies is ectopic
	
	Typical presentation: first-trimester abdominal/pelvic pain and/or vaginal bleeding
	
	Ask about last menstrual period, contraception
	
	Can cause life-threatening hemorrhage
	
	Risk factors: history of PID, fertility treatment, prior ectopic pregnancies or tubal surgery, increasing age, current IUD (unlikely to get pregnant; however, if pregnancy occurs, 53% chance of ectopic)
		CBC, type and screen
		
		Serum hCG
		- If patient has pregnancy of unknown location and is stable, repeat hCG q48-72h to assess if hCG is rising appropriately
		- In normal early pregnancy, hCG should double in 48-72 h (varies by gestational age)
		- Slow increase in hCG may indicate an ectopic pregnancy
		
		Transvaginal U/S—useful for identifying intrauterine pregnancy vs determining location of an ectopic pregnancy, may demonstrate fluid in pelvis
		
		FAST—can be used in unstable patient with suspected ruptured ectopic to assess for intra-abdominal hemorrhage
		- Intra-abdominal hemorrhage in a woman of reproductive age without known trauma is highly suspicious for ruptured ectopic pregnancy
			Initiate resuscitation if patient is in hemorrhagic shock
			
			Methotrexate (MTX) is the medical treatment option for ectopic pregnancy
			- Can be used in stable patients with unruptured ectopic pregnancy
			- Patient must be reliable and able to return to care to trend hCG after treatment and in case of treatment failure or rupture
			- Relative contraindications: hCG > 5000, ectopic > 4 cm, fetal cardiac activity
			
			Surgical intervention required for some patients
			- Hemodynamically unstable patients, ruptured ectopic, patients with contraindication to MTX, advanced gestation (hCG > 5000, fetal cardiac activity, ectopic > 4 cm), or if patient elects surgical management
			- Salpingostomy vs salpingectomy
			  ◦ If fallopian tube is not ruptured, can do tubal salpingostomy
			  ◦ If fallopian tube damaged/ruptured or there is persistent tubal bleeding, then salpingectomy preferred
			- Rh(-) woman should receive anti-D immunoglobulin (Rhogam) within 72 h to prevent alloimmunization
				Laparoscopic salpingostomy:
				- Lift the fallopian tube with atraumatic grasper
				- Inject vasopressin solution along the mesosalpinx beneath the ectopic pregnancy
				- Make a 1-2 cm longitudinal incision with monopolar cautery along the site of ectopic
				- Use hydrodissection or gentle blunt dissection to remove the ectopic
				- Obtain hemostasis, leave tubal incision open
				
				Laparoscopic salpingectomy:
				- Lift the fallopian tube with atraumatic grasper
				- Use bipolar electrocautery to seal and cut along the mesosalpinx distally to proximally and ultimately excise the tube near the uterine cornua
					After treatment for an ectopic pregnancy, follow hCG level until it is undetectable (unless patient underwent salpingectomy and pathology confirms products of conception)
					- If increasing, need to evaluate for persistent ectopic pregnancy
						Risk of recurrent ectopic pregnancy after previous ectopic is ~10% (increases to >25% after 2 ectopic pregnancies)
						
						Additional reading:
						American College of Obstetricians and Gynecologists. ACOG Practice Bulletin No. 193: Tubal ectopic pregnancy. *Obstet Gynecol*. 2018 Mar; 131(3), 91–103.
						
						Hoffman BL, Schorge JO, Bradshaw KD, Halvorson LM, Schaffer JI, Corton, MM. *Williams Gynecology* (3rd ed.). McGraw-Hill Education; 2016.

Disease Process	Relevant H&P	Work-up/Staging	Treatment	Key Surgical Steps	Post-Op Care	Tips & Tidbits
Pelvic inflammatory disease (PID) (core)	Female patient may present with pelvic or lower abdominal pain, vaginal discharge, dyspareunia, N/V, fevers, and/ or chills Risk factors: unprotected sex with multiple partners, young age (most common in patients 15-25 yo), history of previous PID Bimanual exam—assess for cervical motion, uterine, and adnexal tenderness Speculum exam—assess for cervical mucopurulent discharge	Diagnosis of PID can be made on basis of H&P alone, empiric treatment should not be delayed Pregnancy test to rule out ectopic pregnancy Microscopy of vaginal discharge—looking for increased WBC Most common organisms are gonorrhoeae and chlamydia; typically polymicrobial Nucleic acid amplification tests for *N. gonorrhoeae* and *C. trachomatis* HIV screening and serologic testing for syphilis Get imaging if patient is acutely ill, has atypical symptoms, or does not improve with first 72 h of initial therapy - Pelvic U/S is first line—helpful in identifying tuboovarian abscess	If PID suspected, initiate empiric antibiotics - Outpatient treatment: ceftriaxone IM x1 dose + doxycycline + metronidazole - Empiric parenteral therapy: ceftriaxone + doxycycline + metronidazole or cefotetan/ cefoxitin + doxycycline Stable patients with contained abscesses may be drained by IR— consider if abscess ≥8 cm or no improvement with IV antibiotics Consider diagnostic laparoscopy in patients who have acute abdomen, fail to improve with antibiotics, or have ruptured tuboovarian abscesses		PID increases risk for chronic pelvic pain, infertility, and ectopic pregnancy	

Disease Process	Relevant H&P	Work-up/Staging	Treatment	Key Surgical Steps	Post-Op Care	Tips & Tidbits
Ovarian cancer (advanced)	Commonly presents at advanced stage due to lack of symptoms in early stage disease - May have ascites, ovarian torsion, bloating, early satiety, dyspnea (from pleural effusion), bowel obstruction Ovarian cancer risk factors: BRCA mutations, family history, older age, nulliparity, white race, early menarche, late menopause Exam should include abdominal, nodal, and pelvic exam	Routine labs, CA-125, coagulation panel Pregnancy test Transvaginal U/S—findings concerning for adnexal malignancy: mass > 10 cm, solid components, thick septations CT scan—may demonstrate peritoneal studding, omental caking, ascites, lymphadenopathy, pleural effusions Obtain fluid cytology (pleural effusion or ascites) or omental/peritoneal biopsy for definitive diagnosis - Biopsy of ovary not recommended due to potential seeding of the abdomen	Refer to gynecologic oncologist Treatment may include surgery (ranging from oophorectomy to TAH/BSO with debulking), chemotherapy and/or radiation depending on type (epithelial, germ cell, stromal, etc) and stage of ovarian cancer	**Total abdominal hysterectomy and bilateral salpingo-oophrectomy (advanced):** - Can be done through vertical midline or Pfannenstiel incision, typically done through vertical midline if further debulking/biopsies/lymphadenectomy needed - Obtain abdominal and pelvic washings - Place Kelly clamps on each uterine cornua to allow for uterine manipulation - Ligate and divide the round ligament - Open the broad ligament anteriorly to develop bladder flap - Identify and preserve the ureter on medial aspect of the posterior broad ligament leaf - Incise the posterior leaf of the broad ligament parallel to the infundibulopelvic ligament - Ligate and divide the infundipulopelvic ligament (with the ovarian vessels) and fallopian tube - Open the vesicouterine space to further develop the bladder flap - Uterine vessels skeletonized, clamped, and cut - Cardinal and uterosacral ligaments ligated and divided - Cut across the upper vagina just inferior to the external os of the cervix - Specimen removed, close the vaginal cuff	Complications: - Risk of ureter injury—most common site of injury is in the pelvis, at the infundibulopelvic ligament or the level of the uterine arteries	BRCA mutation carriers—prophylactic BSO recommended by 35-40 yo for BRCA1 and 40-45 yo for BRCA2, or after childbearing Additional reading: Hoffman BL, Schorge JO, Bradshaw KD, Halvorson LM, Schaffer JI, Corton, MM. *Williams Gynecology* (3rd ed.). McGraw-Hill Education; 2016.

Disease Process	Relevant H&P	Work-up/Staging	Treatment	Key Surgical Steps	Post-Op Care	Tips & Tidbits
Surgical considerations in the pregnant patient (core)	Acute cholecystitis affects 1 in 1000 pregnancies, delayed emptying of the gallbladder secondary to progesterone Women in third trimester with appendicitis may have RUQ pain because appendix is displaced cephalad	Abdominal U/S is first line imaging test in a stable pregnant patient, MRI/CT if needed Elevation of BP at any point during pregnancy is abnormal and should be further evaluated	Involve the OB/GYN team when considering operation on a pregnant patient Per SAGES guidelines, laparoscopy can be safely performed during any trimester of pregnancy when an operation is indicated - During the first trimester, there are potential teratogenic effects of anesthesia; however, single exposure to anesthesia is safe and laparoscopic treatment of acute abdominal disease should not be withheld, if indicated - Second trimester is typically considered optimal timing, if needed - Large uterus may make operating in the third trimester more challenging, adjust port placement as needed When surgery done in the first trimester and early second trimester, fetal heart tones should be confirmed before and after anesthesia When surgery is done in the late second trimester and third trimester, continuous intra-op fetal monitoring should be considered ~23 wk is typically considered the threshold of fetal viability	General tips for surgery in pregnant patient: - Position patient with a left lateral tilt to minimize uterine compression of IVC - During initial abdominal access consider location of the uterus, open cutdown may be preferred ○ A 20-wk uterus is at the level of the umbilicus, therefore access should be obtained supraumbilical **Cesarean section (advanced):** - Pfannenstiel skin incision (vs lower midline laparotomy in emergent setting) - Enter the abdomen - Sharp dissection of the subcutaneous layer and fascia - Sharp superficial, then blunt entry into the uterus via low transverse uterine incision - Deliver the baby, clamp and cut umbilical cord - Remove the placenta - Uterine closure with an initial layer of running, locking suture, consider a second imbricating layer - Assess for hemostasis and close		Dilutional anemia of pregnancy—plasma volume increases by 50% but RBC only increases by 25%. There is also an expected mild leukocytosis associated with pregnancy. Cholangiogram is safe in pregnancy. Place a lead shield under the patient to shield fetus from radiation. ERCP is also acceptable, although it typically results in more radiation exposure than cholangiogram. Additional reading: Pearl JP, et al. SAGES guidelines for the use of laparoscopy during pregnancy. *Surg Endosc.* 2017 Oct;31(10):3767-3782.

15

Urology

Gary Lucas, MD

DISEASES AND CONDITIONS

- Acute urinary retention (c), cystostomy (c)
- Hydrocele (c)
- Iatrogenic ureter injury, ureteroureterostomy, ureteroneocystostomy

GENERAL UROLOGY TIPS

- It is reasonable to ask for a urology consult for these topics. However, it is likely that the examiners will tell you that urology is not available; therefore, you should be able to describe basic management.

(c) = core topic   (a) = advanced topic

Disease Process	Relevant H&P	Work-up/Staging	Treatment	Key Surgical Steps	Post-Op Care	Tips & Tidbits
Acute urinary retention (core)	Risk factors: - History of BPH, elderly, male, post-op patients, infection - Uncontrolled pain, opioids, fluid overload, decreased mobility - Spinal, pelvic, perineal, and inguinal procedures are highest risk Symptoms: inability to void, bladder fullness, pelvic pain, increased urinary frequency with low-volume voids, overflow incontinence May have suprapubic fullness/tenderness to palpation	Bladder U/S with >400-mL volume Consider UA and urine culture, if cause is unclear	Can try intermittent catheterization initially, with Foley placement if patient continues to retain - If unable to place regular Foley, can try Coudé tip catheter and/or or larger sized catheter - If discharged with Foley in place, usually see back in clinic in 5-7 d for void trial If drainage with Foley not possible, may need suprapubic catheter placement - If no prior pelvic or abdominal surgery, prevesical space should be clear → percutaneous cystostomy - In patients with a history of pelvic surgery (ie, radical prostatectomy, TEPP), this space has been violated and may contain bowel → open cystostomy Can start alpha-blocker (tamsulosin) or 5-alpha reductase inhibitor (finasteride) for men with urinary retention due to BPH	**Percutaneous cystostomy placement (core):** - If patient had prior procedure that dissected prevesical space, use intra-op U/S to visualize the bladder and look for overlying bowel ○ If bowel is in the way, open approach is preferred - If able, perform cystoscopy or place a catheter to distend the bladder with saline - Make a 2-cm transverse incision directly cephalad to pubic symphysis - Using Seldinger technique, insert a 22-gauge spinal needle through the incision until bladder access is obtained, distend bladder by filling through spinal needle - Pass guidewire into bladder - Exchange needle with percutaneous dilator system over wire, upsize dilators until 20 Fr dilator and sheath are in place - Place a 16 Fr Foley catheter through peel-away sheath - Inflate Foley balloon and secure catheter to skin with nonabsorbable suture **Open cystostomy placement:** - Place Foley catheter and use it to fill the bladder, if able - Make 4 cm lower midline abdominal incision and enter the space of Retzius - Place full thickness stay sutures in anterior bladder wall and make small incision into bladder - Place a 16 Fr Foley catheter through the incision into the bladder - Inflate balloon and secure the catheter to the bladder wall with purse string sutures - Bring the Foley out through a separate skin incision, close incision	Presence of succus/stool in catheter or peritonitis is concerning for bowel injury Avoid changing suprapubic catheter for 4-6 wk after placement to allow tract to form, then will need to be changed monthly to prevent encrustation and bladder stones If there is concern that the catheter has been dislodged, obtain cystogram through the catheter	Chronic suprapubic tubes become colonized with bacteria, only treat UTIs if symptomatic

Disease Process	Relevant H&P	Work-up/Staging	Treatment	Key Surgical Steps	Post-Op Care	Tips & Tidbits
Hydrocele (core)	Painless, enlarged unilateral or bilateral scrotal bulge Examine the bilateral groins and scrotum - Hydrocele transilluminates (unlike inguinal hernia) - Non-communicating hydroceles are nonreducible - Communicating hydroceles fluctuate in size Non-communicating hydroceles are more common in adults, communicating hydroceles are more common in pediatrics	Inguinal and scrotal U/S	Most non-communicating hydroceles in infants resolve spontaneously and can be observed Communicating hydroceles/hernias in pediatric patients rarely resolve spontaneously and should be repaired (see inguinal hernia section in pediatric surgery chapter) Pursue operative repair in adults, if symptomatic—can do Lord's plication or Jaboulay bottleneck repair	**Lord's plication repair:** - Scrotal incision lateral to median raphe - Bluntly free up hydrocele/tunica vaginalis from surrounding tissue - Make incision in sac to drain fluid and open tunica, avoid injury to testicular vessels, epididymis, or vas deferens - Place plication sutures all around the edges of the tunica vaginalis so that that sac is everted and shrunken - Close Dartos fascia, then skin	Monitor for scrotal hematoma, wound infection, recurrence	

Disease Process	Relevant H&P	Work-up/Staging	Treatment	Key Surgical Steps	Post-Op Care	Tips & Tidbits
Iatrogenic ureter injury	Typically occurs during surgery, such as hysterectomy, colectomy, or other pelvic surgery Timing of injury detection is important (intra-op vs post-op) Delayed presentation of ureteral injury may include increased drain output, hematuria, peritonitis, leukocytosis, flank pain, and/or fever	Intra-op injury: - Consult urology, may be able to perform intra-op cystoscopy and/or retrograde pyelogram to localize injury and possibly place stent or repair operatively - Can give IV methylene blue or ICG to help localize injury Delayed injury detection: - Check drain creatinine and compare to serum creatinine - CT with IV contrast and delayed images - Cystoscopy and retrograde pyelogram, if not localized on CT	Ideally injury is noted at the time it occurs → immediate repair If identified within 5 d of injury → cystoscopy with stent or take back to OR to repair If identified 10 d or more after injury → percutaneous nephrostomy tube placement and delayed repair Surgical repair: - Injuries to distal 1/3 of ureter (pelvic brim and lower)—repair with ureteroneocystostomy +/- psoas hitch - Injuries to proximal and middle 1/3—manage with ureteroureterostomy over stent 　○ If unable to perform ureteroureterostomy due to reach issue or unsuitable distal segment, may require psoas hitch +/- Boari bladder flap, transureteroureterostomy, or ureteral ligation and percutaneous nephrostomy	**Ureteroureterostomy:** - Debride any devitalized tissue on the ends of the ureter - Mobilize short segment of proximal and distal ureter so that the ends meet without tension - Spatulate ends of the ureter - Create end-to-end primary anastomosis with interrupted full-thickness sutures using 4-0 or 5-0 absorbable suture with heel of one spatulated end to the toe of the other spatulated end - Place stent across anastomosis prior to finishing anastomosis - Leave drain adjacent to anastomosis, leave Foley in place **Ureteroneocystostomy +/- Psoas hitch:** - Identify distal end of ureter, debride back to healthy tissue, mobilize as needed - Spatulate end of the ureter - Fill bladder with sterile fluid via Foley - Mobilize the bladder by dissecting the space of Retzius - Suture superior portion of bladder to psoas tendon with 2-0 nonabsorbable sutures to pull bladder up toward ureter - Make anterior cystotomy, then bring ureter into bladder via submucosal tunnel from separate bladder incision - Create ureteroneocystostomy anastomosis with interrupted 4-0 absorbable suture with full-thickness bites of ureter and mucosal bites of bladder, place ureteral stent across anastomosis, place second outer layer of 3-0 absorbable suture - Close anterior cystotomy - Consider leaving drain, leave Foley in place	- Leave Foley in for 1-2-wk post-op, then get cystogram/ureterogram to confirm no leak prior to removal - Ureteral stents removed 4-6-wk post-op	Transureteroureterostomy is typically not a good idea as it involves taking the injured ureter and sewing it to the otherwise uninjured ureter Boari flap—tongue of bladder used to create neo-distal ureter that can be sewn to remaining distal ureter

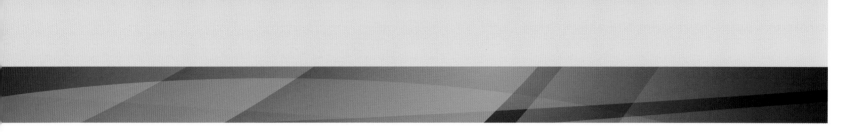

Last-Minute Review Sheet

BIRADS—used to classify mammography findings and determine next steps based on risk of malignancy

- 0 – insufficient ⟶ need more imaging
- 1 – negative ⟶ routine follow-up
- 2 – benign ⟶ routine follow-up
- 3 – likely benign ⟶ short interval follow-up
- 4 – suspicious ⟶ CNB
- 5 – highly suspicious for malignancy ⟶ CNB
- 6 – biopsy proven malignancy ⟶ treat accordingly

Per Dr. Hayes: BIRADS 3, you need to see (get follow-up imaging)! BIRADS 4, you need a core (CNB)!

Bethesda Classification—standardized thyroid cytopathology reporting for FNA of thyroid nodules

- 1 – nondiagnostic ⟶ repeat FNA
- 2 – benign ⟶ follow-up imaging in 12 mo
- 3 – AUS/FLUS ⟶ repeat FNA or obtain molecular testing
- 4 – follicular neoplasm ⟶ diagnostic lobectomy vs molecular testing
- 5 – suspicious for malignancy ⟶ lobectomy vs total thyroidectomy
- 6 – malignant ⟶ treat malignancy accordingly

Types of choledochal cysts and their treatment:

- 1 – dilation of the CBD ⟶ cyst excision with Roux-en-Y hepaticojejunostomy
- 2 – diverticulum off of the CBD ⟶ resection of diverticulum off of the CBD
- 3 – choledochocele ⟶ endoscopic sphincterotomy vs trans-duodenal excision and sphincteroplasty
- 4a – intrahepatic and extrahepatic cysts ⟶ cyst excision followed by Roux-en-Y hepaticojejunostomy or hepaticoduodenostomy, consider partial hepatectomy if cysts are limited to one lobe
- 4b – extrahepatic cysts ⟶ cyst excision followed by Roux-en-Y hepaticojejunostomy or hepaticoduodenostomy
- 5 – intrahepatic cysts (Caroli's disease) - partial hepatectomy (if cysts limited to one lobe) vs liver transplant

Biochemical work-up for adrenal mass:

- To evaluate for aldosteronoma—BMP, aldosterone, renin
- To evaluate for hypercortisolism—24 h urine cortisol, ACTH, low-dose dexamethasone suppression test
- To evaluate for pheochromocytoma—plasma/urine metanephrines
- DHEA-sulfate—can be elevated with adrenal cortical carcinoma

Concerning imaging findings for an adrenal mass:

- >4 cm
- >10 HFU
- Delayed washout
- Irregular borders

Anticoagulation reversal agents

- Heparin—protamine
- Enoxaparin—protamine
- Warfarin—Vit K, PCC, FFP
- Xa inhibitors—Xarelto (rivaroxaban), Eliquis (apixaban)
  - Andexanet alfa—recombinant factor Xa
  - PCC
- IIa inhibitors—Pradaxa (dabigatran)
  - Praxbind (idarucizumab)—monoclonal antibody
  - Dialysis

Type of Cancer	Staging Work-Up
Always get basic labs when a new cancer is diagnosed (CBC, BMP, LFTs)	
Well-differentiated thyroid cancer (follicular, papillary)	Thyroid U/S with biopsy Cervical U/S with of FNA of suspicious nodes CT/MRI used in select patients with clinical suspicion for advanced disease
Medullary thyroid cancer	Thyroid U/S with biopsy Cervical U/S with FNA of suspicious nodes Calcitonin, CEA RET proto-oncogene testing Hyperparathyroidism and pheochromocytoma screening (Ca, PTH, plasma metanephrines) If elevated CEA or very high calcitonin, obtain staging CT neck, chest, and liver
Esophageal	EGD with biopsy EUS CT C/A/P PET Bronchoscopy if tumor is proximal to carina to assess for airway involvement +/- Diagnostic laparoscopy—recommended for Siewart II/III tumors
Gastric adenocarcinoma	EGD with biopsy EUS CT C/A/P PET Diagnostic lap with peritoneal washings for ≥ T1b
Gallbladder cancer	CT C/A/P Tumor markers +/- staging laparoscopy
Cholangiocarcinoma	MRI/CT liver, CT chest Tumor markers +/- ERCP/EUS with brushings and/or FNA
Pancreatic adenocarcinoma	CA 19-9 CT C/A/P, CT pancreas protocol +/- EUS with FNA, ERCP with stent, brushings
PNET	CT C/A/P Consider DOTATATE scan—can help localize and detect metastatic disease Biochemical testing (insulin, C peptide, gastrin, etc), chromogranin A, pancreatic polypeptide +/- EUS with FNA for tissue biopsy PNET graded and staged based on Ki67, mitotic rate, behavior (invasion, mets)
Colon cancer	CT C/A/P CEA Colonoscopy with biopsy, test for MMR deficiency

Rectal cancer	CT C/A/P
	Pelvic MRI
	CEA
	Colonoscopy with biopsy, test for MMR deficiency
	Rigid sigmoidoscopy—determine accurate distance from dentate line
Anal SCC	CT C/A ⟶ rule out M1 disease
	CT or MRI pelvis to evaluate inguinal nodes—FNA any abnormal inguinal LN
	HIV testing
	Pelvic exam in female patients
	Colonoscopy, if indicated
	+/- PET—indicated for N+ and ≥ T2 disease
Breast	Full staging only indicated for locally advanced (T3+ or N2+) breast cancers, inflammatory breast cancer, or those with concerning symptoms
	CT C/A/P
	Bone scan
	+/- PET and brain/spine MRI, if concerning symptoms
Melanoma	Full staging only indicated if patient has N+ disease or concerning symptoms:
	CT C/A/P and/or PET
	Brain MRI
	BRAF testing
	LDH (for stage IV)

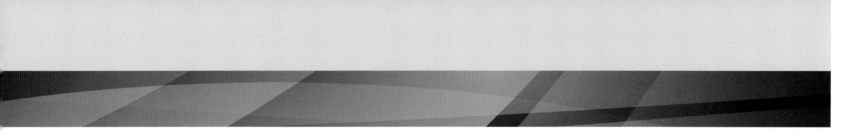

Index

Note: Page numbers followed by *f* denote figures; by *t*, tables.